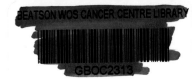
AMERICAN JOINT COMMITTEE ON CANCER

D1330291

CAN   3

Second Edition

EDITORS

CAROLYN C. COMPTON, MD, PhD, FCAP
Critical Path Institute
Tucson, Arizona

DAVID R. BYRD, MD, FACS
University of Washington School of Medicine
Seattle, Washington

JULIO GARCIA-AGUILAR, MD, PhD, FACS
Memorial Sloan-Kettering Cancer Center
New York, New York

SCOTT H. KURTZMAN, MD, FACS
Waterbury Hospital
Waterbury, Connecticut

ALEXANDER OLAWAIYE, MD, MRCOG, FACOG
Magee-Womens Hospital of UPMC
Pittsburgh, Pennsylvania

MARY KAY WASHINGTON, MD, PhD, FCAP
Vanderbilt University Medical Center
Nashville, Tennessee

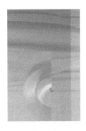

AJCC CANCER STAGING ATLAS

A Companion to the Seventh Editions of the
AJCC Cancer Staging Manual and Handbook
Second Edition

AMERICAN JOINT COMMITTEE ON CANCER
Executive Office
633 North Saint Clair Street
Chicago, Illinois 60611

MEMBER ORGANIZATIONS
American Cancer Society
American College of Physicians
American College of Radiology
American College of Surgeons
American Head and Neck Society
American Society of Clinical Oncology
American Society of Colon and Rectal Surgeons
American Society for Radiation Oncology
American Urological Association
Canadian Partnership Against Cancer
Centers for Disease Control and Prevention
College of American Pathologists
National Cancer Institute
National Cancer Registrars Association
National Comprehensive Cancer Network
North American Association of Central Cancer Registries
Society of Gynecologic Oncologists
Society of Surgical Oncology
Society of Urologic Oncology

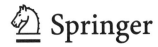

**CD-ROM
Included**

Editors

Carolyn C. Compton, MD, PhD, FCAP
Critical Path Institute
Tucson, AZ, USA

David R. Byrd, MD, FACS
Department of Surgery
University of Washington School of Medicine
Seattle, WA, USA

Julio Garcia-Aguilar, MD, PhD, FACS
Department of Surgery
Memorial Sloan-Kettering Cancer Center
New York, NY, USA

Scott H. Kurtzman, MD, FACS
Department of Surgery
Waterbury Hospital
Waterbury, CT, USA

Alexander Olawaiye, MD, MRCOG, FACOG
Department of OB/GYN
Division of Gynecologic
Oncology Magee-Womens Hospital
University of Pittsburgh Medical Center
Pittsburgh, PA, USA

Mary Kay Washington, MD, PhD, FCAP
Gastrointestinal and Hepatic Pathology
Vanderbilt University Medical Center
Nashville, TN, USA

This publication was prepared and published through the support of the American Cancer Society, the American College of Surgeons, the American Society of Clinical Oncology, and the Centers for Disease Control and Prevention.

ISBN 978-1-4614-2079-8   ISBN 978-1-4614-2080-4 (eBook)
DOI 10.1007/978-1-4614-2080-4
Springer New York Heidelberg Dordrecht London

Library of Congress Control Number: 2012933557

First edition of the *AJCC Cancer Staging Atlas*, published by Springer Science+Business Media, LLC 2006

Printed on acid-free paper

Springer is part of Springer Science+Business Media (www.springer.com)

Preface

The second edition of the AJCC Cancer Staging Atlas has been created as a compendium to the 7th Edition of the AJCC Cancer Staging Manual, which was updated and expanded in 2010 and continues to promulgate the importance of anatomical and pathological staging in the management of cancer. This Atlas has been viewed as a companion to illustrate the TNM classifications of all cancer sites and types that are included in the 7th Edition of the Manual. It is fully illustrated to give meaningful visualization at a glance to the TNM classifications and stage groupings and will serve as a useful reference for clinicians, registrars, students, trainees, and patients alike.

There have been many evidence-based changes in staging strategies in the 7th Edition of the AJCC Cancer Staging Manual, the differences compared to the 6th edition have been highlighted throughout the Atlas. This provides meaningful comparisons as well as a reference for teaching and training.

The 616 illustrations have been developed exclusively for the AJCC Cancer Staging Atlas by Alice Y. Chen, our exceptional medical illustrator. The drawings are specifically designed for simplicity and clarity and have been verified through multi-disciplinary vetting to ensure their accuracy and relevancy for clinical usage. Every illustration provides detailed anatomic depictions to clarify critical structures and to allow the reader to instantly visualize the progressive extent of malignant disease. Appropriate labeling has been incorporated to identify significant anatomic structures, and each illustration is accompanied by a relevant explanatory legend. Throughout all anatomic sites and cancer types, the newly developed illustrations reflect concepts that are more completely discussed in the 7th Edition of the AJCC Cancer Staging Manual and the companion Handbook.

The AJCC Cancer Staging Atlas is an official publication of the American Joint Committee on Cancer and reinforces the AJCC's position as the leader in disseminating state-of-the-art information on TNM staging. The AJCC continues to have as its mission the education of physicians, registrars, and patients and the promotion of evidence-based patient management. The Atlas continues to enhance this mission. This project has been fully supported by our publishing colleagues at Springer and especially Margaret Burns, Richard Lansing, Gregory Sutorius, and Bill Curtis.

The editors of this most recent AJCC project wish to underscore the concept that TNM is a universal language, which must be applied by all clinicians caring for cancer patients. The creation of visual images of clinical and pathological staging parameters serves to clarify and augment this language. We dedicate this work to all of our patients and colleagues and hope that they too will benefit from this illustrated resource.

Carolyn C. Compton, MD, PhD
David R. Byrd, MD
Julio Garcia-Aguilar, MD, PhD
Scott H. Kurtzman, MD
Alexander Olawaiye, MD
Mary Kay Washington, MD, PhD

Acknowledgment of Contributors

The 2nd edition Atlas would not have been possible without the guidance and the help of several individuals who in one way or another contributed their valuable expertise to the illustrations and concepts displayed in this publication. The AJCC and the editors acknowledge and thank the following individuals:

Andreas Andreou, MD
The University of Texas MD Anderson Cancer Center, Houston, TX

Daniel A. Barocas, MD, MPH
Vanderbilt-Ingram Cancer Center, Nashville, TN

Al B. Benson III, MD, FACP
Robert H. Lurie Comprehensive Cancer Center of Northwestern University, Chicago, IL

Karl Bilimoria, MD, MS
Feinberg School of Medicine, Northwestern University, Chicago, IL

Eugene Blackstone, MD
The Cleveland Clinic, Cleveland, OH

George J. Chang, MD, FACS
The University of Texas MD Anderson Cancer Center, Houston, TX

Sam S. Chang, MD, FACS
Vanderbilt-Ingram Cancer Center, Nashville, TN

Bruce D. Cheson, MD, FACP
Georgetown University Hospital, Washington, DC

Peter Goldstraw, MD
Royal Brompton Hospital, London, England

J. Milburn Jessup, MD
National Cancer Institute, Rockville, MD

James M. McKiernan, MD
Columbia University, New York, NY

Raphael Pollock, MD, PhD, FACS
The University of Texas MD Anderson Cancer Center, Houston, TX

Thomas W. Rice, MD, FACS
The Cleveland Clinic, Cleveland, OH

Valerie W. Rusch, MD, FACS
Memorial Sloan-Kettering Cancer Center, New York, NY

Jatin P. Shah, MD, FACS
Memorial Sloan-Kettering Cancer Center, New York, NY

Michael T. Tetzlaff, MD, PhD
The University of Texas MD Anderson Cancer Center, Houston, TX

J. Nicolas Vauthey, MD, FACS
The University of Texas MD Anderson Cancer Center, Houston, TX

STAFF CONTRIBUTORS
Donna M. Gress, RHIT, CTR
Karen A. Pollitt

Contents

PART IV 309
Thorax

PART V 339
Musculoskeletal Sites

PART VI 355
Skin

PART VII 417
Breast

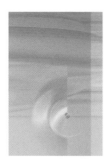

PART I

General Information on Cancer Staging and End-Results Reporting

Purposes and Principles of Cancer Staging

INTRODUCTION AND OVERVIEW

The extent or *stage* of cancer at the time of diagnosis is a key factor that defines prognosis and is a critical element in determining appropriate treatment based on the experience and outcomes of groups of prior patients with similar stage. In addition, accurate staging is necessary to evaluate the results of treatments and clinical trials, to facilitate the exchange and comparison of information among treatment centers, and to serve as a basis for clinical and translational cancer research. At a national and international level, the agreement on classifications of cancer cases provides a method of clearly conveying clinical experience to others without ambiguity.

Several cancer staging systems are used worldwide. Differences among these systems stem from the needs and objectives of users in clinical medicine and in population surveillance. The most clinically useful staging system is the tumor node metastasis (TNM) system maintained collaboratively by the American Joint Committee on Cancer (AJCC) and the International Union for Cancer Control (UICC). The TNM system classifies cancers by the size and extent of the primary tumor (T), involvement of regional lymph node (N), and the presence or absence of distant metastases (M), supplemented in recent years by carefully selected nonanatomic prognostic factors. There is a TNM staging algorithm for cancers of virtually every anatomic site and histology, with the primary exception in this manual being staging of pediatric cancers.

Philosophy of TNM Revision. The AJCC and UICC periodically modify the TNM system in response to newly acquired clinical data and improved understanding of cancer biology and factors affecting prognosis. Revision is one factor that makes the TNM system the most clinically useful staging system and accounts for its use worldwide. However, changes in staging systems may make it difficult to compare outcomes of current and past groups of patients. Because of this, the organizations only make these changes carefully and based on the best possible evidence.

The revision cycle for TNM staging is 6–8 years. This provides sufficient time for implementation of changes in clinical and cancer registry operations and for relevant examination and discussion of data supporting changes in staging. Table 1.1 shows the publication years for each of the versions of the TNM system up through this current seventh edition of the TNM system. The prior sixth edition was used for cases diagnosed on or after January 1, 2003. The seventh edition published in this manual is effective for cancer cases diagnosed on or after January 1, 2010.

Anatomic Staging and Use of Nonanatomic Information. Cancer staging is historically based solely on the anatomic extent of cancer and remains primarily anatomic. However, an increasing number of nonanatomic factors about a cancer and its host provide critical prognostic information and may predict the value of specific therapies. Among those factors known to affect patient outcomes and/or response to therapy are the clinical and pathologic anatomic extent of disease, the reported duration of signs or symptoms, gender, age and health status of the patient, the type and grade of the cancer, and the specific biological properties of the cancer. Clinicians use the pure anatomic extent of disease in defining treatment, but in many cases must supplement TNM with other factors in order to counsel patients and make specific treatment recommendations. As more of these factors are fully validated, it will be necessary to develop strategies to incorporate them into

C.C. Compton et al. (eds.), *AJCC Cancer Staging Atlas: A Companion to the Seventh Editions of the AJCC Cancer Staging Manual and Handbook*, DOI 10.1007/978-1-4614-2080-4_1, © 2012 American Joint Committee on Cancer

prognostic systems for patient management while maintaining the core anatomic structure of staging. The restriction of TNM to anatomic information has led clinicians to develop other prognostic systems and even led some to conclude that TNM is "obsolete" or "anachronistic."

As outlined in this chapter and throughout the *Manual* in many of the revised AJCC staging algorithms, nonanatomic factors are incorporated into stage grouping where needed. This practice started in a limited fashion in prior editions. However, anatomic extent of disease remains central to defining cancer prognosis. Most proposed nonanatomic prognostic factors in use have been validated only for patients with specific types of disease grouped largely on the anatomic stage (e.g., Gleason's score in early stage prostate cancer and genomic profiles that are validated only in women with node-negative breast cancer). Further, it is critical to maintain the ability to report purely anatomic information to allow comparability of patients treated using new prognostic schemas with patients treated in the past using prior anatomic schemas or with current patients for whom new prognostic factors are not obtained because of cost, available expertise, reporting systems, or other logistical issues.

Defining T, N, M and Timing of Staging Data. Stage is determined from information on the tumor T, regional nodes N, and metastases M and by grouping cases with similar prognosis. The criteria for defining anatomic extent of disease are specific for tumors at different anatomic sites and of different histologic types. For example, the size of the tumor is a key factor in breast cancer but has no impact on prognosis in colorectal cancer, where the depth of invasion or extent of the cancer is the primary prognostic feature. Therefore, the criteria for T, N, and M are defined separately for each tumor and histologic type. With certain types of tumors, such as Hodgkin and other lymphomas, a different system for designating the extent of disease and prognosis, and for classifying its groupings, is necessary. In these circumstances, other symbols or descriptive criteria are used in place of T, N, and M, and in the case of lymphoma only the *stage group* is defined. The general rules for defining elements of staging are presented later, and the specifics for each type of disease are in the respective chapters.

Beginning with the sixth edition of the *AJCC Cancer Staging Manual*, TNM adopted a change in the rules for timing of staging data collection to coordinate data collection among the major cancer registry organizations in the USA including the North American Central Registry programs [e.g., the NCI Surveillance Epidemiology and End Results Program (SEER) and the National Program of Cancer Registries (NPCR) of the Center for Disease Control and Prevention], and the National Cancer Data Base, and to accommodate changing practice patterns with increased use of sensitive imaging studies that often were applied during the initial diagnostic phase of care, but occurred after surgery. The timing rules state that:

- *Clinical staging* includes any information obtained about the extent of cancer before initiation of definitive treatment (surgery, systemic or radiation therapy, active surveillance, or palliative care) or within 4 months after the date of diagnosis, whichever is *shorter*, as long as the cancer has not clearly progressed during that time frame.
- *Pathologic staging* includes any information obtained about the extent of cancer through completion of definitive surgery as part of first course treatment or identified within 4 months after the date of diagnosis, whichever is *longer*, as long as there is no systemic or radiation therapy initiated or the cancer has not clearly progressed during that timeframe.

TNM Staging Classification: Clinical, Pathologic, Recurrent, Posttreatment, and Autopsy. Stage may be defined at a number of points in the care of the cancer patient. These include "pretreatment stage" or "clinical stage," and postsurgical or "pathologic stage." In addition, stage may be determined (a) after therapy for those receiving systemic or radiation therapy before surgery (termed neoadjuvant therapy) or as primary treatment without surgery, (b) at the time of recurrence, and (c) for cancers identified at autopsy.

Clinical stage (pretreatment stage) is the extent of disease defined by diagnostic study before information is available from surgical resection or initiation of neoadjuvant therapy, within the required time frame (see previous discussion). The nomenclature for clinical staging is cT, cN, and cM, and the anatomic stage/prognostic groups based on cTNM are termed the clinical stage groups. Clinical staging incorporates information obtained from symptoms; physical examination; endoscopic examinations; imaging studies of the tumor, regional lymph nodes, and metastases; biopsies of the primary tumor; and surgical exploration without resection. When T is classified only clinically (cT), information from biopsy of single or sentinel lymph nodes may be included in clinical node staging (cN). On occasion, information obtained at the time of surgery may be classified as clinical such as when liver metastases that are identified clinically but not biopsied during a surgical resection of an abdominal tumor.

Pathologic stage is defined by the same diagnostic studies used for clinical staging supplemented by findings from surgical resection and histologic examination of the surgically removed tissues. This adds significant additional prognostic information that is more precise than what can be discerned clinically before therapy. This pathologic extent of disease or pathologic stage is expressed as pT, pN, and pM.

Posttherapy stage (yTNM) documents the extent of the disease for patients whose first course of therapy includes systemic or radiation treatment prior to surgical resection or when systemic therapy or radiation is the primary treatment with no surgical resection. The use of so-called *neoadjuvant* therapy is increasingly common in solid tumors including breast, lung, gastrointestinal, head and neck, and other cancers. Posttherapy stage may be recorded as clinical or pathologic depending on the source of posttreatment information. The extent of disease is classified using the same T, N, and M definitions and identified as posttreatment with a "yc" or "yp" prefix (ycT, ycN, ycTNM; ypT, ypN, ypTNM). Note that American registry systems do not have a data element to record "yc" elements, but these may be recorded in the medical record. The measured response to therapy and/or the extent of cancer after therapy may be prognostic. It is also used to guide subsequent surgery or other therapy.

When a patient receives presurgical treatment and has a posttherapy yc- or yp-TNM stage, the *stage* used for surveillance analysis and for comparison purposes is the clinical stage before the start of therapy. Care should be taken not to record the postneoadjuvant therapy stage as the primary stage for comparison of populations or for clinical trials. This could lead to erroneous reports. For example, a patient with a clinical Stage III breast cancer after chemotherapy could have only residual carcinoma in situ. If the final y stage was used as the original stage, the cancer would be erroneously staged as Stage 0. This would be grossly misleading for a case that in fact presented as a locally advanced Stage III cancer.

Two other staging classifications are defined, though there are no data fields reserved for these stages in most cancer registry systems. The first of these is *"Retreatment" classification (rTNM)*. This is used because information gleaned from therapeutic procedures and from extent of disease defined clinically may be prognostic for patients with recurrent cancer after a disease-free interval. Clearly the extent of recurrent disease guides therapy, and this should be recorded in the medical record using the TNM classification. It is important to understand that the rTNM classification does not change the original clinical or pathologic staging of the case. The second of these is the *"Autopsy" classification (aTNM)* used to stage cases of cancer not recognized during life and only identified postmortem.

TNM Groupings. For the purposes of tabulation and analysis of the care of patients with a similar prognosis, T, N, and M are grouped into so-called *anatomic stage/prognostic groups*, commonly referred to as stage groups. Groups are classified by Roman numerals from I to IV with increasing severity of disease. Stage I generally denotes cancers that are smaller or less deeply invasive with negative nodes; Stage II and III define cases with increasing tumor or nodal extent, and Stage IV identifies those who present with distant metastases (M1) at diagnosis. In addition, the term Stage 0 is used to denote carcinoma in situ with no metastatic potential. Stage 0 is almost always determined by pathologic examination.

The primary TNM groupings are purely clinical or pathologic. However, in clinical medicine, it is often expedient to combine clinical and pathologic T, N, and M information to define a mixed stage group for treatment planning. An example of a clinical situation where such "mixed staging" is used clinically is a woman with breast cancer who has had the primary tumor resected providing pathologic T, but for whom there was no lymph node surgery, requiring use of the clinical N. The mixed stage combining clinical and pathologic information is sometimes referred to as *working stage*. However, pure clinical and pathologic stage is still defined for comparative purposes. In addition, clinical M status (M0 or M1) may be mixed with pathologic T and N information to define pathologic stage, and the classification pTis cN0 cM0 may be used to define both clinical and pathologic stage for in situ carcinoma. If there is pathologic evidence of metastases (pM1), it may be used with clinical T and N information to define clinical Stage IV and pathologic Stage IV.

The grouping recommendations in this manual are based primarily on anatomic information. Anatomic extent of disease is supplemented by selected nonanatomic prognostic factors in some disease sites. To denote the significance of this selective use of nonanatomic factors and to underscore the importance of anatomic information, the title of the groupings in the *AJCC Cancer Staging Manual* has been changed to "*Anatomic Stage/Prognostic Groups.*"

Recording Cancer Stage in the Medical Record. All staging classifications, and most importantly clinical and pathologic T, N, and M and stage grouping, should be recorded in the medical record. Clinical stage is used in defining primary therapy (including surgery if surgery is performed), and when surgery is the initial treatment, subsequent systemic or radiation treatment is based on the pathologic stage. Recording clinical stage is also important because it may be the only common denominator among all cancers of a certain anatomic site and histology. Examples include lung cancer, advanced GI tumors, and head and neck cancers where surgery may not be performed, as well as cancers such as prostate cancer and others where surgical resection for limited disease may be omitted. In such scenarios, it may be impossible to compare cases where information is only obtained by clinical means with those where surgical resection is performed. For this reason, clinical stage remains an important component of application of the TNM staging system. This was reinforced in 2008 by the American College of Surgeons Commission on Cancer in its cancer program standards with the requirement that clinical stage be recorded in all cases.

There are many options for recording staging data in the medical record. These include documenting in the initial clinical evaluations, operative reports, discharge summaries, and follow-up reports. Physicians are encouraged to enter the stage of cancer in every record of clinical encounters with the cancer patient. In addition, a paper or electronic staging form may be useful to record stage in the medical record as well as to facilitate communication of staging data to a cancer registry. A simple form for collecting staging data is included for each disease site in this manual.

The Cancer Registry and the Collaborative Stage Data Collection System. Recording stage information in a cancer registry allows analysis of treatment effects and longitudinal population studies. Traditionally registries recorded the staging data provided in the medical record or on a staging form by the physician. With the increasing complexity of staging, the potential to incorporate various nonanatomic factors into staging algorithms, and the need to coordinate staging data collection for hospital- and population-based central registries, there was a need for a more standardized data collection tool for staging data. Such a system, termed the Collaborative Stage Data Collection System (CS), was developed by the AJCC and its cancer surveillance and staging partner organizations and implemented in cancer registries in the USA in 2004. It has also been implemented in parts of Canada with the expectation to implement throughout Canada by 2012.

In the CS system, T, N, and M data plus selected nonanatomic factors are recorded and a computer-based algorithm derives TNM stage as defined in the *AJCC Cancer Staging Manual*. The stage derivation uses the nonanatomic factors if they are available and derives a pure anatomic stage if they are not. In addition, the CS algorithm derives Summary Stage 1977 and 2000. In the CS system, the primary data defining T, N, and M are collected and stored in local registries and transmitted to central registries. T is derived from the size and local extension of disease, N from data elements that describe node status and the number of examined and positive nodes, and M from an element that records the presence or absence of metastases. In addition, the CS system includes "site-specific factors" used to record information beyond the anatomic extent of disease. There are two types of site-specific factors: those that are required for deriving the "Anatomic Stage/Prognostic Group" (e.g., Gleason's Score in prostate cancer) and those that are key prognostic or predictive factors for a given disease (e.g., estrogen receptor and HER2/neu status in breast cancer). Anatomic stage/prognostic groups are calculated from the T, N, and M and relevant site-specific factors. Collaborative stage does not assign a "c" or "p" to the stage grouping but only to the TNM elements. The CS system-derived groups are not necessarily purely clinical or pathologic TNM groups, but represent the best stage that combines clinical and pathologic data.

Importantly, the CS system stores the primary data in an interoperable tagged format that may be exported for other purposes including application in prognostic models and nomograms and for research into new prognostic models. The data elements that are collected in the Collaborative Stage Data Collection System are shown in Table 1.2.

The Collaborative Stage Data Collection System has been revised to accommodate this seventh edition of the *AJCC Cancer Staging Manual*. Key revisions are expansion of the site-specific factors to accommodate added prognostic factors and additional data elements necessary to record the clinical stage used for all cases, and the yp stage after neoadjuvant therapy. This will collect information on pretreatment clinical stage prior to the initiation of therapy and the posttreatment pathologic stage (yp) after completion of neoadjuvant therapy in patients who have resection. Detailed information on the CS system and current CS data element standards is available at http://www.cancerstaging.org/cstage.

NOMENCLATURE OF THE MORPHOLOGY OF CANCER

Cancer treatment requires assessment of the extent and behavior of the tumor and the status of the patient. The most widely used is TNM based on documentation of the anatomic extent of the cancer and selected related nonanatomic factors. The description of the anatomic factors is specific for each disease site. These descriptors and the nomenclature for TNM have been developed and refined over many editions of the *AJCC Cancer Staging Manual* by experts in each disease and cancer registrars who collect the information, taking into consideration the behavior and natural history of each type of cancer.

An *accurate microscopic diagnosis* is essential to the evaluation and treatment of cancer. The histologic and morphologic characteristics of tumors are generally reported by expert pathologists. This is best accomplished using standardized nomenclature in a structured report such as the synoptic reports or cancer protocols defined by the College of American Pathologists (CAP). In addition, for some cancers measurements of other factors including biochemical, molecular, genetic, immunologic, or functional characteristics of the tumor or normal tissues have become important or essential elements in classifying tumors precisely. Techniques that supplement standard histological evaluation including immunohistochemistry, cytogenetics, and genetic characterization are used to characterize tumors and their potential behavior and response to treatment.

Related Classifications. In the interest of promoting international collaboration in cancer research and to facilitate comparison of data among different clinical studies, use of the *WHO International Classification of Tumours* for classification and definition of tumor types, the *International Classifications of Diseases for Oncology (ICD-0)* codes for storage and retrieval of data, CAP protocols for pathology reporting of cancer pathology specimens, and the Collaborative Stage Data Collection System for collecting staging data is recommended. Given here is a summary of relevant related classification and coding systems with source citations.

- *World Health Organization Classification of Tumours, Pathology and Genetics.* Since 1958, the World Health Organization (WHO) has had a program aimed at providing internationally accepted criteria for the histological classification of tumors. The most recent edition is a ten-volume series that contains definitions, descriptions, and illustrations of tumor types and related nomenclature (WHO: World Health Organization Classification of Tumours. Various editions. Lyon, France: IARC Press, 2000–2008).

- *WHO International Classification of Diseases for Oncology (ICD-0), 3rd edition.* ICD-0 is a numerical classification and coding system by topography and morphology (WHO: ICD-O-3 International Classification of Diseases for Oncology. 3rd ed. Geneva: WHO, 2000).

- *Systematized Nomenclature of Medicine (SNOMED).* Published by the CAP, SNOMED provides tumor classification systems compatible with the ICD-O system (http://snomed.org).

- *Collaborative Stage Data Collection System.* This system for collecting cancer staging data was developed through a collaboration of the AJCC and other standard setting organizations. Primary data are recorded on the size and extension of the primary tumor, the status of lymph nodes, and presence of distant metastases and certain "site-specific factors." These data are used to derive TNM stage and Summary Stage (http://www.cancerstaging.org/cstage/index.html).

- *CAP Cancer Protocols.* The CAP publishes standards for pathology reporting of cancer specimens for all cancer types and cancer resection types. These specify the elements necessary for the pathologist to report the extent and characteristics of cancer specimens. These elements are being coordinated with the *Collaborative Stage Data Collection System* to allow direct reporting of pathology elements to cancer registries (http://www.cap.org).

- *caBIG.* The National Cancer Institute of the USA has developed the Cancer Bioinformatics Grid (caBIG) to standardize data elements and integration of these elements for the reporting of information for clinical trials and to annotate biological specimens (http://cabig.cancer.gov).

- *Atlas of Tumor Pathology.* A comprehensive and well-known English language compendium of the macroscopic and microscopic characteristics of tumors and their behavior is the *Atlas of Tumor Pathology* series, published in many volumes by the Armed Forces Institute of Pathology in Washington, DC. These are revised periodically and are used as a basic reference by pathologists throughout the world (*Atlas of Tumor Pathology*, 3rd edition series. Washington, DC: Armed Forces Institute of Pathology, 1991–2002).

- *American College of Radiology Appropriateness Criteria.* The American College of Radiology maintains guidelines and criteria for use of imaging and interventional radiology procedures for many aspects of cancer care. This includes the extent of imaging testing that is recommended for the diagnostic evaluation of the extent of disease of the primary tumor, nodes, and distant metastases in a number of cancer types. The ACR appropriateness criteria are updated regularly (http://www.acr.org/ac).

- *Practice Guidelines of the National Comprehensive Cancer Network (NCCN).* The NCCN provides practice guidelines for most types of cancers. These guidelines are updated at least annually. They include recommendations for diagnostic evaluation and imaging for the primary tumor and screening for metastases for each cancer type that may be useful to guide staging (http://www.nccn.org).

GENERAL RULES FOR TNM STAGING

The TNM system classifies and groups cancers primarily by the anatomic extent of the primary tumor, the status of regional draining lymph nodes, and the presence or absence of distant metastases. The system is in essence a shorthand notation for describing the clinical and pathologic anatomic extent of a tumor. In addition, the AJCC recommends collection of key prognostic factors that either are used to define groupings or are critical to prognosis or defining patient care.

T   The T component is defined by the size or contiguous extension of the primary tumor. The roles of the size component and the extent of contiguous spread in defining T are specifically defined for each cancer site.

N   The N component is defined by the absence, or presence and extent of cancer in the regional draining lymph nodes. Nodal involvement is categorized by the number of positive nodes and for certain cancer sites by the involvement of specific regional nodal groups.

M   The M component is defined by the absence or presence of distant spread or metastases, generally in locations to which the cancer spread by vascular channels, or by lymphatics beyond the nodes defined as "regional."

For each of T, N, and M the use of increasing values denotes progressively greater extent of the cancer as shown later. For some disease sites, subdivisions of the main designators are used to provide more specific prognostic information (e.g., T1mi, T1a, T1b, T1c or N2a, N2b in breast cancer or M1a, M1b, M1c for prostate cancer). Specific definitions for each cancer type are provided in the respective chapters. General designators for T, N, and M are shown later and general rules for applying these designators are shown in the tables. For each designator, the prefix of c, p, yc, yp, r, or a may be applied to denote the classification of stage (see later):

Primary Tumor (T)

T0	No evidence of primary tumor
Tis	Carcinoma in situ
T1, T2, T3, T4	Increasing size and/or local extension of the primary tumor
TX	Primary tumor cannot be assessed (use of TX should be minimized)

Regional Lymph Nodes (N)

N0	No regional lymph node metastases
N1, N2, N3	Increasing number or extent of regional lymph node involvement
NX	Regional lymph nodes cannot be assessed (use of NX should be minimized)

Distant Metastasis (M)

M0	No distant metastases
M1	Distant metastases present

Note: The MX designation has been eliminated from the AJCC/UICC TNM system.

The M1 category may be further specified according to the following notation signifying the location of metastases:

Pulmonary	PUL
Osseous	OSS
Hepatic	HEP
Brain	BRA
Lymph nodes	LYM
Bone marrow	MAR
Pleura	PLE
Peritoneum	PER
Adrenal	ADR
Skin	SKI
Other	OTH

Nonanatomic Prognostic Factors Required for Staging. In some cancer types, nonanatomic factors are required for assigning the anatomic stage/prognostic group. These are clearly defined in each chapter. These factors are collected separately from T, N, and M, which remain purely anatomic, and are used to assign stage groups. Where nonanatomic factors are used in groupings, there is a definition of the groupings provided for cases where the nonanatomic factor is not available (X) or where it is desired to assign a group ignoring the nonanatomic factor.

Use of the Unknown X Designation. The X category is used when information on a specific component is unknown. Cases where T or N is classified as X cannot be assigned a stage (an exception is *Any T* or *Any N M1*, which includes TX or NX, classified as Stage IV – e.g., TX NX M1 or TX N3 M1 are Stage IV). Therefore, the X category for T and N should be used only when absolutely necessary.

The category MX has been eliminated from the AJCC/UICC TNM system. Unless there is clinical or pathologic evidence of distant metastases, the case is classified as clinical M0 (cM0). Because of the requirement for pathologists to assign TNM on cancer pathology reports, and because the pathologist often does not have information to assign M, the CAP has dropped the M component from pathology templates to further discourage use of MX. The elimination of the code MX is a change in the seventh edition of the *AJCC Cancer Staging Manual* and *UICC TNM Cancer Staging Manual*. See later for rules for M classification.

The following general rules apply to application of T, N, and M for all sites and classifications (Table 1.3):

1. Microscopic confirmation: All cases should be confirmed microscopically for classification by TNM (including clinical classification). Rare cases that do not have any biopsy or cytology of the tumor can be staged, but survival should be analyzed separately. These cases should not be included in overall disease survival analyses.
2. Eligible time period for determination of staging:
   a. *Clinical staging* includes any information obtained about the extent of cancer before initiation of definitive treatment (surgery, systemic or radiation therapy, active surveillance, or palliative care) or within 4 months after the date of diagnosis, whichever is *shorter*, as long as the cancer has not clearly progressed during that time frame.
   b. *Pathologic staging* includes any information obtained about the extent of cancer up through completion of definitive surgery as part of first course treatment or identified within 4 months

after the date of diagnosis, whichever is *longer*, as long as there is no systemic or radiation therapy initiated or the cancer has not clearly progressed during that time frame.

3. Staging with neoadjuvant or primary systemic or radiation therapy: Cases with neoadjuvant, or primary systemic or radiation, therapy may have a second stage defined from information obtained after therapy that is recorded using a yc or yp prefix (ycTNM or ypTNM; y must always be modified as yc or yp). However, these patients should also have clinical stage recorded as this is the stage used for comparative purposes. Clinical stage includes only information collected prior to the start of treatment.

4. Progression of disease: In cases where there is documented progression of cancer prior to the initiation of therapy or surgery, only information obtained prior to documented progression is used for staging.

5. If uncertain, classify or stage using the lower category: If there is uncertainty in assigning a T, N, or M classification, a stage modifying factor (i.e., in clinical situations where it is unclear if the lymph nodes are N2 or N1), or anatomic stage/prognostic group, default to the lower (lesser) of the two categories in the uncertain range.

6. Nonanatomic factor not available: If a nonanatomic factor required for grouping is not available, the case is assigned to the group assuming that factor was the lowest or least advanced (e.g., lower Gleason's score in prostate cancer).

Stage Classifications. Five stage classifications may be described for each site (Table 1.4):

- Clinical stage/pretreatment stage, designated as cTNM or TNM
- Pathologic stage, designated as pTNM
- Post therapy or postneoadjuvant therapy stage, designated as ycTNM or ypTNM
- Retreatment or recurrence classification, designated as rTNM
- Autopsy classification, designated as aTNM

Clinical Classification. Clinical classification is based on evidence acquired before the initiation of primary treatment (definitive surgery, or neoadjuvant radiation or systemic therapy). The clinical stage (pretreatment stage) is essential to selecting primary therapy. In addition, the clinical stage is critical for comparison of groups of cases because differences in the use of primary therapy may make such comparisons based on pathologic assessment impossible, such as in situations where some patients are treated with primary surgery and others are treated with neoadjuvant chemotherapy or with no therapy.

Clinical assessment uses information available from clinical history, physical examination, imaging, endoscopy, biopsy of the primary site, surgical exploration, or other relevant examinations. Observations made at surgical exploration where a biopsy of the primary site is performed without resection or where pathologic material is not obtained are classified as clinical, unless the biopsy provides pathologic material on the highest possible T category in which case it is classified at pT (see pathologic staging later). Pathologic examination of a single node in the absence of pathologic evaluation of the primary tumor is classified as clinical (cN) (e.g., if sentinel node biopsy is performed prior to neoadjuvant therapy in breast cancer). Extensive imaging is not necessary to assign clinical classifications. Guides to the generally accepted standards for diagnostic evaluations of individual cancer types include the American College of Radiology Appropriateness Standards (http://www.acr.org/ac) and the NCCN Practice Guidelines (http://www.nccn.org). The clinical (pretreatment) stage assigned on the basis of information obtained prior to cancer-directed treatment is not changed on the basis of subsequent information obtained from the pathologic examination of resected tissue or from information obtained after initiation of definitive therapy. In the case of treatment with palliative care or active surveillance (watchful waiting), the information for staging is that defined prior to making the decision for no active treatment or that which occurs within

4 months of diagnosis, whichever is shorter. Any information obtained after the decision for active surveillance or palliative care may not used in clinical staging. Classification of T, N, and M by clinical means is denoted by use of a lower case c prefix (cT, cN, cM).

Clinical staging of metastases warrants special consideration. A case where there are no symptoms or signs of metastases is classified as clinically M0. There is no MX classification. The only evaluation necessary to classify a case as clinically M0 is history and physical examination. It is not necessary to do extensive imaging studies to classify a case as clinically M0. The optimal extent of testing required in many cancer types is provided in guidelines of the American College of Radiology Appropriateness Criteria (http://www.acr.org/ac) and in the National Comprehensive Cancer Network practice guidelines (http://www.nccn.org). The classification pM0 does not exist and may not be assigned on the basis of a negative biopsy of a suspected metastatic site. Cases with clinical evidence of metastases by examination, invasive procedures including exploratory surgery, and imaging, but without a tissue biopsy confirming metastases are classified as cM1. If there is a positive biopsy of a metastatic site (pM1) and T and N are staged only clinically, then the case may be staged as clinical and pathologic Stage IV.

Pathologic Classification. The pathologic classification of a cancer is based on information acquired before treatment supplemented and modified by the additional evidence acquired during and from surgery, particularly from pathologic examination of resected tissues. The pathologic classification provides additional precise and objective data. Classification of T, N, and M by pathologic means is denoted by use of a lower case p prefix (pT, pN, pM).

Pathologic T. The pathologic assessment of the *primary tumor (pT)* generally is based on resection of the primary tumor generally from a single specimen (Table 1.5). Resection of the tumor with several partial removals at the same or separate operations necessitates an effort at reasonable estimates of the size and extension of the tumor to assign the correct or highest pT category. Tumor size should be recorded in whole millimeters. If the size is reported in smaller units such as a tenth or hundredth of a millimeter, it should be rounded to the nearest whole millimeter for reporting stage. Rounding is performed as follows: one through four are rounded down, and five through nine are rounded up. For example, a breast tumor reported as 1.2 mm in size should be recorded for staging as a 1-mm tumor, and a 1.7-mm tumor should be recorded as a 2-mm tumor. If the tumor is not resected, but a biopsy of the primary tumor is performed that is adequate to evaluate the highest pT category, the pT classification is assigned. Some disease sites have specific rules to guide assignment of pT category in such cases.

Pathologic N. The pathologic assessment of *regional lymph nodes (pN)* ideally requires resection of a minimum number of lymph nodes to assure that there is sufficient sampling to identify positive nodes if present (Table 1.6). This number varies among diseases sites, and the expected number of lymph nodes is defined in each chapter. The recommended number generally does not apply in cases where sentinel node has been accepted as accurate for defining regional node involvement and a sentinel node procedure has been performed. However, in cases where lymph node surgery results in examination of fewer than the ideal minimum number, the N category is still generally classified as pathologic N according to the number of positive nodes and/or location of the most advanced pathologic node resected. At least one node with presence or absence of cancer documented by pathologic examination is required for pathologic staging N. The impact of use of pathologic N classification with fewer than the minimum resected nodes may be subsequently defined by review of the number of resected nodes as recorded in a cancer registry.

Pathologic assessment of T (pT) is generally necessary to assign pathologic assessment of lymph nodes. In conjunction with pT, it is not necessary to have pathologic confirmation of the status of the highest N category to assign pN. However, if N is based on microscopic confirmation of the highest N category, it is pN regardless of whether T is pT or cT. For example, in the case of breast cancer with pT defined by resection, pN may be assigned solely on the basis of resected level I or II nodes, or a level I sentinel node without biopsy of level III or supraclavicular nodes. However, if there is microscopic confirmation of supraclavicular node involvement, the case may also be classified as pN3.

Specialized pathologic techniques such as immunohistochemistry or molecular techniques may identify limited metastases in lymph nodes that may not have been identified without the use of the special diagnostic techniques. Single tumor cells or small clusters of cells are classified as *isolated tumor cells* (ITC). The standard definition for ITC is a cluster of cells not more than 0.2 mm in greatest diameter. The appropriate N classification for cases with nodes only involved by ITC's is defined in the disease site chapters for those cancers where this commonly occurs. In most of such chapters, these cases with ITC only in lymph nodes or distant sites are classified as pN0 or cM0. This rule also generally applies to cases with findings of tumor cells or their components by nonmorphologic techniques such as flow cytometry or DNA analysis. There are specific designators to identify such cases by disease site [e.g., N0 (i+) in breast cancer to denote nodes with ITC only].

Pathologic M. The pathologic assignment of the presence of *metastases* (*pM1*) requires a biopsy positive for cancer at the metastatic site (Table 1.7). Pathologic M0 is an undefined concept and the category pM0 may not be used. Pathologic classification of the absence of distant metastases can only be made at autopsy. However, the assessment of metastases to group a patient by pathologic TNM groupings may be either clinical (cM0 or cM1) or pathologic (pM1) (e.g., pTNM = pT; pN; cM or pM). Cases with a biopsy of a possible metastatic site that shows ITC such as circulating tumor cells (CTCs) or disseminated tumor cells (DTCs), or bone marrow micrometastases detected by IHC or molecular techniques are classified as cM0(i+) to denote the uncertain prognostic significance of these findings and to classify the stage group according to the T and N and M0.

Pathologic staging depends on the proven anatomic extent of disease, whether or not the primary lesion has been completely removed. If a primary tumor cannot be technically removed, or when it is unreasonable to remove it, and if the highest T and N categories or the M1 category of the tumor can be confirmed microscopically, the criteria for pathologic classification and staging have been satisfied without total removal of the primary tumor. Note that microscopic confirmation of the highest T and N does not necessarily require removal of that structure and may entail biopsy only.

Posttherapy or Postneoadjuvant Therapy Classification (yTNM). Cases where systemic and/or radiation therapy are given before surgery (*neoadjuvant*) or where no surgery is performed may have the extent of disease assessed at the conclusion of the therapy by clinical or pathologic means (if resection performed). This classification is useful to clinicians because the extent of response to therapy may provide important prognostic information to patients and help direct the extent of surgery or subsequent systemic and/or radiation therapy. T and N are classified using the same categories as for clinical or pathologic staging for the disease type, and the findings are recorded using the prefix designator y (e.g., ycT; ycN; ypT; ypN). The yc prefix is used for the clinical stage after therapy, and the yp prefix is used for the pathologic stage for those cases that have surgical resection after neoadjuvant therapy. Both the ycTNM and ypTNM may be recorded in the medical record, though cancer registries will in general only record the ypTNM in cases where surgery is performed. The M component should be classified by the M status defined clinically or pathologically prior to therapy. If a biopsy of a metastatic site is positive, the case is classified as clinical and pathologic Stage IV. The estimate of disease prior to therapy is recorded using the clinical designator as described earlier (cTNM). The stage used for case comparisons and population purposes in these cases should be the clinical (cTNM) one.

Retreatment Classification. The retreatment classification (rTNM) is assigned when further treatment is planned for a cancer that recurs after a disease-free interval. The original stage assigned at the time of initial diagnosis and treatment does not change when the cancer recurs or progresses. The use of this staging for retreatment or recurrence is denoted using the r prefix (rTNM). All information available at the time of retreatment should be used in determining the rTNM stage. Biopsy confirmation of recurrent cancer is important if clinically feasible. However, this may not be appropriate for each component, so clinical evidence for the T, N, or M component by clinical, endoscopic, radiologic, or related methods may be used.

Autopsy Classification. TNM classification of a cancer may be performed by postmortem examination for a patient where cancer was not evident prior to death. This autopsy classification (aTNM) is denoted using the a prefix (aTNM) and should include all clinical and pathologic information obtained at the time of death and autopsy.

Stage Groupings. Cases of cancers with similar prognosis are grouped based on the assigned cT, cN, and cM and/or pT, pN and c/pM categories, and disease-specific groups of T, N, and M are defined. In select disease sites nonanatomic factors are required to supplement T, N, and M to define these groups. Termed *anatomic stage/prognostic groups*, and commonly referred to as stage groups, these form a reproducible and easily communicated summary of staging information (Table 1.8).

Groups are assigned increasing values that correlate with worsening prognosis. Stage I is usually assigned to tumors confined to the primary site with a better prognosis, stages II and III for tumors with increasing local and regional nodal involvement, and stage IV to cases with distant metastatic disease. In addition, a group termed stage 0 is assigned to cases of carcinoma in situ (CIS). Groupings may be expanded into subsets (e.g., stage II can become stage IIA, stage IIB) for more refined prognostic information.

Generally, a pure clinical group and pure pathologic group are defined for each case, using the classifications discussed earlier. In the clinical setting, it is appropriate to combine clinical and pathologic data when only partial information is available in either the pathologic or clinical classification, and this may be referred to as the *working* stage.

Carcinoma in situ (CIS) is an exception to the stage grouping guidelines. By definition, CIS has not involved any structures in the primary organ that would allow tumor cells to spread to regional nodes or distant sites. Therefore, pTis cN0 cM0 should be reported as both clinical and pathologic stage 0.

The clinical, pathologic, and if applicable, posttherapy and retreatment, groups are recorded in the medical record. Once assigned according to the appropriate rules and timing, the stage group recorded in the medical record does not change. The rule applied to T, N, or M that in cases with uncertainty about the classification the cases are assigned the lower (less advanced) category also applies to grouping. One specific circumstance requires special comment. When there has been a complete pathologic response and the ypTNM is ypT0 ypN0 cM0, this is not a "stage 0" case as this would denote in situ disease, and as in every case, the stage for comparison of cases is the pretreatment clinical stage.

Multiple Tumors. When there are multiple simultaneous tumors of the same histology in one organ, the tumor with the highest T category is the one selected for classification and staging, and the multiplicity or the number of tumors is indicated in parentheses: for example, T2(m) or T2(5). For simultaneous bilateral cancers in paired organs, the tumors are classified separately as independent tumors in different organs. For tumors of the thyroid, liver, and ovary, multiplicity is a criterion of the T classification. Most registry software systems have a mechanism to record the m descriptor.

Metachronous Primaries. Second or subsequent primary cancers occurring in the same organ or in different organs are staged as a new cancer using the TNM system described in this manual. Second cancers are not staged using the y prefix unless the treatment of the second cancer warrants this use.

Unknown Primary. In cases where there is no evidence of a primary tumor or the site of the primary tumor is unknown, staging may be based on the clinical suspicion of the primary tumor with the T category classified as T0. For example, a case with metastatic adenocarcinoma in axillary lymph nodes that is pathologically consistent with breast cancer, but in which there is no apparent primary breast tumor may be classified as breast cancer – T0 N1 M0 (Table 1.9).

HISTOPATHOLOGIC TYPE, GRADE, AND OTHER DESCRIPTORS

Histopathologic Type. The histopathologic type is a *qualitative* assessment whereby a tumor is categorized according to the normal tissue type or cell type it most closely resembles (e.g., hepatocellular or cholangiocarcinoma, osteosarcoma, squamous cell carcinoma). The *World Health Organization Classification of Tumours* published in numerous anatomic site-specific editions may be used for histopathologic typing. Each chapter in the *AJCC Cancer Staging Manual* includes the applicable ICD-O-3 histopathologic codes expressed as individual codes or ranges of codes. If a specific histology is not listed, the case should not be staged using the AJCC classification in that chapter.

Grade. The grade of a cancer is a qualitative assessment of the degree of differentiation of the tumor. Grade may reflect the extent to which a tumor resembles the normal tissue at that site. Historically, histologic stratification of solid tumors has been dominated by the description of differentiation with grade expressed as the overall histologic differentiation of the cancer in numerical grades from the most or well differentiated (grade 1) to the least differentiated (grade 3 or 4). This system is still used in some cancer types. For many cancer types, more precise and reproducible grading systems have been developed. These incorporate more specific and objective criteria based on single or multiple characteristics of the cancers. These factors include such characteristics as nuclear grade, the number of mitoses identified microscopically (mitotic count), measures of histologic differentiation (e.g., tubule formation in breast cancer), and others. For some cancer types these systems have been fully validated and largely implemented worldwide. Examples include the Gleason's scoring system for prostate cancer and the Scarff–Bloom–Richardson (Nottingham) grading system for breast cancer.

The recommended grading system for each cancer type is specified in the site-specific chapters. In general, when there is no specific grading system for a cancer type, it should be noted if a two-grade, three-grade, or four-grade system was used. For some anatomic sites, grade 3 and grade 4 are combined into a single grade – for example, poorly differentiated to undifferentiated (G3–4). The use of grade 4 is reserved for those tumors that show no specific differentiation that would identify the cancer as arising from its site of origin. In some sites, the WHO histologic classification includes undifferentiated carcinomas. For these, the tumor is graded as undifferentiated – grade 4. Some histologic tumor types are by definition listed as grade 4 for staging purposes but are not to be assigned a grade of undifferentiated in ICD-O-3 coding for cancer registry purposes. These include the following:

- Small cell carcinoma, any site
- Large cell carcinoma of lung
- Ewing's sarcoma of bone and soft tissue
- Rhabdomyosarcoma of soft tissue

The grade should be recorded for each cancer. Two data elements should be recorded: the grade and whether a two, three, or four-grade system was used for grading. If there is evidence of more than one grade of level or differentiation of the tumor, the least differentiated (highest grade) is recorded.

Residual Tumor and Surgical Margins. The absence or presence of residual tumor after treatment is described by the symbol R. cTNM and pTNM describe the extent of cancer in general without consideration of treatment. cTNM and pTNM can be supplemented by the R classification, which deals with the tumor status after treatment. In some cases treated with surgery and/or with neoadjuvant therapy there will be residual tumor at the primary site after treatment because of incomplete resection or local and regional disease that extends beyond the limit or ability of resection. The presence of residual tumor may indicate the effect of therapy, influence further therapy, and be a strong predictor of prognosis. In addition, the presence or absence of disease at the margin of resection may be a predictor of the risk of recurrent cancer. The presence of residual disease or positive margins may be more likely with more advanced T or N category tumors. The R category is not incorporated into TMM staging itself. However, the absence or presence of residual tumor and status of the margins may be recorded in the medical record and cancer registry.

The absence or presence of residual tumor at the primary tumor site after treatment is denoted by the symbol R. The R categories for the primary tumor site are as follows:

R0   No residual tumor
R1   Microscopic residual tumor
R2   Macroscopic residual tumor
RX   Presence of residual tumor cannot be assessed

The margin status may be recorded using the following categories:

- Negative margins (tumor not present at the surgical margin)
- Microscopic positive margin (tumor not identified grossly at the margin, but present microscopically at the margin)
- Macroscopic positive margin (tumor identified grossly at the margin)
- Margin not assessed

Lymph-Vascular Invasion. Indicates whether microscopic lymph-vascular invasion (LVI) is identified in the pathology report. This term includes lymphatic invasion, vascular invasion, or lymph-vascular invasion (synonymous with "lymphovascular").

ORGANIZATION OF THE *AJCC CANCER STAGING MANUAL* AND ANATOMIC SITES AND REGIONS

In general, the anatomic sites for cancer in this manual are listed by primary site code number according to the International Classification of Diseases for Oncology (ICD-O, third edition, WHO, 2000). Each disease site or region is discussed and the staging classification is defined in a separate chapter. There are a number of new chapters and disease sites in this seventh edition of the *AJCC Cancer Staging Manual*.

Each chapter includes a discussion of information relevant to staging that cancer type, the data supporting the staging, and the specific rationale for changes in staging. In addition, it includes definition of key prognostic factors including those required for staging and those recommended for collection in cancer registries. Each chapter ends with the specific definitions of T, N, M, site-specific factors, and anatomic stage/prognostic groups (Table 1.10).

Cancer Staging Data Form. Each site chapter includes a staging data form that may be used by providers and registrars to record the TNM classifications and the stage of the cancer. The form provides for entry of data on T, N, M, site-specific prognostic factors, cancer grade, and anatomic stage/prognostic groups. This form may be useful for recording information in the medical record and for communication of information from providers to the cancer registrar.

The staging form may be used to document cancer stage at different points in the course of therapy, including before the initiation of therapy, after surgery and completion of all staging evaluations, or at the time of recurrence. It is best to use a separate form at each point. If all time points are recorded on a single form, the staging basis for each element should be clearly identified.

The cancer staging form is a specific additional document in the patient records. It is not a substitute for documentation of history, physical examination, and staging evaluation, nor for documenting treatment plans or follow-up. The data forms in this manual may be duplicated for individual or institutional use without permission from the AJCC or the publisher. Incorporation of these forms into electronic record systems requires appropriate permission from the AJCC and the publisher.

TABLE 1.1. *AJCC Cancer Staging Manual editions*

Edition	Publication	Dates effective for cancer diagnosed
1	1977	1978–1983
2	1983	1984–1988
3	1988	1989–1992
4	1992	1993–1997
5	1997	1998–2002
6	2002	2003–2009
7	2009	2010–

TABLE 1.2. *Collaborative stage data collection system data elements*

Tumor	CS tumor size (primary tumor size in mm)
	CS extension (direct extension of the primary tumor)
	CS tumor size/extension eval (method of evaluating T)[a]
Nodes	CS lymph nodes (regional lymph node involvement)
	CS lymph nodes eval (method of evaluating N)[a]
	Regional nodes positive (number nodes positive)
	Regional nodes examined (number nodes examined)
Metastases	CS Mets at Dx (distant metastases present at time of diagnosis)
	CS Mets Eval (method of evaluating M)[a]
Site-specific factors	CS site-specific factors (specific number defined by disease)[b]

[a] Method of evaluation fields: Define source of data – clinical (c) or pathologic (p); response to neoadjuvant therapy utilizing pathologic information (yp).

[b] Site-specific factors: Additional items necessary for (a) defining cancer stage group or (b) key prognostic factors including anatomic disease modifiers and nonanatomic factors (e.g., grade and tumor markers). Most disease sites use only a few of the available site-specific factor fields.

These tumor, node, and metastases fields for best stage are duplicated as needed for pretreatment and posttreatment stages.

For full description of Collaborative Stage Data Collection System, see http://www.cancerstaging.org/cstage/index.html.

TABLE 1.3. *General rules for TNM staging*

General rules for staging	
Microscopic confirmation	Microscopic confirmation required for TNM classification Rare cases without microscopic confirmation should be analyzed separately
	Cancers classified by ICD-O-3 Recommend pathology reporting using CAP cancer protocols
Timing of data eligible for clinical staging	Data obtained before definitive treatment as part of primary treatment or within 4 months of diagnosis, whichever is shorter
	The time frame for collecting clinical stage data also ends when a decision is made for active surveillance ("watchful waiting") without therapy
Timing data eligible for pathologic staging	Data obtained through definitive surgery as part of primary treatment or within 4 months of diagnosis, whichever is longer
Timing of data eligible for staging with neoadjuvant therapy	Stage in cases with neoadjuvant therapy is (a) clinical as defined earlier before initiation of therapy and (b) clinical or pathologic using data obtained after completion of neoadjuvant therapy (ycTNM or ypTNM)
Staging in cases with uncertainty among T, N, or M categories	Assign the lower (less advanced) category of T, N, or M, prognostic factor, or stage group
Absence of staging-required nonanatomic prognostic factor	Assign stage grouping by the group defined by the lower (less advanced) designation for that factor
Multiple synchronous primary tumors in single organ	Stage T by most advanced tumor; use "m" suffix or the number of tumors in parentheses, e.g., pT3(m)N0M0 or pT3(4)N0M0
Synchronous primary tumors in paired organs	Stage and report independently
Metachronous primary tumors in single organ (not recurrence)	Stage and report independently
T0 staging – unknown primary	Stage based on clinical suspicion of primary tumor (e.g., T0 N1 M0 Group IIA breast cancer)

TABLE 1.4. *Staging classifications*

Classification	*Data source*	*Usage*
Clinical (pretreatment) (cTNM)	Diagnostic data including symptoms, physical examination, imaging, endoscopy; biopsy of primary site; resection of single node/sentinel node(s) with clinical T; surgical exploration without resection; other relevant examinations	Define prognosis and initial therapy Population comparisons
Pathologic (pTNM)	Diagnostic data and data from surgical resection and pathology	Most precise prognosis estimates Define subsequent therapy
Posttherapy (ycTNM or ypTNM)	Clinical and pathologic data after ystemic or radiation before surgery or as primary therapy denoted with a yc (clinical) or yp (pathologic) prefix	Determine subsequent therapy Identify response to therapy
Retreatment (rTNM)	Clinical and pathologic data at time of retreatment for recurrence or progression	Define treatment
Autopsy (aTNM)	Clinical and pathologic data as determined at autopsy	Define cancer stage on previously undiagnosed cancer identified at autopsy

TABLE 1.5. *T classification rules*

T determined by site-specific rules based on size and/or local extension

Clinical assessment of T (cT) based on physical examination, imaging, endoscopy, and biopsy and surgical exploration without resection

Pathologic assessment of T (pT) entails a resection of the tumor or may be assigned with biopsy only if it assigns the highest T category

pT generally based on resection in single specimen. If resected in > 1 specimen, make reasonable estimate of size/extension. Disease-specific rules may apply

Tumor size should be recorded in whole millimeters. If the size is reported in smaller units such as a tenth or hundredth of a millimeter, it should be rounded to the nearest whole millimeter for reporting stage. Rounding is performed as follows: one through four are rounded down, and five through nine are rounded up

If not resected, and highest T and N category can be confirmed microscopically; case may be classified by pT or pN without resection

TABLE 1.6. *N classification rules*

Categorize N by disease-specific rules based on number and location of positive regional nodes

Minimum expected number and location of nodes to examine for staging defined by disease type

If lymph node surgery is performed, classify N category as pathologic even if minimum number is not examined

Pathologic assessment of the primary tumor (pT) is necessary to assign pathologic assessment of nodes (pN) except with unknown primary (T0). If pathologic T (pT) is available, then any microscopic evaluation of nodes is pN

In cases with only clinical T in the absence of pT excision of a single node or sentinel node(s) is classified as clinical nodal status (cN)

Microscopic examination of a single node or nodes in the highest N category is classified as pN even in the absence of pathologic information on other nodes

Sentinel lymph node biopsy is denoted with (sn), e.g., pN0(sn); pN1 (sn)

Lymph nodes with ITC only generally staged as pN0; disease-specific rules may apply (e.g., melanoma)

Direct extension of primary tumor into regional node classified as node positive

Tumor nodule with smooth contour in regional node area classified as positive node

When size is the criterion for N category, stage by size of metastasis, not size of node when reported (unless specified in disease-specific rules)

TABLE 1.7. *M classification rules*

Clinical M classification only requires history and examination

Imaging of distant organ sites not required to assign cM0

Infer status as clinical M0 status unless known clinical M1

"MX" is not a valid category and may not be assigned

Elimination of "MX" is new with AJCC/UICC, 7th edition

Pathologic M classification requires a positive biopsy of the metastatic site (pM1)

Pathologic M0 ("pM0") is not a valid category and may not be assigned

Stage a case with a negative biopsy of suspected metastatic site as cM0

Case with pathologic T and N may be grouped as pathologic TNM using clinical M designator (cM0 or cM1) (e.g., pT1 pN0 cM0 = pathologic stage I)

Case with pathologic M1 (pM1) may be grouped as clinical and pathologic Stage IV regardless of "c" or "p" status of T and N (e.g., cT1 cN1 pM1 = clinical or pathologic stage IV)

ITC in metastatic sites (e.g., bone marrow)

Or circulating or DTCs classified as cM0(i+)

Disease-specific rules may apply

TABLE 1.8. *Anatomic stage/prognostic grouping rules*

Define separate clinical and pathologic group for each case

May combine clinical and pathologic information as a "working stage" in either the pathologic or clinical classification when only partial information is available – this may be necessary for clinical care

Minimize use of TX and NX

Use of "X" for any component makes case unstageable

Case will not be usable in comparison analyses (exception: any combination of T and N including TX or NX with M1 is stage IV)

For groupings that require a nonanatomic factor, if factor is missing, stage using lowest category for that factor

Case with pT and pN and cM0 or cM1 staged as pathologic stage group

Case with cT and cN and pM1 staged as clinical and pathologic stage group

Carcinoma in situ, stage pTis cN0 cM0 as both clinical and pathologic stage 0

TABLE 1.9. *Special classification/designator rules*

ycTNM or ypTNM	Posttherapy classification: "y" prefix to utilize with "c" or "p" for denoting extent of cancer after neoadjuvant or primary systemic and/or radiationtherapy	Assess clinical stage prior to initiation of therapy (cTNM)
		Use cTNM for comparison of cases and population surveillance
		Denote posttherapy T and N stage using "y" prefix – ycT; ycN; ypT; ypN
		yc is used for clinical information postprimary therapy systemic or radiation therapy, or postneoadjuvant therapy before surgery
		yp is used for pathologic
		postneoadjuvant systemic or radiation therapy followed by surgical resection
		Use clinical/pretreatment M status
rTNM	Retreatment classification	The original stage assigned at initial diagnosis and treatment should not be changed at the time of recurrence or progression
		Assign for cases where treatment is planned for cancer that recurs after a disease-free interval
		Use all information available at time of retreatment or recurrence (c or p)
		Biopsy confirmation desirable if feasible, but not required
aTNM	Autopsy classification	Applied for cases where cancer is not evident prior to death
		Use all clinical and pathologic
		information obtained at the time of death and at postmortem examination
m suffix	Multiple primary tumors	Multiple simultaneous tumors in one organ: Assign T by the tumor with the highest T category. Indicate multiplicity by "(m)" or "(number)" in parentheses – e.g., T2(m) or T2(5)

TABLE 1.10. *Chapter outline for the seventh edition of the AJCC Cancer Staging Manual*

Staging at a Glance	Summary of anatomic stage/prognostic grouping and major changes
Changes in Staging	Table summarizing changes in staging from the 6th edition
Introduction	Overview of factors affecting staging and outcome for the disease
Anatomic Considerations	Primary tumor
	Regional lymph nodes
	Metastatic sites
Rules for Classification	Clinical
	Pathologic
Prognostic Features	Identification and discussion of nonanatomic prognostic factors important in each disease
Definitions of TNM	T: Primary tumor
	N: Regional lymph nodes
	M: Distant metastases
Anatomic Stage/Prognostic Groups	
Prognostic Factors	(a) Required for staging
(Site-Specific Factors)	(b) Clinically significant
Grade	
Histopathologic Type	
Bibliography	
Staging Form	

Cancer Survival Analysis

2

Analysis of cancer survival data and related outcomes is necessary to assess cancer treatment programs and to monitor the progress of regional and national cancer control programs. The appropriate use of data from cancer registries for outcomes analyses requires an understanding of the correct application of appropriate quantitative tools and the limitations of the analyses imposed by the source of data, the degree to which the available data represent the population, and the quality and completeness of registry data. In this chapter the most common survival analysis methodology is illustrated, basic terminology is defined, and the essential elements of data collection and reporting are described. Although the underlying principles are applicable to both, the focus of this discussion is on the use of survival analysis to describe data typically available in cancer registries rather than to analyze research data obtained from clinical trials or laboratory experimentation. Discussion of statistical principles and methodology will be limited. Persons interested in statistical underpinnings or research applications are referred to textbooks that explore these topics at length.

BASIC CONCEPTS

A *survival rate* is a statistical index that summarizes the probable frequency of specific outcomes for a group of patients at a particular point in time. A *survival curve* is a summary display of the pattern of survival rates over time. The basic concept is simple. For example, for a certain category of patient, one might ask what proportion is likely to be alive at the end of a specified interval, such as 5 years. The greater the proportion surviving, the lower the *risk* for this category of patients. Survival analysis, however, is somewhat more complicated than it first might appear. If one were to measure the length of time between diagnosis and death or record the vital status when last observed for every patient in a selected patient group, one might be tempted to describe the survival of the group as the proportion alive at the end of the period under investigation. This simple measure is informative only if all of the patients were observed for the same length of time.

In most real situations, not all members of the group are observed for the same amount of time. Patients diagnosed near the end of the study period are more likely to be alive at last contact and will have been followed for less time than those diagnosed earlier. Even though it was not possible to follow these persons as long as the others, their survival might eventually prove to be just as long or longer. Although we do not know the complete survival time for these individuals, we do know a minimum survival time (time from diagnosis to last known contact date), and this information is still valuable in estimating survival rates. Similarly, it is usually not possible to know the outcome status of all of the patients who were in the group at the beginning. People may be lost to follow-up for many reasons: they may move, change names, or change physicians. Some of these individuals may have died and others could be still living. Thus, if a survival rate is to describe the outcomes for an entire group accurately, there must be some means to deal with the fact that different people in the group are observed for different lengths of time and that for others, their vital status is not known at the time of analysis. In the language of survival analysis, subjects who are observed until they reach the endpoint of interest (e.g., recurrence or death) are called *uncensored* cases, and those who survive beyond the end of the follow-up or who are lost to follow-up at some point are termed *censored* cases.

C.C. Compton et al. (eds.), *AJCC Cancer Staging Atlas: A Companion to the Seventh Editions of the AJCC Cancer Staging Manual and Handbook*, DOI 10.1007/978-1-4614-2080-4_2,

Two basic survival procedures that enable one to determine overall group survival, taking into account both censored and uncensored observations, are the life table method and the Kaplan–Meier method. The life table method was the first method generally used to describe cancer survival results, and it came to be known as the actuarial method because of its similarity to the work done by actuaries in the insurance industry. It is most useful when data are only available in grouped categories as described in the next section. The Kaplan–Meier estimate utilizes individual survival times for each patient and is preferable when data are available in this form.

The specific method of computation, that is, life table or Kaplan–Meier, used for a specific study should always be clearly indicated in the report to avoid any confusion associated with the use of less precise terminology. Rates computed by different methods are not directly comparable, and when the survival experiences of different patient groups are compared, the different rates must be computed by the same method.

The concepts of survival analysis are illustrated in this chapter. These illustrations are based on data obtained from the public-use files of the National Cancer Institute's Surveillance, Epidemiology, and End Results (SEER) Program. The cases selected are a 1% random sample of the total number for the selected sites and years of diagnosis. Follow-up of these patients continued through the end of 1999. Thus, for the earliest patients, there can be as many as 16 years of follow-up, but for those diagnosed at the end of the study period, there can be as little as 1 year of follow-up. These data are used both because they are realistic in terms of the actual survival rates they yield and because they encompass a number of cases that might be seen in a single large tumor registry over a comparable number of years. They are intended only to illustrate the methodology and concepts of survival analysis. SEER results from 1973 to 1997 are more fully described elsewhere. These illustrations are not intended and should not be used or cited as an analysis of patterns of survival in breast and lung cancer in the USA.

THE LIFE TABLE METHOD

The life table method involves dividing the total period over which a group is observed into fixed intervals, usually months or years. For each interval, the proportion surviving to the end of the interval is calculated on the basis of the number known to have experienced the endpoint event (e.g., death) during the interval and the number estimated to have been at risk at the start of the interval. For each succeeding interval, a cumulative survival rate may be calculated. The cumulative survival rate is the probability of surviving the most recent interval multiplied by the probabilities of surviving all of the prior intervals. Thus, if the percent of the patients surviving the first interval is 90% and is the same for the second and third intervals, the cumulative survival percentage is 72.9% $(0.9 \times 0.9 \times 0.9 = 0.729)$.

Results from the life table method for calculating survival for the breast cancer illustration are shown in Figure 2.1. Two-thousand eight-hundred nineteen (2,819) patients diagnosed between 1983 and 1998 were followed through 1999. Following the life table calculation method for each year after diagnosis, the 1-year survival rate is 95.6%. The 5-year cumulative survival rate is 76.8%. At 10 years, the cumulative survival is 61.0 %.

The lung cancer data show a much different survival pattern (Figure 2.2). At 1 year following diagnosis, the survival rate is only 41.8%. By 5 years it has fallen to 12.0%, and only 6.8% of lung cancer patients are estimated to have survived for 10 years following diagnosis. For lung cancer patients the *median survival time* is 10.0 months. Median survival time is the point at which half of the patients have experienced the endpoint event and half of the patients remain event-free. If the cumulative survival does not fall below 50% it is not possible to estimate median survival from the data, as is the case in the breast cancer data.

In the case of breast cancer, the 10-year survival rate is important because such a large proportion of patients live more than 5 years past their diagnosis. The 10-year time frame for lung cancer is less meaningful because such a large proportion of this patient group dies well before that much time passes.

An important assumption of all actuarial survival methods is that censored cases do not differ from the entire collection of uncensored cases in any systematic manner that would affect their survival. For example, if the more recently diagnosed cases in Figure 2.1, that is, those who were most likely not to have died yet, tended to be detected with earlier-stage disease than the uncensored cases or if they were treated differently, the assumption about comparability of censored and uncensored cases would not be met, and the result for the group as a whole would be inaccurate. Thus, it is important, when patients are included in a life table analysis, that one be reasonably confident that differences in the amount of information available about survival are not related to differences that might affect survival.

THE KAPLAN–MEIER METHOD

If individual patient data are available, these same data can be analyzed using the Kaplan–Meier method. It is similar to the life table method but calculates the proportion surviving to each point that a death occurs, rather than at fixed intervals. The principal difference evident in a survival curve is that the stepwise changes in the cumulative survival rate appear to occur independently of the intervals on the "Years Following Diagnosis" axis. Where available, this method provides a more accurate estimate of the survival curve.

PATIENT-, DISEASE-, AND TREATMENT-SPECIFIC SURVIVAL

Although overall group survival is informative, comparisons of the overall survival between two groups often are confounded by differences in the patients, their tumors, or the treatments they received. For example, it would be misleading to compare the overall survival depicted in Figure 2.1 for the sample of all breast cancer cases with the overall survival for a sample of breast cancer patients who were diagnosed with more advanced disease, whose survival would be presumed to be poorer. The simplest approach to accounting for possible differences between groups is to provide survival results that are specific to the categories of patient, disease, or treatment that may affect results. In most cancer applications, the most important variable by which survival results should be subdivided is the stage of disease. Figure 2.3 shows the *stage-specific* 5-year survival curves of the same breast cancer patients described earlier. These data show that breast cancer patient survival differs markedly according to the stage of the tumor at the time of diagnosis.

Almost any variable can be used to subclassify survival rates, but some are more meaningful than others. For example, it would be possible to provide season-of-diagnosis-specific (i.e., spring, summer, winter, and fall) survival rates, but the season of diagnosis probably has no biologic association with the length of a breast cancer patient's survival. On the other hand, the race-specific and age-specific survival rates shown in Figures 2.4 and 2.5 suggest that both of these variables are related to breast cancer survival. Caucasians have the highest survival rates and African-Americans the lowest. In the case of age, these data suggest that only the oldest patients experience poor survival and that it would be helpful to consider the effects of other causes of death that affect older persons using adjustments to be described.

Although the factors that affect survival may be unique to each type of cancer, it has become conventional that a basic description of survival for a specific cancer should include stage-, age-, and race-specific survival results. Treatment is a factor by which survival is commonly subdivided, but it must be kept in mind that selection of treatment is usually related to other factors that exert influence on survival. For example, in cancer care the choice of treatment is often dependent on the stage of disease at diagnosis. Comparison of survival curves by treatment is most appropriately accomplished within the confines of randomized clinical trials.

CAUSE-ADJUSTED SURVIVAL RATE

The survival rates depicted in the illustrations account for all deaths, regardless of cause. This is known as the *observed survival rate*. Although observed survival is a true reflection of total mortality in the patient group, we frequently are interested in describing mortality attributable only to the disease under investigation. In the past, this was most often calculated using the *cause-adjusted survival rate*, defined as the proportion of the initial patient group that escaped death due to a specific cause (e.g., cancer) if no other cause of death was operating. This technique requires that reliable information on cause of death is available and makes an adjustment for deaths due to causes other than the disease under study. This was accomplished by treating patients who died without the disease of interest as censored observations.

COMPETING RISKS/CUMULATIVE INCIDENCE

The treatment of deaths from other causes as censored is controversial, since statistical methods used in survival analysis settings assume that censoring is independent of outcome. This means that if the patient was followed longer, one could eventually observe the outcome of interest. This makes sense for patients lost to follow-up (if we located them, we might eventually observe their true survival time). However, if a patient dies due to another cause, we will never observe their death due to the cancer of interest. Estimation of the adjusted rate as described previously does not appropriately distinguish between patients who are still alive at last known contact date and those known to have died from another cause. These latter events are called *competing risks*.

When competing risks are present, an alternative to the Kaplan–Meier estimate is the cumulative incidence method. This technique is similar to the Kaplan–Meier estimate in its treatment of censored observations and is identical to the Kaplan–Meier estimate if there are no competing risks. However, in the presence of competing risks, the other causes of death are handled in a different manner.

RELATIVE SURVIVAL

Information on cause of death is sometimes unavailable or unreliable. Under such circumstances, it is not possible to compute a *cause*-adjusted survival rate. However, it is possible to adjust partially for differences in the risk of dying from causes other than the disease under study. This can be done by means of the *relative survival rate*, which is the ratio of the observed survival rate to the expected rate for a group of people in the general population similar to the patient group with respect to race, sex, and age. The relative survival rate is calculated using a procedure described by Ederer et al.

The relative survival rate represents the likelihood that a patient will not die from causes associated specifically with the cancer at some specified time after diagnosis. It is always greater than the observed survival rate for the same group of patients. If the group is sufficiently large and the patients are roughly representative of the population of the USA (taking race, sex, and age into account), the relative survival rate provides a useful estimate of the probability of escaping death from the specific cancer under study. However, if reliable information on cause of death is available, it is preferable to use the *cause*-adjusted rate. This is particularly true when the series is small or when the patients are largely drawn from a particular socioeconomic segment of the population. Relative survival rates may be derived from life table or Kaplan–Meier results.

REGRESSION METHODS

Examining survival within specific patient, disease, or treatment categories is the simplest way of studying multiple factors possibly associated with survival. This approach, however, is limited to factors into which patients may be broadly grouped. This approach does not lend itself to studying the effects of measures that vary on an interval scale. There are many examples of interval variables in cancer, such as age, number of positive nodes, cell counts, and laboratory marker values. If the patient population were to be divided up into each interval value, too few subjects would be in each analysis to be meaningful. In addition, when more than one factor is considered, the number of curves that result provides so many comparisons that the effects of the factors defy interpretation.

Conventional multiple regression analysis investigates the joint effects of multiple variables on a single outcome, but it is incapable of dealing with censored observations. For this reason, other statistical methods are used to assess the relationship of survival time to a number of variables simultaneously. The most commonly used is the Cox proportional hazards regression model. This model provides a method for estimating the influence of multiple covariates on the survival distribution from data that include censored observations. Covariates are the multiple factors to be studied in association with survival. In the Cox proportional hazards regression model, the covariates may be categorical variables such as race, interval measures such as age, or laboratory test results.

Specifics of these methods are beyond the scope of this chapter. Fortunately, many readily accessible computer packages for statistical analysis now permit the methods to be applied quite easily by the knowledgeable analyst. Although much useful information can be derived from multivariate survival models, they generally require additional assumptions about the shape of the survival curve and the nature of the effects of the covariates. One must always examine the appropriateness of the model that is used relative to the assumptions required.

STANDARD ERROR OF A SURVIVAL RATE

Survival rates that describe the experience of the specific group of patients are frequently used to generalize to larger populations. The existence of true population values is postulated, and these values are estimated from the group under study, which is only a sample of the larger population. If a survival rate was calculated from a second sample taken from the same population, it is unlikely that the results would be exactly the same. The difference between the two results is called the sampling variation (chance variation or sampling error). The *standard error* is a measure of the extent to which sampling variation influences the computed survival rate. In repeated observations under the same conditions, the true or population survival rate will lie within the range of two standard errors on either side of the computed rate approximately 95 times in 100. This range is called the *95% confidence interval*.

COMPARISON OF SURVIVAL BETWEEN PATIENT GROUPS

In comparing survival rates of two patient groups, the statistical significance of the observed difference is of interest. The essential question is, "What is the probability that the observed difference may have occurred by chance?" The standard error of the survival rate provides a simple means for answering this question. If the 95% confidence intervals of two survival rates do not overlap, the observed difference would customarily be considered statistically significant, that is, unlikely to be due to chance. This latter statement is generally true, although it is possible for a formal statistical test to yield a significant difference even with overlapping confidence intervals. Moreover, comparisons at any single time point must be made with care; if a specific time (5 years, for example) is known to be of interest when the study is planned, such a comparison may be valid; however, identification of a time based on inspection of the curves and selection of the widest difference make any formal assessment of difference invalid.

It is possible that the differences between two groups at each comparable time of follow-up do not differ significantly but that when the survival curves are considered in their entirety, the individual insignificant differences combine to yield a significantly different pattern of survival. The most common statistical test that examines the whole pattern of differences between survival curves is the *log rank test*. This test equally weights the effects of differences occurring throughout the follow-up and is the appropriate choice for most situations. Other tests weight the differences according to the numbers of persons at risk at different points and can yield different results depending on whether deaths tend more to occur early or later in the follow-up.

Care must be exercised in the interpretation of tests of statistical significance. For example, if differences exist in the patient and disease characteristics of two treatment groups, a statistically significant difference in survival results may primarily reflect differences between the two patient series, rather than differences in efficacy of the treatment regimens. The more definitive approach to therapy evaluation requires a randomized clinical trial that helps to ensure comparability of the patient characteristics and the disease characteristics of the two treatment groups.

Definition of Study Starting Point. The starting time for determining survival of patients depends on the purpose of the study. For example, the starting time for studying the natural history of a particular cancer might be defined in reference to the appearance of the first symptom. Various reference dates are commonly used as starting times for evaluating the effects of therapy. These include (1) date of diagnosis, (2) date of first visit to physician or clinic, (3) date of hospital admission, (4) date of treatment initiation, date of randomization in a clinical trial evaluating treatment efficacy, and (5) others. The specific reference date used should be clearly specified in every report.

Vital Status. At any given time, the vital status of each patient is defined as alive, dead, or unknown (i.e., lost to follow-up). The endpoint of each patient's participation in the study is (1) a specified *terminal event* such as death, (2) survival to the completion of the study, or (3) loss to follow-up. In each case, the observed follow-up time is the time from the starting point to the terminal event, to the end of the study, or to the date of last observation. This observed follow-up may be further described in terms of patient status at the endpoint, such as the following:

- Alive; tumor-free; no recurrence
- Alive; tumor-free; after recurrence
- Alive with persistent, recurrent, or metastatic disease
- Alive with primary tumor
- Dead; tumor-free
- Dead; with cancer (primary, recurrent, or metastatic disease)
- Dead; postoperative
- Unknown; lost to follow-up

Completeness of the follow-up is crucial in any study of survival, because even a small number of patients lost to follow-up may lead to inaccurate or biased results. The maximum possible effect of bias from patients lost to follow-up may be ascertained by calculating a maximum survival rate, assuming that all lost patients lived to the end of the study. A minimum survival rate may be calculated by assuming that all patients lost to follow-up died at the time they were lost.

Time Intervals. The total survival time is often divided into intervals in units of weeks, months, or years. The survival curve for these intervals provides a description of the population under study with respect to the dynamics of survival over a specified time. The time interval used should be selected with regard to the natural history of the disease under consideration. In diseases with a long natural history, the duration of study could be 5–20 years, and survival intervals of 6–12 months will provide a meaningful description of the survival dynamics. If the population being studied has a very poor prognosis (e.g., patients with carcinoma of the esophagus or pancreas), the total duration of study may be 2–3 years, and the survival intervals may be described in terms of 1–3 months. In interpreting survival rates, one must also take into account the number of individuals entering a survival interval.

SUMMARY

This chapter has reviewed the rudiments of survival analysis as it is often applied to cancer registry data and to the analysis of data from clinical trials. Complex analysis of data and exploration of research hypotheses demand greater knowledge and expertise than could be conveyed herein. Survival analysis is now performed automatically in many different registry data management and statistical analysis programs available for use on personal computers. Persons with access to these programs are encouraged to explore the different analysis features available to demonstrate for themselves the insight on cancer registry data that survival analysis can provide and to understand the limitations of these analyses and how their validity is affected by the characteristics of the patient cohorts and the quality and completeness of data.

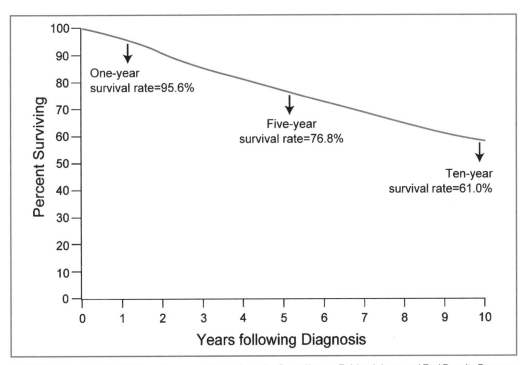

FIGURE 2.1. *Survival of 2,819 breast cancer patients from the Surveillance, Epidemiology, and End Results Program of the National Cancer Institute, 1983–1998. Calculated by the life table method.*

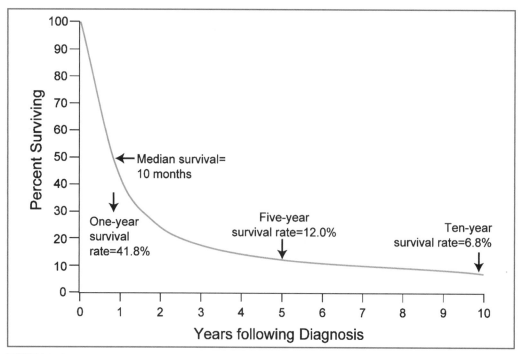

FIGURE 2.2. *Survival of 2,347 lung cancer patients from the Surveillance, Epidemiology, and End Results Program of the National Cancer Institute, 1983–1998. Calculated by the life table method.*

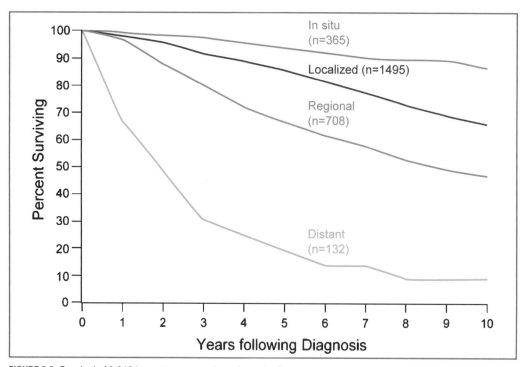

FIGURE 2.3. *Survival of 2,819 breast cancer patients from the Surveillance, Epidemiology, and End Results Program of the National Cancer Institute, 1983–1998. Calculated by the life table method and stratified by historic stage of disease. Note: Excludes 119 patients with unknown stage of disease. SEER uses extent of disease (EOD) staging.*

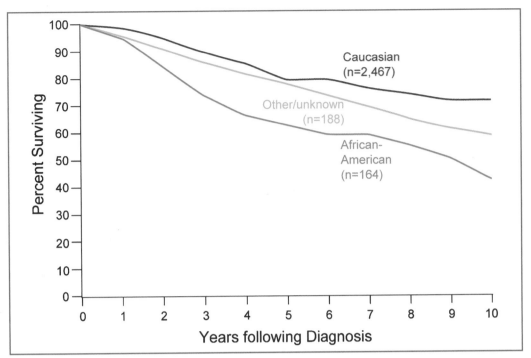

FIGURE 2.4. *Survival of 2,819 breast cancer patients from the Surveillance, Epidemiology, and End Results Program of the National Cancer Institute, 1983–1998. Calculated by the life table method and stratified by race.*

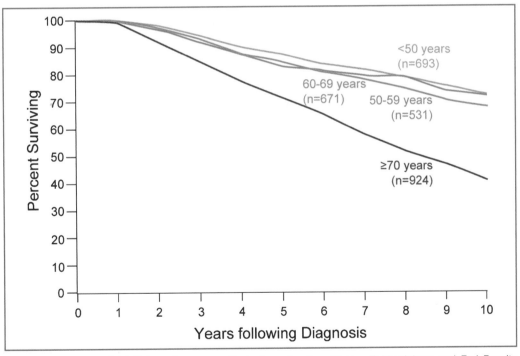

FIGURE 2.5. *Survival of 2,819 breast cancer patients from the Surveillance, Epidemiology, and End Results Program of the National Cancer Institute, 1983–1998. Calculated by the life table method and stratified by age at diagnosis.*

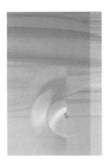

PART II
Head and Neck

Regional Lymph Nodes. The status of the regional lymph nodes in head and neck cancer is of such prognostic importance that the cervical nodes must be assessed for each patient and tumor. The lymph nodes may be subdivided into specific anatomic subsites and grouped into seven levels for ease of description (Tables II.1 and II.2 and Figure II.1).

Other groups:
Suboccipital (Figure II.2)
Retropharyngeal (Figure II.3)
Parapharyngeal
Buccinator (facial) (Figure II.2)
Preauricular (Figure II.2)
Periparotid and intraparotid (Figure II.2)

The pattern of the lymphatic drainage varies for different anatomic sites. However, the location of the lymph node metastases has prognostic significance in patients with squamous cell carcinoma of the head and neck. Survival is significantly worse when metastases involve lymph nodes beyond the first echelon of lymphatic drainage and, particularly, lymph nodes in the lower regions of the neck, that is, level IV and level VB (supraclavicular region). Consequently, it is recommended that each N staging category be recorded to show whether the nodes involved are located in the upper (U) or lower (L) regions of the neck, depending on their location above or below the lower border of the cricoid cartilage.

Extracapsular spread (ECS) has been recognized to worsen the adverse outcome associated with nodal metastasis. ECS can be diagnosed clinically by a matted mass of nodes adherent to overlying skin, adjacent soft tissue, or clinical evidence of cranial nerve invasion. Radiologic signs of ECS include amorphous, spiculated margins of a metastatic node and stranding of the perinodal soft tissue in previously untreated patients. The absence or presence of clinical/radiologic ECS is designated E– or E+, respectively. Surgically resected metastatic nodes should be examined for the presence and extent of ECS. Gross ECS (Eg) is defined as tumor apparent to the naked eye, beyond the confines of the nodal capsule. Microscopic ECS (Em) is defined as the presence of metastatic tumor beyond the capsule of the lymph node. ECS evident on clinical/radiologic examination is designated E+or E–, while ECS on histopathologic examination is designated En (no extranodal extension), Em (microscopic ECS), and Eg (gross ECS). These descriptors will not affect current nodal staging.

The natural history and response to treatment of cervical nodal metastases from nasopharynx primary sites are different, in terms of their impact on prognosis, so they justify a different N classification scheme. Regional node metastases from well-differentiated thyroid cancer do not significantly affect the ultimate prognosis in most patients and therefore also justify a unique staging system for thyroid cancers. Nonmelanoma skin cancers in the head and neck have similar behavior as elsewhere in the body. Therefore, nodal staging for these (NMSC) is different than that for mucosal cancers and is similar to that in the axilla and groin for cutaneous cancers.

Histopathologic examination is necessary to exclude the presence of tumor in lymph nodes. No imaging study (as yet) can identify microscopic tumor foci in regional nodes or distinguish between small reactive nodes and small malignant nodes.

When enlarged lymph nodes are detected, the actual size of the nodal mass(es) should be measured. It is recognized that most masses over 3 cm in diameter are not single nodes but are confluent nodes or tumor in soft tissues of the neck. Pathologic examination is necessary for documentation of tumor extent in terms of the location or level of the lymph node(s) involved, the number of nodes that contain metastases, and the presence or absence of ECS of tumor, designated as En (not present), Em (microscopic), or Eg (gross).

Distant Metastases. The most common sites of distant spread are in the lungs and bones; hepatic and brain metastases occur less often. Mediastinal lymph node metastases are considered distant metastases, except level VII lymph nodes (anterior superior mediastinal lymph nodes cephalad to the innominate artery).

Regional Lymph Nodes (N) (Figure II.4)

NX	Regional lymph nodes cannot be assessed
N0	No regional lymph node metastasis
N1*	Metastasis in a single ipsilateral lymph node, 3 cm or less in greatest dimension
N2*	Metastasis in a single ipsilateral lymph node, more than 3 cm but not more than 6 cm in greatest dimension; or in multiple ipsilateral lymph nodes, none more than 6 cm in greatest dimension; or in bilateral or contralateral lymph nodes, none more than 6 cm in greatest dimension
N2a*	Metastasis in single ipsilateral lymph node more than 3 cm but not more than 6 cm in greatest dimension
N2b*	Metastasis in multiple ipsilateral lymph nodes, none more than 6 cm in greatest dimension
N2c*	Metastasis in bilateral or contralateral lymph nodes, none more than 6 cm in greatest dimension
N3*	Metastasis in a lymph node more than 6 cm in greatest dimension

*Note: A designation of "U" or "L" may be used for any N stage to indicate metastasis above the lower border of the cricoid (U) or below the lower border of the cricoid (L). Similarly, clinical/radiological ECS should be recorded as E– or E+, and histopathologic ECS should be designated En, Em, or Eg.

Distant Metastasis (M)

M0	No distant metastasis
M1	Distant metastasis

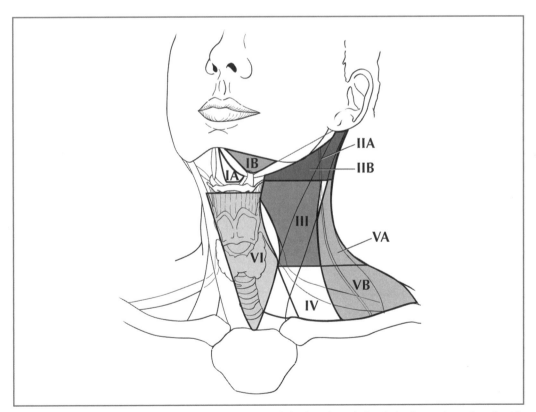

FIGURE II.1. *Schematic diagram indicating the location of the lymph node levels in the neck as described in Tables II.1 and II.2.*

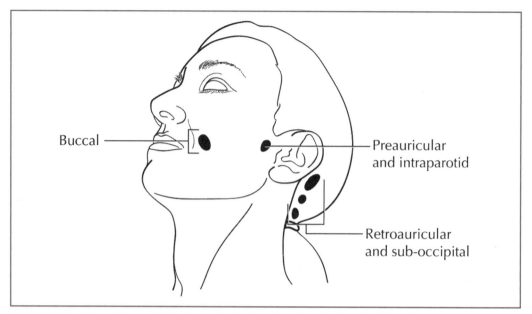

FIGURE II.2. *Location of intraparotid and preauricular, buccal, retroauricular and sub-occipital nodes.*

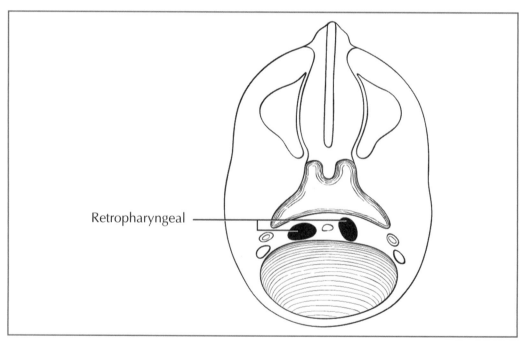

FIGURE II.3. *Location of retropharyngeal nodes.*

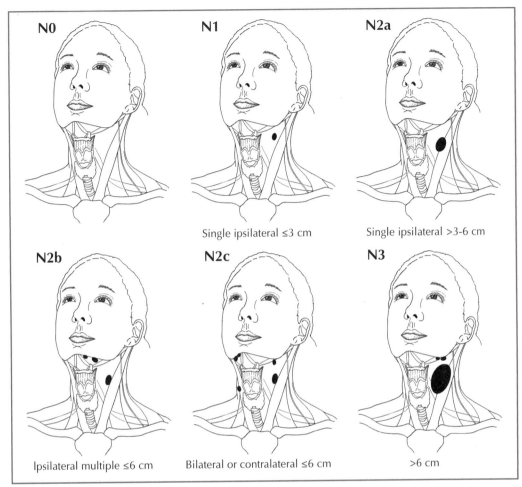

FIGURE II.4. *Regional lymph node (N) classification for all head and neck cancer sites except nasopharynx and thyroid cancers.*

TABLE II.1. *Anatomical structures defining the boundaries of the neck levels and sublevels*

Boundary Level	Superior	Inferior	Anterior (medial)	Posterior (lateral)
IA	Symphysis of mandible	Body of hyoid	Anterior belly of contralateral digastric muscle	Anterior belly of ipsilateral digastric muscle
IB	Body of mandible	Posterior belly of diagastric muscle	Anterior belly of digastric muscle	Stylohyoid muscle
IIA	Skull base	Horizontal plane defined by the inferior border of the hyoid bone	The stylohyoid muscle	Vertical plane defined by the spinal accessory nerve
IIB	Skull base	Horizontal plane defined by the inferior body of the hyoid bone	Vertical plane defined by the spinal accessory nerve	Lateral border of the sternocleido-mastoid muscle
III	Horizontal plane defined by the inferior body of hyoid	Horizontal plane defined by the inferior border of the cricoid cartilage	Lateral border of the sternohyoid muscle	Lateral border of the sterno-cleidomastoid or sensory branches of cervical plexus
IV	Horizontal plane defined by the inferior border of the cricoid cartilage	Clavicle	Lateral border of the sternohyoid muscle	Lateral border of the sterno-cleidomastoid or sensory branches of cervical plexus
VA	Apex of the convergence of the sterno-cleidomastoid and trapezius muscles	Horizontal plane defined by the lower border of the cricoid cartilage	Posterior border of the sternocleidomas-toid muscle or sensory branches of cervical plexus	Anterior border of the trapezius muscle
VB	Horizontal plane defined by the lower border of the cricoid cartilage	Clavicle	Posterior border of the sterno-cleidomastoid muscle	Anterior border of the trapezius muscle
VI	Hyoid bone	Suprasternal notch	Common carotid artery	Common carotid artery
VII	Suprasternal notch	Innominate artery	Sternum	Trachea, esophagus, and prevertebral fascia

Modified from Robbins KT, Clayman G, Levine PA, et al. American Head and Neck Society; American Academy of Otolaryngology – Head and Neck Surgery. Neck dissection classification update: revisions proposed by the American Head and Neck Society and the American Academy of Otolaryngology-Head and Neck Surgery. Arch Otolaryngol Head Neck Surg. 2002;128(7):751–8, with permission of the American Medical Association.

TABLE II.2. *Lymph node groups found within the seven levels and sublevels of the neck*

Lymph node group	Description
Submental (sublevel IA)	Lymph nodes within the triangular boundary of the anterior belly of the digastric muscles and the hyoid bone. These nodes are at greatest risk for harboring metastases from cancers arising from the floor of mouth, anterior oral tongue, anterior mandibular alveolar ridge, and lower lip.
Submandibular (sublevel IB)	Lymph nodes within the boundaries of the anterior and posterior bellies of the digastric muscle, the stylohyoid muscle, and the body of the mandible. It includes the preglandular and the postglandular nodes and the prevascular and postvascular nodes. The submandibular gland is included in the specimen when the lymph nodes within the triangle are removed. These nodes are at greatest risk for harboring mestastases from cancers arising from the oral cavity, anterior nasal cavity, skin, and soft tissue structures of the midface, and submandibular gland.
Upper jugular (includes sublevels IIA and IIB)	Lymph nodes located around the upper third of the internal jugular vein and adjacent spinal accessory nerve extending from the level of the skull base (above) to the level of the inferior border of the hyoid bone (below). The anterior (medial) boundary is stylohyoid muscle (the radiologic correlate is the vertical plane defined by the posterior surface of the submandibular gland) and the posterior (lateral) boundary is the posterior border of the sternocleidomastoid muscle. Sublevel IIA nodes are located anterior (medial) to the vertical plane defined by the spinal accessory nerve. Sublevel IIB nodes are located posterior lateral to the vertical plane defined by the spinal accessory nerve. (The radiologic correlate is the lateral border of the internal jugular on a contrast-enhanced CT scan.) The upper jugular nodes are at greatest risk for harboring metastases from cancers arising from the oral cavity, nasal cavity, nasopharynx, oropharynx, hypopharynx, larynx, and parotid gland.
Middle jugular (level III)	Lymph nodes located around the middle third of the internal jugular vein extending from the inferior border of the hyoid bone (above) to the inferior border of the cricoid cartilage (below). The anterior (medial) boundary is the lateral border of the sternohyoid muscle, and the posterior (lateral) boundary is the posterior border of the sternocleidomastoid muscle. These nodes are at greatest risk for harboring metastases from cancers arising from the oral cavity, nasophyarynx, orophar-ynx, hypopharynx, and larynx.
Lower jugular (level IV)	Lymph nodes located around the lower third of the internal jugular vein extending from the inferior border of the cricoid cartilage (above) to the clavicle below. The anterior (medial) boundary is the lateral border of the sternohyoid muscle and the posterior (lateral) boundary is the posterior border of the sternocleidomastoid muscle. These nodes are at greatest risk for harboring metastases from cancers arising from the hypopharynx, thyroid, cervical esophagus, and larynx.

(continued)

TABLE II.2. *(continued)*

Lymph node group	Description
Posterior triangle group (includes sublevels VA and VB)	This group is composed predominantly of the lymph nodes located along the lower half of the spinal accessory nerve and the transverse cervical artery. The supraclavicular nodes are also included in posterior triangle group. The superior boundary is the apex formed by convergence of the sternocleidomastoid and trapezius muscles; the inferior boundary is the clavicle; the anterior (medial) boundary is the posterior border of the sternocleidomastoid muscle, and the posterior (lateral) boundary is the anterior border of the trapezius muscle. Thus, sublevel VA includes the spinal accessory nodes, whereas sublevel VB includes the nodes following the transverse cervical vessels and the supraclavicular nodes, with the exception of the Virchow node, which is located in level IV. The posterior triangle nodes are at greatest risk for harboring metastases from cancers arising from the nasopharynx, oropharynx, and cutaneous structures of the posterior scalp and neck.
Anterior Compartment group (level VI)	Lymph nodes in this compartment include the pretracheal and paratracheal nodes, precricoid (Delphian) node, and the perithyroidal nodes including the lymph nodes along the recurrent laryngeal nerves. The superior boundary is the hyoid bone; the inferior boundary is the suprasternal notch, and the lateral boundaries are the common carotid arteries. These nodes are at greatest risk for harboring metastases from cancers arising from the thyroid gland, glottic and subglottic larynx, apex of the piriform sinus, and cervical esophagus.
Superior mediastinal group (level VII)	Lymph nodes in this group include pretracheal, paratracheal, and esophageal groove lymph nodes, extending from the level of the suprasternal notch cephalad and up to the innominate artery caudad. These nodes are at greatest risk of involvement by thyroid cancer and cancer of the esophagus.

Modified from Robbins KT, Clayman G, Levine PA, et al. American Head and Neck Society; American Academy of Otolaryngology – Head and Neck Surgery. Neck dissection classification update: revisions proposed by the American Head and Neck Society and the American Academy of Otolaryngology-Head and Neck Surgery. Arch Otolaryngol Head Neck Surg. 2002;128(7):751–8, with permission of the American Medical Association.

Lip and Oral Cavity

(Nonepithelial tumors such as those of lymphoid tissue, soft tissue, bone, and cartilage are not included. Staging for mucosal melanoma of the lip and oral cavity is not included in this chapter – see Chap. 9.)

3

SUMMARY OF CHANGES

- T4 lesions have been divided into T4a (moderately advanced local disease) and T4b (very advanced local disease), leading to the stratification of Stage IV into Stage IVA (moderately advanced local/regional disease), Stage IVB (very advanced local/regional disease), and Stage IVC (distant metastatic disease)

ICD-O-3 TOPOGRAPHY CODES

C00.0	External upper lip
C00.1	External lower lip
C00.2	External lip, NOS
C00.3	Mucosa of upper lip
C00.4	Mucosa of lower lip
C00.5	Mucosa of lip, NOS
C00.6	Commissure of lip
C00.8	Overlapping lesion of lip
C00.9	Lip, NOS
C02.0	Dorsal surface of tongue, NOS
C02.1	Border of tongue
C02.2	Ventral surface of tongue, NOS
C02.3	Anterior two-thirds of tongue, NOS
C02.8	Overlapping lesion of tongue
C02.9	Tongue, NOS
C03.0	Upper gum
C03.1	Lower gum
C03.9	Gum,NOS
C04.0	Anterior floor of mouth
C04.1	Lateral floor of mouth
C04.8	Overlapping lesion of floor of mouth
C04.9	Floor of mouth, NOS
C05.0	Hard palate
C05.8	Overlapping lesion of palate
C05.9	Palate, NOS
C06.0	Cheek mucosa
C06.1	Vestibule of mouth
C06.2	Retromolar area
C06.8	Overlapping lesion of other and unspecified parts of mouth
C06.9	Mouth, NOS

ICD-O-3 HISTOLOGY CODE RANGES

8000–8576, 8940–8950, 8980–8981

ANATOMY

Primary Site. The oral cavity extends from the skin–vermilion junction of the lips to the junction of the hard and soft palate above and to the line of circumvallate papillae below (Figures 3.1, 3.2, 3.3, and 3.4) and is divided into the following specific sites:

Mucosal Lip. The lip begins at the junction of the vermilion border with the skin and includes only the vermilion surface or that portion of the lip that comes into contact with the opposing lip. It is well defined into an upper and lower lip joined at the commissures of the mouth.

Buccal Mucosa. This includes all the membranous lining of the inner surface of the cheeks and lips from the line of contact of the opposing lips to the line of attachment of mucosa of the alveolar ridge (upper and lower) and pterygomandibular raphe.

Lower Alveolar Ridge. This refers to the mucosa overlying the alveolar process of the mandible, which extends from the line of attachment of mucosa in the lower gingivobuccal sulcus to the line of free mucosa of the floor of the mouth. Posteriorly it extends to the ascending ramus of the mandible.

Upper Alveolar Ridge. This refers to the mucosa overlying the alveolar process of the maxilla, which extends from the line of attachment of mucosa in the upper gingivobuccal sulcus to the junction of the hard palate. Its posterior margin is the upper end of the pterygopalatine arch.

Retromolar Gingiva (Retromolar Trigone). This is the attached mucosa overlying the ascending ramus of the mandible from the level of the posterior surface of the last molar tooth to the apex superiorly, adjacent to the tuberosity of the maxilla.

Floor of the Mouth. This is a semilunar space overlying the mylohyoid and hyoglossus muscles, extending from the inner surface of the lower alveolar ridge to the undersurface of the tongue. Its posterior boundary is the base of the anterior pillar of the tonsil. It is divided into two sides by the frenulum of the tongue and contains the ostia of the submandibular and sublingual salivary glands.

Hard Palate. This is the semilunar area between the upper alveolar ridge and the mucous membrane covering the palatine process of the maxillary palatine bones. It extends from the inner surface of the superior alveolar ridge to the posterior edge of the palatine bone.

Anterior Two-Thirds of the Tongue (Oral Tongue). This is the freely mobile portion of the tongue that extends anteriorly from the line of circumvallate papillae to the undersurface of the tongue at the junction of the floor of the mouth. It is composed of four areas: the tip, the lateral borders, the dorsum, and the undersurface (nonvillous ventral surface of the tongue). The undersurface of the tongue is considered a separate category by the World Health Organization.

CHARACTERISTICS OF TUMOR

Endophytic. The tumor thickness measurement using an ocular micrometer is taken perpendicular from the surface of the invasive squamous cell carcinoma (A) to the deepest area of involvement (B) and recorded in millimeters. The measurement should not be done on tangential sections or in lesions without a clearly recognizable surface component (Figures 3.5A, B, C).

Exophytic. The measurement that is better characterized as tumor thickness rather than depth of invasion is taken from the surface (A) to the deepest area (B).

Ulcerated. The thickness measurement is taken from the ulcer base (A) to the deepest area (B), as well as from the surface of the most lateral extent of the invasive carcinoma (C) to the deepest area (D). Depth of tumor invasion (mm) should be recorded. Depth is *not* used for T staging.

Although the grade of the tumor does not enter into staging of the tumor, it should be recorded. The pathologic description of any lymphadenectomy specimen should describe the size, number, and level of involved lymph node(s) and the presence or absence of extracapsular extension.

Regional Lymph Nodes. Mucosal cancer of the oral cavity may spread to regional lymph node(s). Tumors of each anatomic site have their own predictable patterns of regional spread. The risk of regional metastasis is generally related to the T category and, probably more important, to the depth of infiltration of the primary tumor. Cancer of the lip carries a low metastatic risk and initially involves adjacent submental and submandibular nodes, then jugular nodes. Cancers of the hard palate and alveolar ridge likewise have a low metastatic potential and involve buccinator, submandibular, jugular, and occasionally retropharyngeal nodes. Other oral cancers spread primarily to submandibular and jugular nodes and uncommonly to posterior triangle/supraclavicular nodes. Cancer of the anterior oral tongue may occasionally spread directly to lower jugular nodes. The closer to the midline is the primary, the greater is the risk of bilateral cervical nodal spread. The patterns of regional lymph node metastases are predictable, and sequential progression of disease occurs beyond first echelon lymph nodes. Any previous treatment to the neck, surgical and/or radiation, may alter normal lymphatic drainage patterns, resulting in unusual distribution of regional spread of disease to the cervical lymph nodes. In general, cervical lymph node involvement from oral cavity primary sites is predictable and orderly, spreading from the primary to upper, then middle, and subsequently lower cervical nodes. However, disease in the anterior oral cavity may also spread directly to the mid-cervical lymph nodes. The risk of distant metastasis is more dependent on the N than on the T status of the head and neck cancer. In addition to the components to describe the N category, regional lymph nodes should also be described according to the level of the neck that is involved. It is recognized that the level of involved nodes in the neck is prognostically significant (lower is worse), as is the presence of extracapsular extension of metastatic tumor from individual nodes. Midline nodes are considered ipsilateral. Imaging studies showing amorphous spiculated margins of involved nodes or involvement of internodal fat resulting in loss of normal oval-to-round nodal shape strongly suggest extracapsular (extranodal) tumor spread; however, pathologic examination is necessary for documentation of the extent of such disease. No imaging study (as yet) can identify microscopic foci of cancer in regional nodes or distinguish between small reactive nodes and small malignant nodes (unless central radiographic inhomogeneity is present). For pN, a selective neck dissection will ordinarily include six or more lymph nodes, and a radical or modified radical neck dissection will ordinarily include ten or more lymph nodes. Negative pathologic examination of a lesser number of nodes still mandates a pN0 designation.

Extracapsular spread (ECS) has been recognized to worsen the adverse outcome associated with nodal metastasis. The presence of ECS can be diagnosed clinically by the presence of a "matted" mass of nodes, fixity to overlying skin, adjacent soft tissue, or clinical signs of cranial nerve invasion. Radiologic imaging is capable of detecting clinically undetectable ECS, but histopathologic examination is the only reliable technique currently available for detecting microscopic ECS. Radiologic signs of ECS include amorphous spiculated margins of a metastatic node and stranding of the perinodal soft tissue in previously untreated patients. The absence or presence of clinical/radiologic ECS is designated E – or E+, respectively. Surgically resected metastatic nodes should be examined for the presence and extent of ECS. Gross ECS (Eg) is defined as tumor apparent to the naked eye beyond the confines of the nodal capsule. Microscopic ECS (Em) is defined as the presence of metastatic tumor beyond the capsule of the lymph node with desmoplastic reaction in the surrounding stromal tissue. The absence of ECS on histopathologic examination is designated En.

Distant Metastases. The lungs are the commonest site of distant metastases; skeletal and hepatic metastases occur less often. Mediastinal lymph node metastases are considered distant metastases, except level VII lymph nodes (anterior superior mediastinal lymph nodes cephalad to the innominate artery).

PROGNOSTIC FEATURES

In addition to the importance of the TNM factors outlined previously, the overall health of these patients clearly influences outcome. An ongoing effort to better assess prognosis using both tumor and nontumor-related factors is underway. Chart abstraction will continue to be performed by cancer registrars to obtain important information regarding specific factors related to prognosis. These data will then be used to further hone the predictive power of the staging system in future revisions.

Comorbidity can be classified by specific measures of additional medical illnesses. Accurate reporting of all illnesses in the patients' medical record is essential to assessment of these parameters. General performance measures are helpful in predicting survival. The AJCC strongly recommends the clinician report performance status using the ECOG, Zubrod, or Karnofsky performance measures along with standard staging information. An interrelationship between each of the major performance tools exists.

ZUBROD/ECOG PERFORMANCE SCALE

0. Fully active, able to carry on all predisease activities without restriction (Karnofsky 90–100)
1. Restricted in physically strenuous activity but ambulatory and able to carry work of a light or sedentary nature. For example, light housework, office work (Karnofsky 70–80)
2. Ambulatory and capable of all self-care but unable to carry out any work activities. Up and about more than 50% of waking hours (Karnofsky 50–60)
3. Capable of only limited self-care, confined to bed or chair 50% or more of waking hours (Karnofsky 30–40)
4. Completely disabled. Cannot carry on self-care. Totally confined to bed (Karnofsky 10–20)
5. Death (Karnofsky 0)

Lifestyle factors such as tobacco and alcohol abuse negatively influence survival. Accurate recording of smoking in pack years and alcohol in number of days drinking per week and number of drinks per day will provide important data for future analysis. Nutrition is important to prognosis and will be indirectly measured by weight loss of >10% of body weight. Depression adversely impacts quality of life and survival. Notation of a previous or current diagnosis of depression should be recorded in the medical record.

DEFINITIONS OF TNM

Primary Tumor (T)

TX	Primary tumor cannot be assessed
T0	No evidence of primary tumor
Tis	Carcinoma in situ
T1	Tumor 2 cm or less in greatest dimension (Figures 3.6A, B)
T2	Tumor more than 2 cm but not more than 4 cm in greatest dimension (Figures 3.7A, B)
T3	Tumor more than 4 cm in greatest dimension (Figures 3.8A, B, C)
T4a	Moderately advanced local disease* (lip) Tumor invades through cortical bone, inferior alveolar nerve, floor of mouth, or skin of face, that is, chin or nose (Figure 3.9) (oral cavity) Tumor invades adjacent structures only (e.g., through cortical bone [mandible or maxilla] into deep [extrinsic] muscle of tongue [genioglossus, hyoglossus, palatoglossus, and styloglossus], maxillary sinus, skin of face) (Figure 3.10)
T4b	Very advanced local disease Tumor invades masticator space, pterygoid plates, or skull base and/or encases internal carotid artery (Figure 3.11)

*Note: Superficial erosion alone of bone/tooth socket by gingival primary is not sufficient to classify a tumor as T4.

Regional Lymph Nodes (N) (See Part II Head and Neck Figures II.1–II.4)

NX	Regional lymph nodes cannot be assessed
N0	No regional lymph node metastasis
N1	Metastasis in a single ipsilateral lymph node, 3 cm or less in greatest dimension
N2	Metastasis in a single ipsilateral lymph node, more than 3 cm but not more than 6 cm in greatest dimension; or in multiple ipsilateral lymph nodes, none more than 6 cm in greatest dimension; or in bilateral or contralateral lymph nodes, none more than 6 cm in greatest dimension
N2a	Metastasis in single ipsilateral lymph node more than 3 cm but not more than 6 cm in greatest dimension
N2b	Metastasis in multiple ipsilateral lymph nodes, none more than 6 cm in greatest dimension
N2c	Metastasis in bilateral or contralateral lymph nodes, none more than 6 cm in greatest dimension
N3	Metastasis in a lymph node more than 6 cm in greatest dimension

Distant Metastasis (M)

M0	No distant metastasis
M1	Distant metastasis

ANATOMIC STAGE/PROGNOSTIC GROUPS

Stage 0	Tis	N0	M0
Stage I	T1	N0	M0
Stage II	T2	N0	M0
Stage III	T3	N0	M0
	T1	N1	M0
	T2	N1	M0
	T3	N1	M0
Stage IVA	T4a	N0	M0
	T4a	N1	M0
	T1	N2	M0
	T2	N2	M0
	T3	N2	M0
	T4a	N2	M0
Stage IVB	Any T	N3	M0
	T4b	Any N	M0
Stage IVC	Any T	Any N	M1

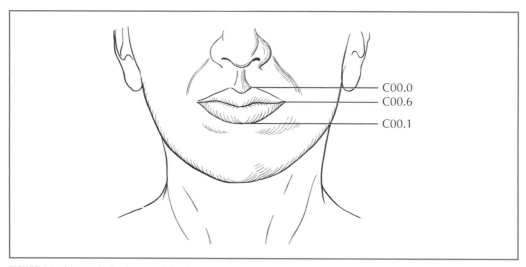

FIGURE 3.1. *Anatomical subsites of the lip.*

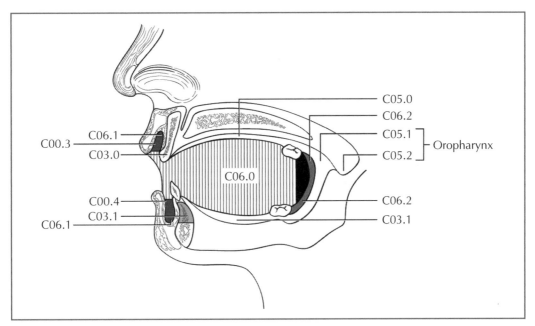

FIGURE 3.2. *Anatomical sites and subsites of the oral cavity.*

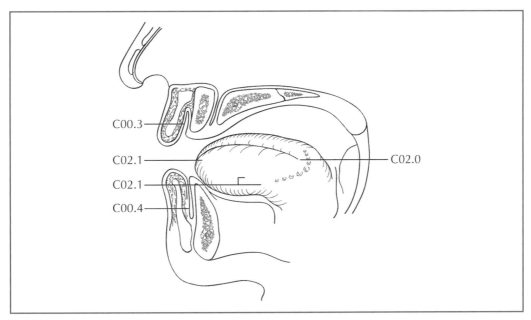

FIGURE 3.3. *Anatomical sites and subsites of the oral cavity.*

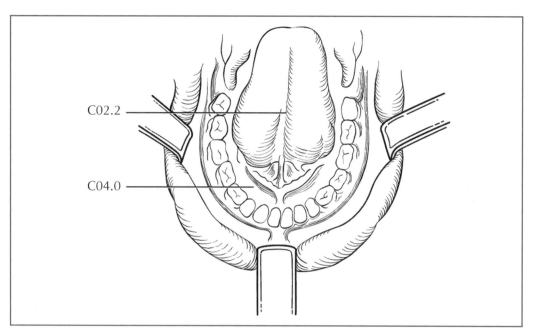

C02.2

C04.0

FIGURE 3.4. *Anatomical sites and subsites of the oral cavity.*

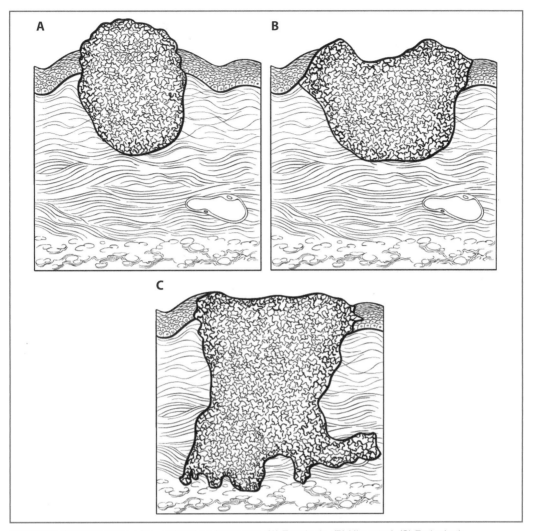

FIGURE 3.5. *Characteristics of lip and oral cavity tumors. (A) Exophytic. (B) Ulcerated. (C) Endophytic.*

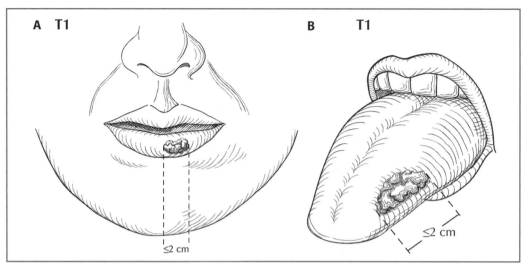

FIGURE 3.6. *(A) T1 is defined as tumor 2 cm or less in greatest dimension. (B) T1 is defined as tumor 2 cm or less in greatest dimension.*

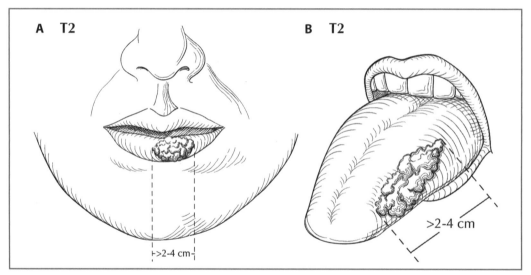

FIGURE 3.7. *(A) T2 is defined as tumor more than 2 cm but not more than 4 cm in greatest dimension. (B) T2 is defined as tumor more than 2 cm but not more than 4 cm in greatest dimension.*

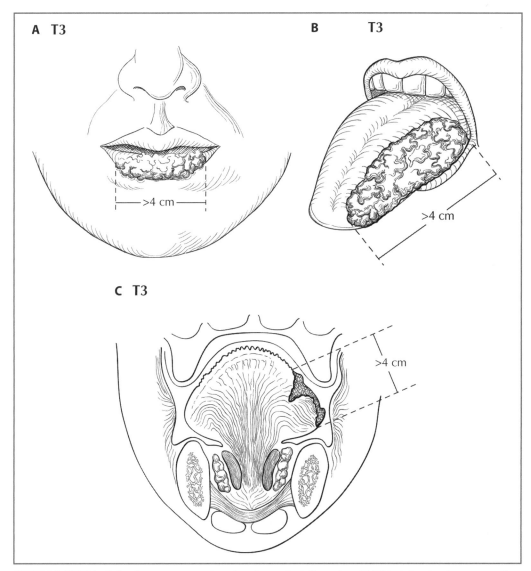

FIGURE 3.8. *(A) T3 is defined as tumor more than 4 cm in greatest dimension. (B) T3 is defined as tumor more than 4 cm in greatest dimension. (C) T3 is defined as tumor more than 4 cm in greatest dimension.*

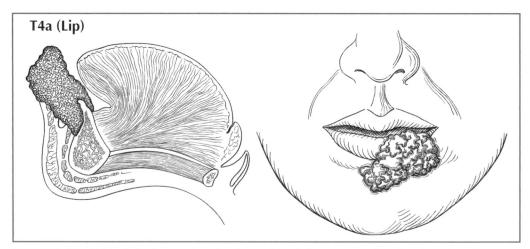

T4a (Lip)

FIGURE 3.9. *T4a (lip) is defined as moderately advanced local disease, tumor invading through cortical bone, inferior alveolar nerve, floor of mouth, or skin of face, i.e., chin or nose (as shown).*

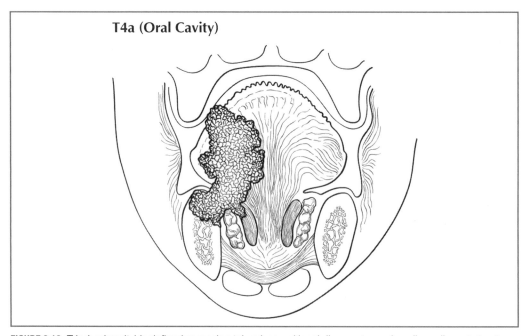

T4a (Oral Cavity)

FIGURE 3.10. *T4a (oral cavity) is defined as moderately advanced local disease, tumor invading adjacent structures only (e.g., through cortical bone [mandible or maxilla] into deep [extrinsic] muscle of tongue (genioglossus, hyoglossus, palatoglossus, and styloglossus), maxillary sinus, or skin of face.*

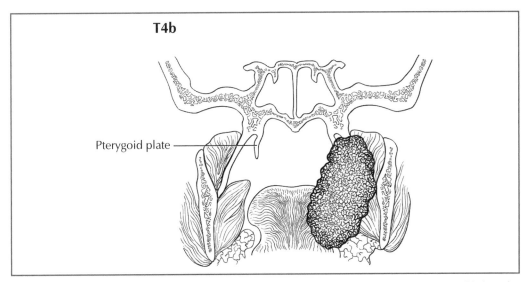

FIGURE 3.11. *T4b is defined as very advanced local disease, tumor involves masticator space, pterygoid plates (as shown), or skull base and/or encases internal carotid artery.*

PROGNOSTIC FACTORS (SITE-SPECIFIC FACTORS)
(Recommended for Collection)

Required for staging	None
Clinically significant	Size of lymph nodes
	Extracapsular extension from lymph nodes for head and neck
	Head and neck lymph nodes levels I–III
	Head and neck lymph nodes levels IV–V
	Head and neck lymph nodes levels VI–VII
	Other lymph node group
	Clinical location of cervical nodes
	Extracapsular spread (ECS) clinical
	Extracapsular spread (ECS) pathologic
	Human papillomavirus (HPV) status
	Tumor thickness

Pharynx

(Nonepithelial tumors such as those of lymphoid tissue, soft tissue, bone, and cartilage are not included. Staging of mucosal melanoma of the pharynx is not included – see Chap. 9.)

4

SUMMARY OF CHANGES

- For nasopharynx, T2a lesions will now be designated T1. Stage IIA will therefore be Stage I. Lesions previously staged T2b will be T2 and therefore Stage IIB will now be designated Stage II. Retropharyngeal lymph node(s), regardless of unilateral or bilateral location, is considered N1
- For oropharynx and hypopharynx only, T4 lesions have been divided into T4a (moderately advanced local disease) and T4b (very advanced local disease), leading to the stratification of Stage IV into Stage IVA (moderately advanced local/regional disease), Stage IVB (very advanced local/regional disease), and Stage IVC (distant metastatic disease)

ICD-O-3 TOPOGRAPHY CODES

C01.9	Base of tongue, NOS
C02.4	Lingual tonsil
C05.1	Soft palate, NOS
C05.2	Uvula
C09.0	Tonsillar fossa
C09.1	Tonsillar pillar
C09.8	Overlapping lesion of tonsil
C09.9	Tonsil, NOS
C10.0	Vallecula
C10.2	Lateral wall of oropharynx
C10.3	Posterior pha-ryngeal wall
C10.4	Branchial cleft Overlapping lesion of oropharynx
C10.8	Overlapping lesion of oropharynx
C10.9	Oropharynx, NOS
C11.0	Superior wall of nasopharynx
C11.1	Posterior wall of nasopharynx
C11.2	Lateral wall of nasopharynx
C11.3	Anterior wall of nasopharynx
C11.8	Overlapping lesion of nasopharynx
C11.9	Nasopharynx, NOS
C12.9	Pyriform sinus
C13.0	Postcricoid region
C13.1	Hypopharyn-geal aspect of aryepiglottic fold
C13.2	Posterior wall of hypo-pharynx
C13.8	Overlapping lesion of hypopharynx
C13.9	Hypopharynx, NOS

ICD-O-3 HISTOLOGY CODE RANGES

8000–8576, 8940–8950, 8980–8981

ANATOMY

Primary Sites and Subsites. The pharynx is divided into three regions: nasopharynx, oropharynx, and hypopharynx (Figures 4.1, 4.2, and 4.3). Each region is further subdivided into specific sites as summarized in the following:

Nasopharynx. The nasopharynx begins anteriorly at the posterior choana and extends along the plane of the airway to the level of the free border of the soft palate. It includes the vault, the lateral walls (including the fossae of Rosenmuller and the mucosa covering the torus tubaris forming the eustachian tube orifice), and the posterior wall. The floor is the superior surface of the soft palate. The posterior margins of the choanal orifices and of the nasal septum are included in the nasal fossa. Nasopharyngeal tumors extending to the nasal cavity or oropharynx in the absence of parapharyngeal space (PPS) involvement do not have significantly worse outcome compared with tumors restricted to the nasopharynx. This edition of the staging system has therefore been updated to reflect the prognostic implication of PPS involvement, which is important in staging nasopharynx cancer.

PPS is a triangular space anterior to the styloid process (prestyloid) that extends from the skull base to the level of the angle of the mandible. The PPS is located lateral to the pharynx and medial to the masticator space and parotid spaces. The PPS contains primarily deep lobe of parotid gland, fat, vascular structures, and small branches of the mandibular division of the fifth cranial nerve. The vascular components include the internal maxillary artery, ascending pharyngeal artery, and the pharyngeal venous plexus. Other less commonly recognized components of the PPS are lymph nodes and ectopic rests of minor salivary gland tissue.

Poststyloid space or carotid space (CS) is an enclosed fascial space located posterior to the styloid process and lateral to the retropharyngeal space (RPS) and prevertebral space (PVS). A slip of alar fascia contributes to the medial wall of the CS and helps separate the RPS and PVS from the CS. In the suprahyoid neck, the CS is bordered anteriorly by the styloid process and the PPS, laterally by the posterior belly of the digastric muscle and the parotid space, and medially by the lateral margin of the RPS. The CS contains the internal carotid artery, internal jugular vein, cranial nerves IX–XII, and lymph nodes. The CS extends superiorly to the jugular foramen and inferiorly to the aortic arch.

Masticator space primarily consists of the muscles of mastication. Anatomically, the superficial layer of the deep cervical fascia splits to enclose the muscles of mastication to enclose this space. These muscles are the medial and lateral pterygoid, masseter, and temporalis. The contents of the masticator space also include the additional structures encompassed within these fascial boundaries, which include the ramus of the mandible and the third division of the CN V as it passes through foramen ovale into the suprahyoid neck.

Oropharynx. The oropharynx is the portion of the continuity of the pharynx extending from the plane of the superior surface of the soft palate to the superior surface of the hyoid bone (or vallecula). It includes the base of the tongue, the inferior (anterior) surface of the soft palate and the uvula, the anterior and posterior tonsillar pillars, the glossotonsillar sulci, the pharyngeal tonsils, and the lateral and posterior pharyngeal walls.

Hypopharynx. The hypopharynx is that portion of the pharynx extending from the plane of the superior border of the hyoid bone (or vallecula) to the plane corresponding to the lower border of the cricoid cartilage. It includes the pyriform sinuses (right and left), the lateral and posterior hypopharyngeal walls, and the postcricoid region. The postcricoid area extends from the level of the arytenoid cartilages and connecting folds to the plane of the inferior border of the cricoid cartilage. It connects the two pyriform sinuses, thus forming the anterior wall of the hypopharynx. The pyriform sinus extends from the pharyngoepiglottic fold to the upper end of the esophagus at the lower border of the cricoid cartilage and is bounded laterally by the lateral pharyngeal wall and medially by the lateral surface of the aryepiglottic fold and the arytenoid and cricoid cartilages. The posterior pharyngeal wall extends from the level of the superior surface of the hyoid bone (or vallecula) to the inferior border of the cricoid cartilage and from the apex of one pyriform sinus to the other.

Regional Lymph Nodes. The risk of regional nodal spread from cancers of the pharynx is high. Primary nasopharyngeal tumors commonly spread to retropharyngeal, upper jugular, and spinal accessory nodes, often bilaterally. Nasopharyngeal cancer with retropharyngeal lymph node involvement independent of laterality and without cervical lymph node involvement is staged as N1. Oropharyngeal cancers involve upper and mid-jugular lymph nodes and (less commonly) submental/submandibular nodes. Hypopharyngeal cancers spread to adjacent parapharyngeal, paratracheal, and mid- and lower jugular nodes. Bilateral lymphatic drainage is common.

In clinical evaluation, the maximum size of the nodal mass should be measured. Most masses over 3 cm in diameter are not single nodes but, rather, are confluent nodes or tumor in soft tissues of the neck. There are three categories of clinically involved nodes for the nasopharynx, oropharynx, and hypopharynx: N1, N2, and N3. The use of subgroups a, b, and c is required. Midline nodes are considered ipsilateral nodes. Superior mediastinal lymph nodes are considered regional lymph nodes (level VII). In addition to the components to describe the N category, regional lymph nodes should also be described according to the level of the neck that is involved. The level of involved nodes in the neck is prognostically significant (lower is worse), as is the presence of extracapsular spread (ECS) of metastatic tumor from individual nodes. Imaging studies showing amorphous spiculated margins of involved nodes or involvement of internodal fat resulting in loss of normal oval-to-round nodal shape strongly suggest extracapsular (extranodal) spread of tumor. However, pathologic examination is necessary for documentation of such disease extent. No imaging study (as yet) can identify microscopic foci in regional nodes or distinguish between small reactive nodes and small malignant nodes (unless central radiographic inhomogeneity is present).

For pN, a selective neck dissection will ordinarily include six or more lymph nodes, and a radical or modified radical neck dissection will ordinarily include ten or more lymph nodes. Negative pathologic examination of a lesser number of nodes still mandates a pN0 designation.

Distant Metastases. The lungs are the commonest site of distant metastases; skeletal or hepatic metastases occur less often. Mediastinal lymph node metastases are considered distant metastases, except level VII lymph nodes.

PROGNOSTIC FEATURES

In addition to the importance of the TNM factors outlined previously, the overall health of these patients clearly influences outcome. An ongoing effort to better assess prognosis using both tumor and nontumor-related factors is underway. Chart abstraction will continue to be performed by cancer registrars to obtain important information regarding specific factors related to prognosis. This data will then be used to further hone the predictive power of the staging system in future revisions.

Comorbidity can be classified by specific measures of additional medical illnesses. Accurate reporting of all illnesses in the patients' medical record is essential to assessment of these parameters. General performance measures are helpful in predicting survival. The AJCC strongly recommends the clinician report performance status using the ECOG, Zubrod or Karnofsky performance measures along with standard staging information. An interrelationship between each of the major performance tools exists.

ZUBROD/ECOG PERFORMANCE SCALE

0. Fully active, able to carry on all predisease activities without restriction (Karnofsky 90–100)
1. Restricted in physically strenuous activity but ambulatory and able to carry work of a light or sedentary nature. For example, light housework, office work (Karnofsky 70–80)
2. Ambulatory and capable of all self-care but unable to carry out any work activities. Up and about more than 50% of waking hours (Karnofsky 50–60)
3. Capable of only limited self-care, confined to bed or chair 50% or more of waking hours (Karnofsky 30–40)
4. Completely disabled. Cannot carry on self-care. Totally confined to bed (Karnofsky 10–20)
5. Death (Karnofsky 0)

Lifestyle factors such as tobacco and alcohol abuse negatively influence survival. Accurate recording of smoking in pack years and alcohol in number of days drinking per week and number of drinks per day will provide important data for future analysis. Nutrition is important to prognosis and will be indirectly measured by weight loss of >10% of body weight. Depression adversely impacts quality of life and survival. Notation of a previous or current diagnosis of depression should be recorded in the medical record.

MUCOSAL MELANOMA

Mucosal melanoma of all head and neck sites is staged using a uniform classification discussed in Chap. 9.

DEFINITIONS OF TNM

Primary Tumor (T)	
TX	Primary tumor cannot be assessed
T0	No evidence of primary tumor
Tis	Carcinoma in situ
Nasopharynx	
T1	Tumor confined to the nasopharynx, or tumor extends to oropharynx and/or nasal cavity without parapharyngeal extension* (Figures 4.4, 4.5)
T2	Tumor with parapharyngeal extension*(Figures 4.4, 4.6)
T3	Tumor involves bony structures of skull base and/or paranasal sinuses (Figure 4.7)
T4	Tumor with intracranial extension and/or involvement of cranial nerves, hypopharynx, orbit, or with extension to the infratemporal fossa/masticator space (Figure 4.8A, B)

*Note: Parapharyngeal extension denotes posterolateral infiltration of tumor.

Oropharynx

T1	Tumor 2 cm or less in greatest dimension (Figure 4.9)
T2	Tumor more than 2 cm but not more than 4 cm in greatest dimension (Figure 4.10)
T3	Tumor more than 4 cm in greatest dimension or extension to lingual surface of epiglottis (Figure 4.11)
T4a	Moderately advanced local disease
	Tumor invades the larynx, extrinsic muscle of tongue, medial pterygoid, hard palate, or mandible* (Figure 4.12)
T4b	Very advanced local disease
	Tumor invades lateral pterygoid muscle, pterygoid plates, lateral nasopharynx, or skull base or encases carotid artery (Figure 4.13)

*Note: Mucosal extension to lingual surface of epiglottis from primary tumors of the base of the tongue and vallecula does not constitute invasion of larynx.

Hypopharynx

T1	Tumor limited to one subsite of hypopharynx and 2 cm or less in greatest dimension (Figure 4.14A, B, C)
T2	Tumor invades more than one subsite of hypopharynx or an adjacent site, or measures more than 2 cm but not more than 4 cm in greatest dimension without fixation of hemilarynx (Figure 4.15A, B, C, D, E)
T3	Tumor more than 4 cm in greatest dimension or with fixation of hemilarynx or extension to esophagus (Figures 4.16A, B, C, 4.17A)
T4a	Moderately advanced local disease
	Tumor invades thyroid/cricoid cartilage, hyoid bone, thyroid gland, or central compartment soft tissue* (Figure 4.17B)
T4b	Very advanced local disease
	Tumor invades prevertebral fascia, encases carotid artery, or involves mediastinal structures (Figure 4.18)

*Note: Central compartment soft tissue includes prelaryngeal strap muscles and subcutaneous fat.

Regional Lymph Nodes (N)

Nasopharynx

The distribution and the prognostic impact of regional lymph node spread from nasopharynx cancer, particularly of the undifferentiated type, are different from those of other head and neck mucosal cancers and justify the use of a different N classification scheme.

NX	Regional lymph nodes cannot be assessed
N0	No regional lymph node metastasis
N1	Unilateral metastasis in cervical lymph node(s), 6 cm or less in greatest dimension, above the supraclavicular fossa, and/or unilateral or bilateral, retropharyngeal lymph nodes, 6 cm or less, in greatest dimension* (Figure 4.19)
N2	Bilateral metastasis in cervical lymph node(s), 6 cm or less in greatest dimension, above the supraclavicular fossa* (Figure 4.20)
N3	Metastasis in a lymph node(s)* >6 cm and/or to supraclavicular fossa
N3a	Greater than 6 cm in dimension (Figure 4.21)
N3b	Extension to the supraclavicular fossa** (Figure 4.21)

*Note: Midline nodes are considered ipsilateral nodes.

**Note: Supraclavicular zone or fossa is relevant to the staging of nasopharyngeal carcinoma and is the triangular region originally described by Ho. It is defined by three points: (1) the superior margin of the sternal end of the clavicle, (2) the superior margin of the lateral end of the clavicle, (3) the point where the neck meets the shoulder (see Figure 4.2). Note that this would include caudal portions of levels IV and VB. All cases with lymph nodes (whole or part) in the fossa are considered N3b (Figure 4.22).

Regional Lymph Nodes (N)*(See Part II Head and Neck Figures II.1–II.4)

Oropharynx and Hypopharynx

NX	Regional lymph nodes cannot be assessed
N0	No regional lymph node metastasis
N1	Metastasis in a single ipsilateral lymph node, 3 cm or less in greatest dimension
N2	Metastasis in a single ipsilateral lymph node, more than 3 cm but not more than 6 cm in greatest dimension, or in multiple ipsilateral lymph nodes, none more than 6 cm in greatest dimension, or in bilateral or contralateral lymph nodes, none more than 6 cm in greatest dimension
N2a	Metastasis in a single ipsilateral lymph node more than 3 cm but not more than 6 cm in greatest dimension
N2b	Metastasis in multiple ipsilateral lymph nodes, none more than 6 cm in greatest dimension
N2c	Metastasis in bilateral or contralateral lymph nodes, none more than 6 cm in greatest dimension
N3	Metastasis in a lymph node more than 6 cm in greatest dimension

*Note: Metastases at level VII are considered regional lymph node metastases.

Distant Metastasis (M)

M0	No distant metastasis
M1	Distant metastasis

ANATOMIC STAGE/PROGNOSTIC GROUPS

Nasopharynx

Stage 0	Tis	N0	M0
Stage I	T1	N0	M0
Stage II	T1	N1	M0
	T2	N0	M0
	T2	N1	M0
Stage III	T1	N2	M0
	T2	N2	M0
	T3	N0	M0
	T3	N1	M0
	T3	N2	M0
Stage IVA	T4	N0	M0
	T4	N1	M0
	T4	N2	M0
Stage IVB	Any T	N3	M0
Stage IVC	Any T	Any N	M1

Oropharynx, Hypopharynx

Stage 0	Tis	N0	M0
Stage I	T1	N0	M0
Stage II	T2	N0	M0
Stage III	T3	N0	M0
	T1	N1	M0
	T2	N1	M0
	T3	N1	M0
Stage IVA	T4a	N0	M0
	T4a	N1	M0
	T1	N2	M0
	T2	N2	M0
	T3	N2	M0
	T4a	N2	M0
Stage IVB	T4b	Any N	M0
	Any T	N3	M0
Stage IVC	Any T	Any N	M1

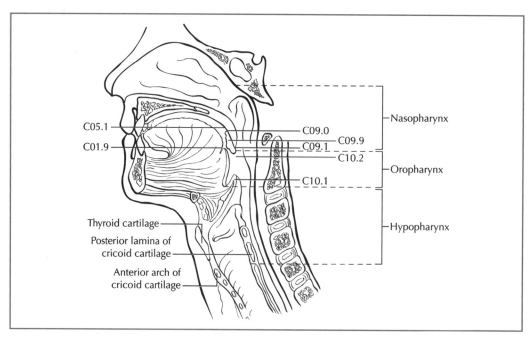

FIGURE 4.1. *Sagittal view of the face and neck depicting the subdivisions of the pharynx as described in the text.*

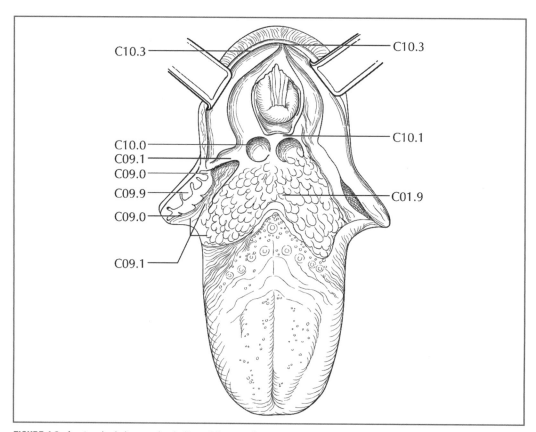

FIGURE 4.2. *Anatomical sites and subsites of the oropharynx.*

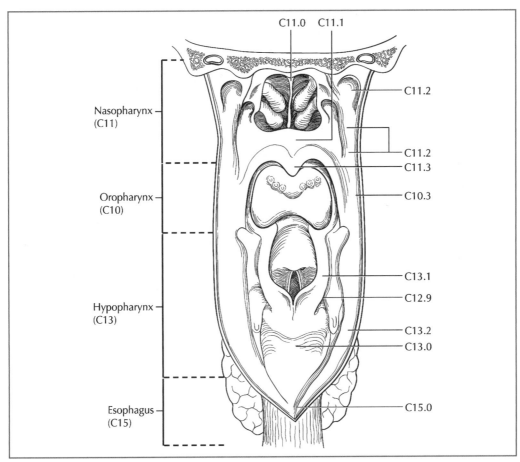

FIGURE 4.3. *Anatomical sites and subsites of the nasopharynx, oropharynx, hypopharynx, and esophagus.*

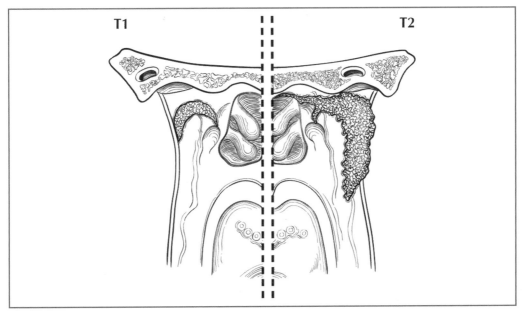

FIGURE 4.4. *For nasopharynx, T1 tumors are defined as tumor confined to the nasopharynx (left) whereas T2 extends to parapharyngeal tissue.*

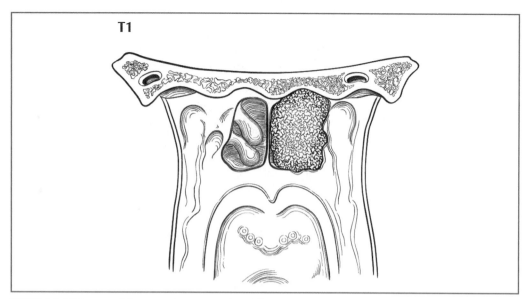

FIGURE 4.5. *T1 tumors of the nasopharynx are also defined as tumor extending to the oropharynx and/or nasal cavity without parapharyngeal extension.*

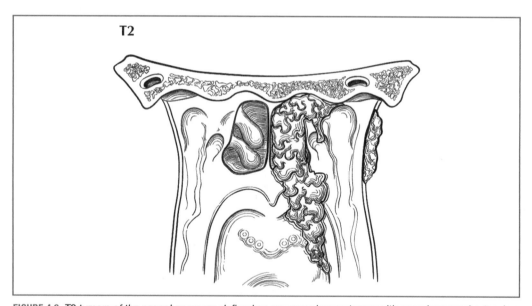

FIGURE 4.6. *T2 tumors of the nasopharynx are defined as any nasopharynx tumor with parapharyngeal extension.*

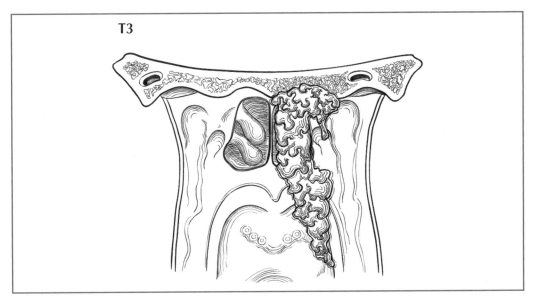

FIGURE 4.7. *T3 tumors of the nasopharynx involve bony structures and/or paranasal sinuses.*

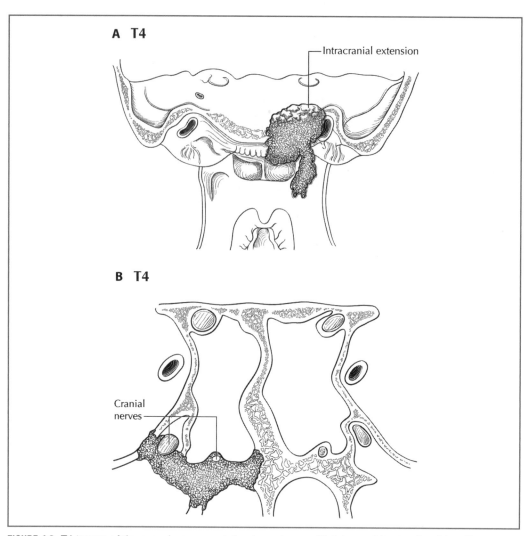

FIGURE 4.8. *T4 tumors of the nasopharynx are defined as a tumor with intracranial extension (A) and/or involvement of cranial nerves (B), hypopharynx, orbit, or with extension to the infratemporal fossa/masticator space.*

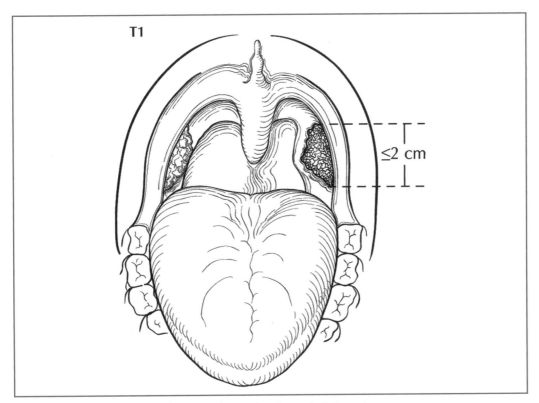

FIGURE 4.9. *T1 tumors of the oropharynx are 2 cm or less in greatest dimension.*

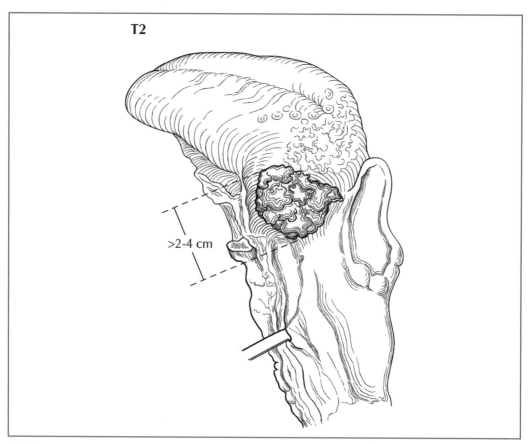

FIGURE 4.10. *T2 tumors of the oropharynx measure more than 2 cm but not more than 4 cm.*

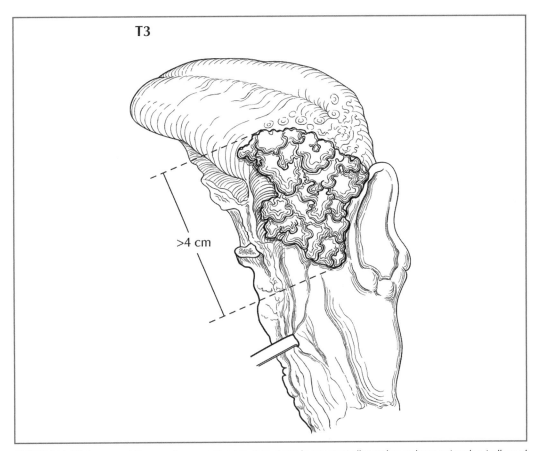

FIGURE 4.11. *T3 tumors of the oropharynx are more than 4 cm in greatest dimension or have extension to lingual surface of epiglottis.*

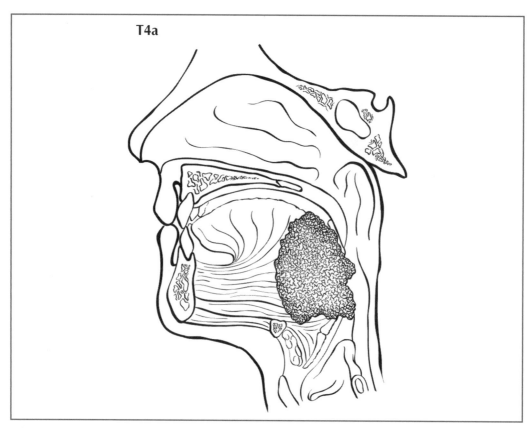

FIGURE 4.12. *T4a tumor of the oropharynx is described as moderately advanced local disease, a tumor that invades the larynx, extrinsic muscle or tongue, medial pterygoid, hard palate, or mandible.*

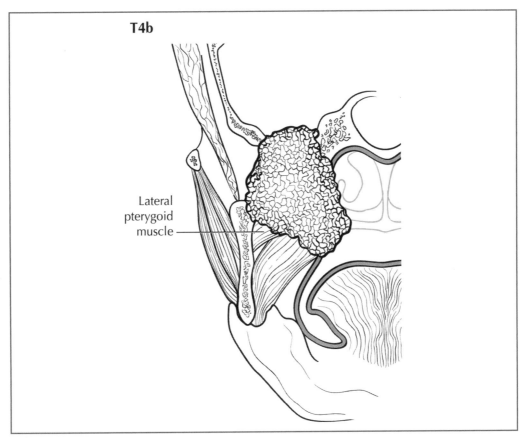

FIGURE 4.13. *T4b tumor of the oropharynx is described as very advanced local disease, a tumor that invades lateral pterygoid muscle, pterygoid plates, lateral nasopharynx, or skull base or encases carotid artery.*

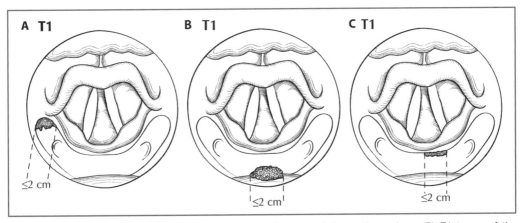

FIGURE 4.14. *(A) T1 tumor of the hypopharynx with involvement of the pyriform sinus. (B) T1 tumor of the hypopharynx with involvement of the posterior wall. (C) T1 tumor of the hypopharynx with involvement of the post-cricoid area.*

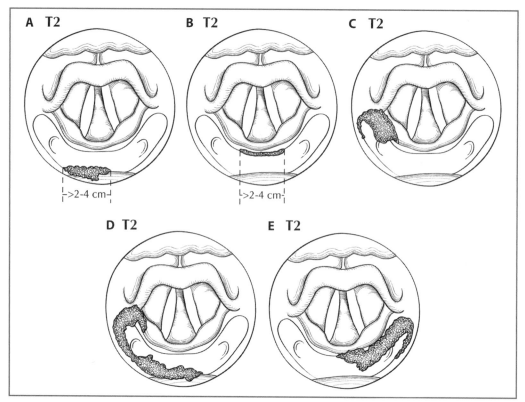

FIGURE 4.15. (A) T2 tumor of the hypopharynx with involvement of the posterior wall of the hypopharynx. (B) T2 tumor of the hypopharynx with involvement of the post-cricoid area. (C) T2 tumor of the hypopharynx with involvement of the pyriform sinus and the aryepiglottic fold. (D) T2 tumor of the hypopharynx with involvement of the pyriform sinus and the posterior wall. (E) T2 tumor of the hypopharynx with involvement of the pyriform sinus and the post-cricoid area.

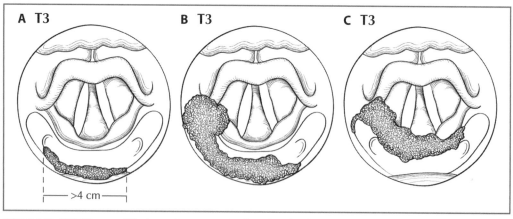

FIGURE 4.16. (A) T3 tumor of the hypopharynx greater than 4 cm in diameter and with involvement of the posterior wall. (B) T3 tumor of the hypopharynx with fixation of the hemilarynx and invasion of the pyriform sinus, aryepiglottic fold, and posterior wall. (C) T3 tumor of the hypopharynx with fixation of the hemilarynx with invasion of the pyriform sinus and post-cricoid area.

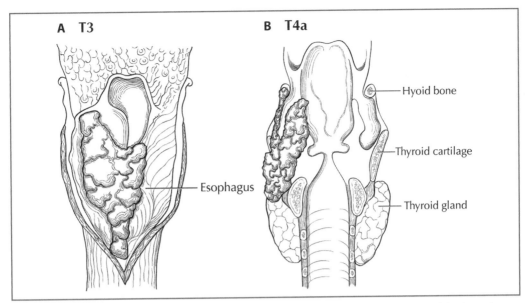

FIGURE 4.17. A. T3 tumor of the hypopharynx with invasion of the esophagus. (B) T4a tumor of the hypopharynx which is moderately advanced local disease, with invasion of the hyoid bone, thyroid/cricoid cartilage, thyroid gland, or central compartment soft tissue.

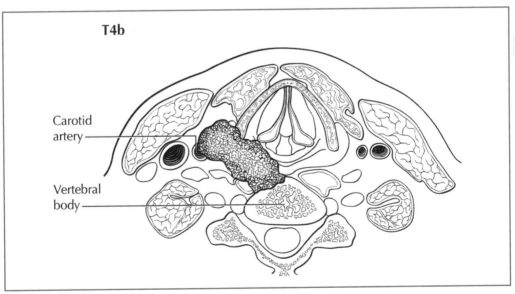

FIGURE 4.18. T4b tumor of the hypopharynx, which is very advanced local disease, with invasion of the prevertebral fascia, encases carotid artery, or that involves mediastinal structures.

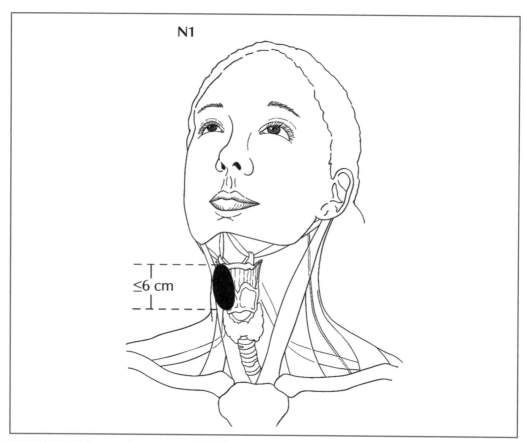

FIGURE 4.19. *N1 for nasopharynx cancer is defined as unilateral metastasis in cervical lymph node(s), 6 cm or less in greatest dimension, above the supraclavicular fossa, and/or unilateral or bilateral, retropharyngeal lymph nodes, 6 cm or less in greatest dimension.*

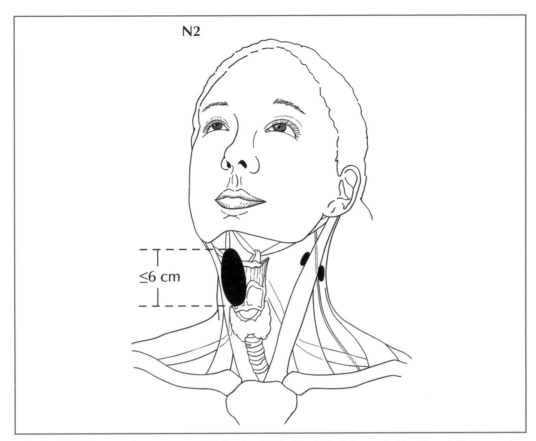

FIGURE 4.20. *N2 for nasopharynx cancer is defined as bilateral metastasis in cervical lymph node(s), 6 cm or less in greatest dimension, above the supraclavicular fossa.*

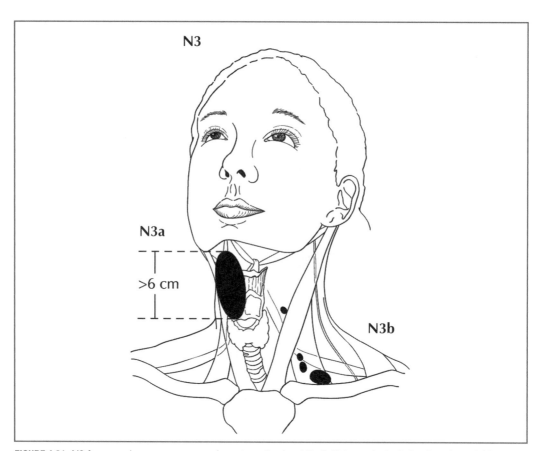

FIGURE 4.21. *N3 for nasopharynx cancer may be categorized as N3a (left) for metastasis in a lymph node(s) greater than 6 cm in dimension and/or N3b (right) metastatic to the supraclavicular fossa.*

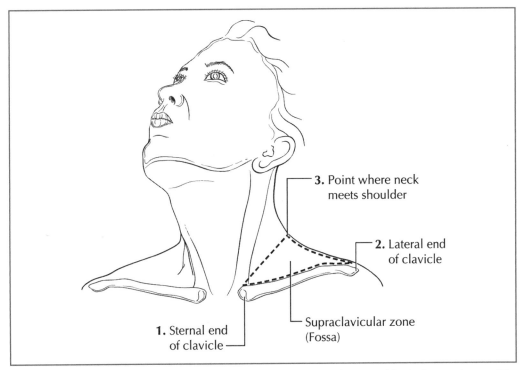

FIGURE 4.22. *Shaded triangular area corresponds to the supraclavicular fossa used in staging carcinoma of the nasopharynx.*

PROGNOSTIC FACTORS (SITE-SPECIFIC FACTORS)	
(Recommended for Collection)	
Required for staging	None
Clinically significant	Size of lymph nodes
	Extracapsular extension from lymph nodes for head and neck
	Head and neck lymph nodes levels I–III
	Head and neck lymph nodes levels IV–V
	Head and neck lymph nodes levels VI–VII
	Other lymph nodes group
	Clinical location of cervical nodes
	ECS clinical
	ECS pathologic
	Human papillomavirus (HPV) status

Larynx

(Nonepithelial tumors such as those of lymphoid tissue, soft tissue, bone, and cartilage are not included)

5

ICD-O-3 TOPOGRAPHY CODES

C10.1   Anterior (lingual) surface of epiglottis
C32.0   Glottis
C32.1   Supraglottis (laryngeal surface)
C32.2   Subglottis
C32.8* Overlapping lesion of larynx
C32.9* Larynx, NOS
*Stage by location of tumor bulk or epicenter

ICD-O-3 HISTOLOGY CODE RANGES

8000–8576, 8940–8950, 8980–8981

ANATOMY

Primary Site. The following anatomic definition of the larynx allows classification of carcinomas arising in the encompassed mucous membranes but excludes cancers arising on the lateral or posterior pharyngeal wall, pyriform fossa, postcricoid area, or base of tongue.

The anterior limit of the larynx is composed of the anterior or lingual surface of the suprahyoid epiglottis, the thyrohyoid membrane, the anterior commissure, and the anterior wall of the subglottic region, which is composed of the thyroid cartilage, the cricothyroid membrane, and the anterior arch of the cricoid cartilage.

The posterior and lateral limits include the laryngeal aspect of the aryepiglottic folds, the arytenoid region, the interarytenoid space, and the posterior surface of the subglottic space, represented by the mucous membrane covering the surface of the cricoid cartilage.

The superolateral limits are composed of the tip and the lateral borders of the epiglottis. The inferior limits are made up of the plane passing through the inferior edge of the cricoid cartilage.

For purposes of this clinical stage classification, the larynx is divided into three regions: supraglottis, glottis, and subglottis (Figures 5.1 and 5.2). The supraglottis is composed of the epiglottis (both its lingual and laryngeal aspects), aryepiglottic folds (laryngeal aspect), arytenoids, and ventricular bands (false cords). The epiglottis is divided for staging purposes into suprahyoid and infrahyoid portions by a plane at the level of the hyoid bone. The inferior boundary of the supraglottis is a horizontal plane passing through the lateral margin of the ventricle at its junction with the superior surface of the vocal cord. The glottis is composed of the superior and inferior surfaces of the true vocal cords, including the anterior and posterior commissures. It occupies a horizontal plane 1 cm in thickness, extending inferiorly from the lateral margin of the ventricle. The subglottis is the region extending from the lower boundary of the glottis to the lower margin of the cricoid cartilage.

The division of the larynx is summarized as follows:

Site	Subsite
Supraglottis	Suprahyoid epiglottis
	Infrahyoid epiglottis
	Aryepiglottic folds (laryngeal aspect); arytenoids
	Ventricular bands (false cords)
Glottis	True vocal cords, including anterior and posterior commissures
Subglottis	Subglottis

Regional Lymph Nodes. The incidence and distribution of cervical nodal metastases from cancer of the larynx vary with the site of origin and the T classification of the primary tumor. The true vocal cords are nearly devoid of lymphatics, and tumors of that site alone rarely spread to regional nodes. By contrast, the supraglottis has a rich and bilaterally interconnected lymphatic network, and primary supraglottic cancers are commonly accompanied by regional lymph node spread. Glottic tumors may spread directly to adjacent soft tissues and prelaryngeal, pretracheal, paralaryngeal, and paratracheal nodes, as well as to upper, mid, and lower jugular nodes. Supraglottic tumors commonly spread to upper and midjugular nodes, considerably less commonly to submental or submandibular nodes, and occasionally to retropharyngeal nodes. The rare subglottic primary tumors spread first to adjacent soft tissues and prelaryngeal, pretracheal, paralaryngeal, and paratracheal nodes, then to mid- and lower jugular nodes. Contralateral lymphatic spread is common.

In clinical evaluation, the physical size of the nodal mass should be measured. Most masses over 3 cm in diameter are not single nodes but, rather, are confluent nodes or tumor in soft tissues of the neck. There are three categories of clinically positive nodes: N1, N2, and N3. Midline nodes are considered ipsilateral nodes. In addition to the components to describe the N category, regional lymph nodes should also be described according to the level of the neck that is involved. Pathologic examination is necessary for documentation of such disease extent. Imaging studies showing amorphous spiculated margins of involved nodes or involvement of internodal fat resulting in loss of normal oval-to-round nodal shape strongly suggest extracapsular (extranodal) tumor spread. No imaging study (as yet) can identify microscopic foci in regional nodes or distinguish between small reactive nodes and small malignant nodes without central radiographic inhomogeneity.

Distant Metastases. Distant spread is common only for patients who have bulky regional lymphadenopathy. When distant metastases occur, spread to the lungs is most common; skeletal or hepatic metastases occur less often. Mediastinal lymph node metastases are considered distant metastases, except level VII, lymph nodes (in the anterior superior mediastinum, cephalad to the innominate artery).

MUCOSAL MELANOMA

Mucosal melanoma of all head and neck sites is staged using a uniform classification discussed in Chap. 9.

DEFINITIONS OF TNM

Primary Tumor (T)

TX   Primary tumor cannot be assessed

T0   No evidence of primary tumor

Tis   Carcinoma in situ

Supraglottis

T1   Tumor limited to one subsite of supraglottis with normal vocal cord mobility (Figure 5.3A, B)

T2   Tumor invades mucosa of more than one adjacent subsite of supraglottis or glottis or region outside the supraglottis (e.g., mucosa of base of tongue, vallecula, medial wall of pyriform sinus) without fixation of the larynx (Figure 5.4A, B)

T3   Tumor limited to larynx with vocal cord fixation and/or invades any of the following: postcricoid area, preepiglottic space, paraglottic space, and/or inner cortex of thyroid cartilage (Figure 5.5A, B)

T4a   Moderately advanced local disease

Tumor invades through the thyroid cartilage and/or invades tissues beyond the larynx (e.g., trachea, soft tissues of neck including deep extrinsic muscle of the tongue, strap muscles, thyroid, or esophagus) (Figure 5.6)

T4b   Very advanced local disease

Tumor invades prevertebral space, encases carotid artery, or invades mediastinal structures (Figure 5.7)

Glottis

T1   Tumor limited to the vocal cord(s) (may involve anterior or posterior commissure) with normal mobility (Figure 5.8)

T1a   Tumor limited to one vocal cord (Figure 5.8)

T1b   Tumor involves both vocal cords (Figure 5.8)

T2   Tumor extends to supraglottis and/or subglottis, and/or with impaired vocal cord mobility (Figure 5.9)

T3   Tumor limited to the larynx with vocal cord fixation and/or invasion of paraglottic space, and/or inner cortex of the thyroid cartilage (Figure 5.10)

T4a   Moderately advanced local disease

Tumor invades through the outer cortex of the thyroid cartilage and/or invades tissues beyond the larynx (e.g., trachea, soft tissues of neck including deep extrinsic muscle of the tongue, strap muscles, thyroid, or esophagus) (Figure 5.11)

T4b   Very advanced local disease

Tumor invades prevertebral space, encases carotid artery, or invades mediastinal structures

Subglottis

T1   Tumor limited to the subglottis (Figure 5.12)

T2   Tumor extends to vocal cord(s) with normal or impaired mobility (Figure 5.13)

T3   Tumor limited to larynx with vocal cord fixation (Figure 5.14)

(continued)

Primary Tumor (T) (*continued*)

T4a   Moderately advanced local disease

Tumor invades cricoid or thyroid cartilage and/or invades tissues beyond the larynx (e.g., trachea, soft tissues of neck including deep extrinsic muscles of the tongue, strap muscles, thyroid, or esophagus) (Figure 5.15)

T4b   Very advanced local disease

Tumor invades prevertebral space, encases carotid artery, or invades mediastinal structures

Regional Lymph Nodes (N)* (See Part II Head and Neck Figures II.1–II.4)

NX   Regional lymph nodes cannot be assessed N0; no regional lymph node metastasis

N1   Metastasis in a single ipsilateral lymph node, 3 cm or less in greatest dimension

N2   Metastasis in a single ipsilateral lymph node, more than 3 cm but not more than 6 cm in greatest dimension, or in multiple ipsilateral lymph nodes, none more than 6 cm in greatest dimension, or in bilateral or contralateral lymph nodes, none more than 6 cm in greatest dimension

N2a   Metastasis in a single ipsilateral lymph node, more than 3 cm but not more than 6 cm in greatest dimension

N2b   Metastasis in multiple ipsilateral lymph nodes, none more than 6 cm in greatest dimension

N2c   Metastasis in bilateral or contralateral lymph nodes, none more than 6 cm in greatest dimension

N3   Metastasis in a lymph node, more than 6 cm in greatest dimension

*Note: Metastases at level VII are considered regional lymph node metastases.

Distant Metastasis (M)

M0   No distant metastasis

M1   Distant metastasis

ANATOMIC STAGE/PROGNOSTIC GROUPS

Stage 0	Tis	N0	M0
Stage I	T1	N0	M0
Stage II	T2	N0	M0
Stage III	T3	N0	M0
	T1	N1	M0
	T2	N1	M0
	T3	N1	M0
Stage IVA	T4a	N0	M0
	T4a	N1	M0
	T1	N2	M0
	T2	N2	M0
	T3	N2	M0
	T4a	N2	M0
Stage IVB	T4b	Any N	M0
	Any T	N3	M0
Stage IVC	Any T	Any N	M1

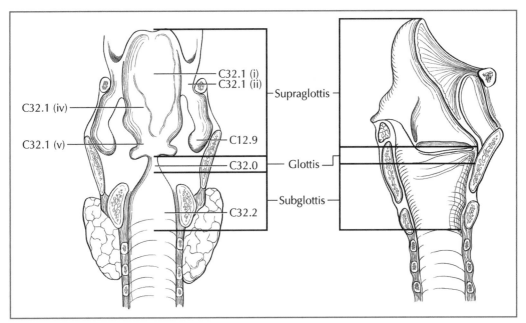

FIGURE 5.1. *Anatomical sites and subsites of the three regions of the larynx: supraglottis, glottis, and subglottis. Supraglottis (C32.1) subsites include suprahyoid epiglottis (i), aryepiglottic fold, laryngeal aspect (ii), infrahyoid epiglottis (iv), and ventricular bands or false cords (v).*

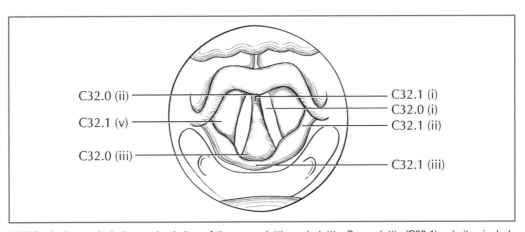

FIGURE 5.2. *Anatomical sites and subsites of the supraglottis and glottis. Supraglottis (C32.1) subsites include suprahyoid epiglottis (i), aryepiglottic fold, laryngeal aspect (ii), arytenoids (iii), and ventricular bands or false cords (v). Glottis (C32.0) subsites include vocal cords (i), anterior commissure (ii), and posterior commissure (iii).*

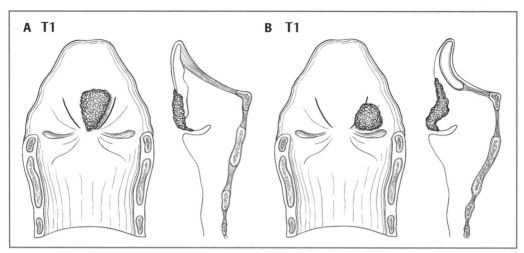

FIGURE 5.3. *(A) T1 for the supraglottis is defined as tumor limited to one subsite of supraglottis (shown here in the epiglottis) with normal vocal cord mobility. (B) T1 for the supraglottis is defined as tumor limited to one subsite of supraglottis (shown here in the ventricular bands) with normal vocal cord mobility.*

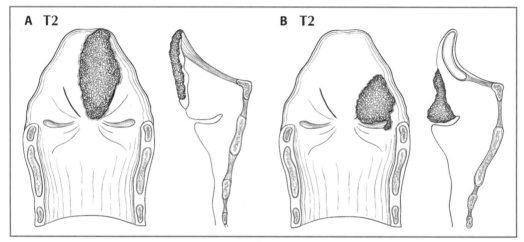

FIGURE 5.4. *(A) T2 for the supraglottis is defined as tumor invading the mucosa of more than one adjacent subsite of supraglottis or glottis or region outside the supraglottis (e.g., mucosa of base of tongue, vallecula, medial wall of pyriform sinus) without fixation of the larynx (shown here with tumor involvement in the suprahyoid and mucosa of the infrahyoid epiglottis). (B) T2 for the supraglottis with invasion of ventricular bands (false cords) and the epiglottis.*

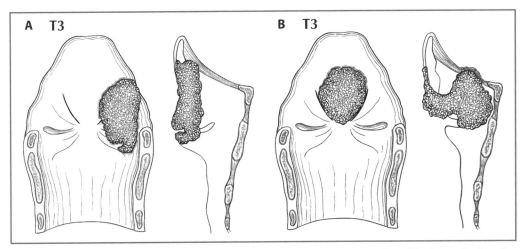

FIGURE 5.5. (A) T3 for the supraglottis is defined as tumor limited to larynx with vocal cord fixation and/or invading any of the following: postcricoid area, pre-epiglottic tissues, paraglottic space, and/or inner cortex of thyroid cartilage, here with invasion of the supraglottis and vocal cord with vocal cord fixation. (B) T3 for the supraglottis with invasion of the pre-epiglottic tissues with vocal cord fixation.

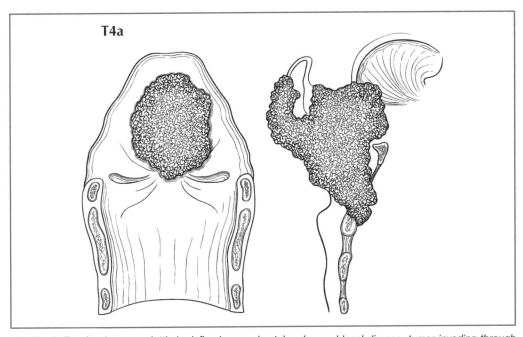

FIGURE 5.6. T4a for the supraglottis is defined as moderately advanced local disease, tumor invading through the thyroid cartilage and/or invading tissues beyond the larynx (e.g., trachea, soft tissues of neck including deep extrinsic muscle of the tongue, strap muscles, thyroid, or esophagus). Here, tumor has invaded beyond the larynx into the vallecula and base of the tongue as well as into soft tissues of the neck.

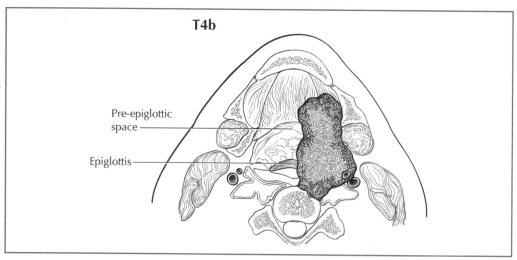

FIGURE 5.7. *Cross-sectional illustration of T4b tumor for the supraglottis, which is defined as very advanced local disease, invading prevertebral space, encasing the carotid artery (shown), or invading mediastinal structures.*

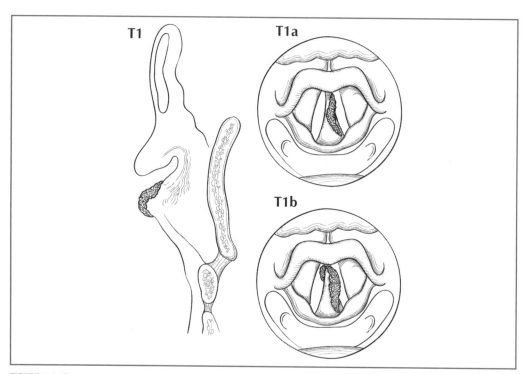

FIGURE 5.8. *T1 tumors of the glottis are limited to the vocal cord(s) with normal mobility (may involve anterior or posterior commissure). T1a tumors are limited to one vocal cord (top right) and T1b tumors involve both vocal cords (bottom right).*

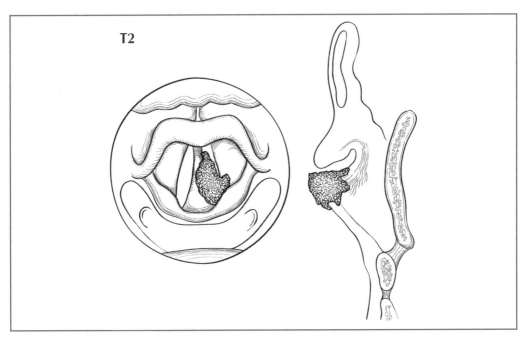

FIGURE 5.9. *T2 tumors of the glottis extend to supraglottis and/or subglottis, and/or with impaired vocal cord mobility.*

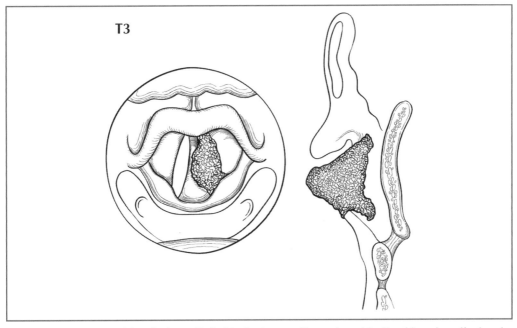

FIGURE 5.10. *T3 tumors of the glottis are limited to the larynx with vocal cord fixation (shown), and/or invades paraglottic space, and/or inner cortex of the thyroid cartilage.*

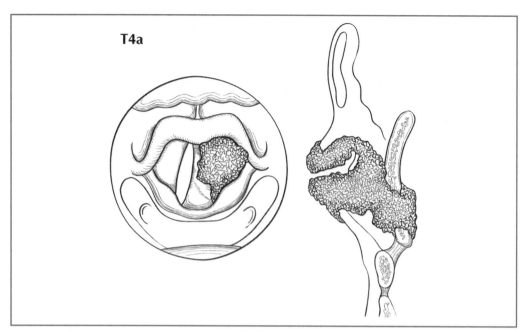

FIGURE 5.11. *T4a tumors of the glottis are moderately advanced local disease and invade through the outer cortex of the thyroid cartilage and/or invade tissues beyond the larynx (e.g., trachea, soft tissues of neck including deep extrinsic muscle of the tongue, strap muscles, thyroid, or esophagus).*

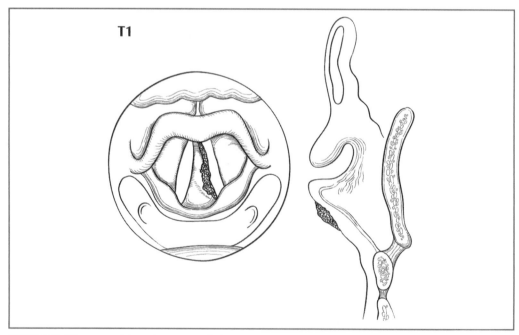

FIGURE 5.12. *T1 tumors of the subglottis are limited to subglottis.*

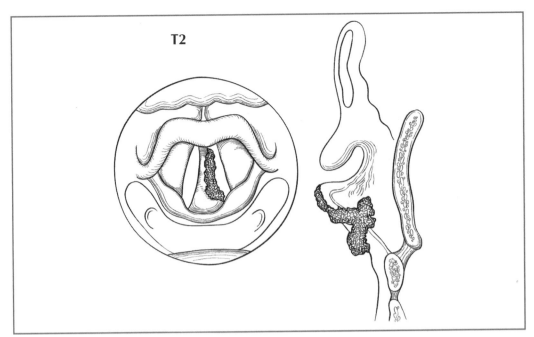

FIGURE 5.13. *T2 tumors of the subglottis extend to vocal cord(s), with normal or impaired mobility.*

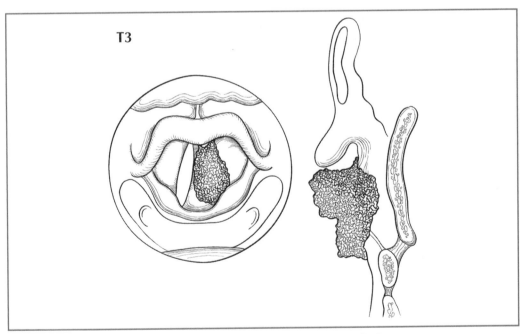

FIGURE 5.14. *T3 tumors of the subglottis are limited to larynx with vocal cord fixation.*

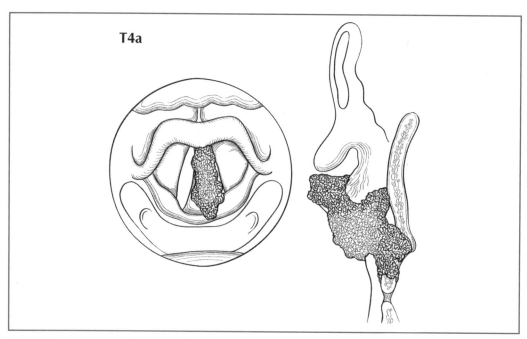

FIGURE 5.15. *T4a tumors of the subglottis are moderately advanced local disease and invade cricoid or thyroid cartilage and/or invade tissues beyond the larynx (e.g., trachea, soft tissues of neck including deep extrinsic muscles of the tongue, strap muscles, thyroid, or esophagus).*

PROGNOSTIC FACTORS (SITE SPECIFIC FACTORS)
(Recommended for Collection)

Required for staging	None
Clinically significant	Size of lymph nodes
	Extracapsular extension from lymph nodes for head and neck
	Head and neck lymph nodes levels I–III
	Head and neck lymph nodes levels IV–V
	Head and neck lymph nodes levels VI–VII
	Other lymph nodes group
	Clinical location of cervical nodes
	Extracapsular spread (ECS) clinical
	Extracapsular spread (ECS) pathologic
	Human papillomavirus (HPV) status

Nasal Cavity and Paranasal Sinuses

6

(Nonepithelial tumors such as those of lymphoid tissue, soft tissue, bone, and cartilage are not included. Staging for mucosal melanoma of the nasal cavity and paranasal sinuses is not included in this chapter – see Chap. 9.)

SUMMARY OF CHANGES

- T4 lesions have been divided into T4a (moderately advanced local disease) and T4b (very advanced local disease), leading to the stratification of Stage IV into Stage IVA (moderately advanced local/regional disease), Stage IVB (very advanced local/regional disease), and Stage IVC (distant metastatic disease)

ICD-O-3 TOPOGRAPHY CODES

C30.0   Nasal cavity
C31.0   Maxillary sinus
C31.1   Ethmoid sinus

ICD-O-3 HISTOLOGY CODE RANGES

8000–8576, 8940–8950, 8980–8981

ANATOMY

Primary Sites. Cancer of the maxillary sinus is the most common of the sinonasal malignancies. Ethmoid sinus and nasal cavity cancers are equal in frequency but considerably less common than maxillary sinus cancers. Tumors of the sphenoid and frontal sinuses are rare.

The location as well as the extent of the mucosal lesion within the maxillary sinus has prognostic significance. Historically, a plane, connecting the medial canthus of the eye to the angle of the mandible, represented by Ohngren's line, is used to divide the maxillary sinus into an anteroinferior portion (infrastructure), which is associated with a good prognosis, and a posterosuperior portion (suprastructure), which has a poor prognosis (Figure 6.1). The poorer outcome associated with suprastructure cancers reflects early invasion by these tumors to critical structures, including the eye, skull base, pterygoids, and infratemporal fossa.

For the purpose of staging, the nasoethmoidal complex is divided into two sites: nasal cavity and ethmoid sinuses. The ethmoids are further subdivided into two subsites: left and right, separated by the nasal septum (perpendicular plate of ethmoid). The nasal cavity is divided into four subsites: the septum, floor, lateral wall, and vestibule.

Site	Subsite
Maxillary sinus	Left/right
Nasal cavity	Septum
	Floor
	Lateral wall
	Vestibule (edge of naris to mucocutaneous junction)
Ethmoid sinus	Left/right

Regional Lymph Nodes. Regional lymph node spread from cancer of nasal cavity and paranasal sinuses is relatively uncommon. Involvement of buccinator, submandibular, upper jugular, and (occasionally) retropharyngeal nodes may occur with advanced maxillary sinus cancer, particularly those extending beyond the sinus walls to involve adjacent structures, including soft tissues of the cheek, upper alveolus, palate, and buccal mucosa. Ethmoid sinus cancers are less prone to regional lymphatic spread. When only one side of the neck is involved, it should be considered ipsilateral. Bilateral spread may occur with advanced primary cancer, particularly with spread of the primary beyond the midline.

In clinical evaluation, the physical size of the nodal mass should be measured. Most masses over 3 cm in diameter are not single nodes but, rather, are confluent nodes or tumor in soft tissues of the neck. There are three categories of clinically positive nodes: N1, N2, and N3. The use of subgroups a, b, and c is required. Midline nodes are considered ipsilateral nodes. In addition to the components to describe the N category, regional lymph nodes should also be described according to the level of the neck that is involved. Pathologic examination is necessary for documentation of such disease extent. Imaging studies showing amorphous spiculated margins of involved nodes or involvement of internodal fat resulting in loss of normal oval-to-round nodal shape strongly suggest extracapsular (extranodal) tumor spread. No imaging study (as yet) can identify microscopic foci in regional nodes or distinguish between small reactive nodes and small malignant nodes without central radiographic inhomogeneity.

For pN, a selective neck dissection will ordinarily include six or more lymph nodes, and a radical or modified radical neck dissection will ordinarily include ten or more lymph nodes. Negative pathologic examination of a lesser number of lymph nodes still mandates a pN0 designation.

Distant Metastases. Distant spread usually occurs to lungs but occasionally there is spread to bone.

PROGNOSTIC FEATURES

In addition to the importance of the TNM factors outlined previously, the overall health of these patients clearly influences outcome. An ongoing effort to better assess prognosis using both tumor and nontumor related factors is underway. Chart abstraction will continue to be performed by cancer registrars to obtain important information regarding specific factors related to prognosis. This data will then be used to further hone the predictive power of the staging system in future revisions.

Comorbidity can be classified by specific measures of additional medical illnesses. Accurate reporting of all illnesses in the patients' medical record is essential to assessment of these parameters. General performance measures are helpful in predicting survival. The AJCC strongly recommends the clinician report performance status using the ECOG, Zubrod, or Karnofsky performance measures along with standard staging information. An interrelationship between each of the major performance tools exists.

ZUBROD/ECOG PERFORMANCE SCALE

0. Fully active, able to carry on all predisease activities without restriction (Karnofsky 90–100).
1. Restricted in physically strenuous activity but ambulatory and able to carry work of a light or sedentary nature. For example, light housework, office work (Karnofsky 70–80).
2. Ambulatory and capable of all self-care but unable to carry out any work activities. Up and about more than 50% of waking hours (Karnofsky 50–60).
3. Capable of only limited self-care, confined to bed or chair 50% or more of waking hours (Karnofsky 30–40).
4. Completely disabled. Cannot carry on self-care. Totally confined to bed (Karnofsky 10–20).
5. Death (Karnofsky 0).

Lifestyle factors such as tobacco and alcohol abuse negatively influence survival. Accurate recording of smoking in pack years and alcohol in number of days drinking per week and number of drinks per day will provide important data for future analysis. Nutrition is important to prognosis and will be indirectly measured by weight loss of >10% of body weight. Depression adversely impacts quality of life and survival. Notation of a previous or current diagnosis of depression should be recorded in the medical record.

Mucosal Melanoma. Mucosal melanoma of all head and neck sites is staged using a uniform classification as discussed in Chap. 9.

DEFINITIONS OF TNM

Primary Tumor (T)

TX	Primary tumor cannot be assessed
T0	No evidence of primary tumor
Tis	Carcinoma in situ

Maxillary Sinus

T1	Tumor limited to maxillary sinus mucosa with no erosion or destruction of bone (Figure 6.2)
T2	Tumor causing bone erosion or destruction including extension into the hard palate and/or middle nasal meatus, except extension to posterior wall of maxillary sinus and pterygoid plates (Figure 6.3)
T3	Tumor invades any of the following: bone of the posterior wall of maxillary sinus, subcutaneous tissues, floor or medial wall of orbit, pterygoid fossa, ethmoid sinuses (Figure 6.4)
T4a	Moderately advanced local disease
	Tumor invades anterior orbital contents, skin of cheek, pterygoid plates, infratemporal fossa, cribriform plate, sphenoid or frontal sinuses (Figure 6.5A, B)
T4b	Very advanced local disease
	Tumor invades any of the following: orbital apex, dura, brain, middle cranial fossa, cranial nerves other than maxillary division of trigeminal nerve (V2), nasopharynx, or clivus (Figure 6.6)

Nasal Cavity and Ethmoid Sinus

T1	Tumor restricted to any one subsite, with or without bony invasion (Figure 6.7)
T2	Tumor invading two subsites in a single region or extending to involve an adjacent region within the nasoethmoidal complex, with or without bony invasion (Figure 6.8)
T3	Tumor extends to invade the medial wall or floor of the orbit, maxillary sinus, palate, or cribriform plate (Figure 6.9)

(continued)

Primary Tumor (T) (*continued*)

T4a   Moderately advanced local disease

Tumor invades any of the following: anterior orbital contents, skin of nose or cheek, minimal extension to anterior cranial fossa, pterygoid plates, sphenoid or frontal sinuses (Figure 6.10)

T4b   Very advanced local disease

Tumor invades any of the following: orbital apex, dura, brain, middle cranial fossa, cranial nerves other than (V2), nasopharynx, or clivus (Figure 6.11)

Regional Lymph Nodes (N) (See Part II Head and Neck Figures II.1–II.4)

NX   Regional lymph nodes cannot be assessed

N0   No regional lymph node metastasis

N1   Metastasis in a single ipsilateral lymph node, 3 cm or less in greatest dimension

N2   Metastasis in a single ipsilateral lymph node, more than 3 cm but not more than 6 cm in greatest dimension, or in multiple ipsilateral lymph nodes, none more than 6 cm in greatest dimension, or in bilateral or contralateral lymph nodes, none more than 6 cm in greatest dimension

N2a   Metastasis in a single ipsilateral lymph node, more than 3 cm but not more than 6 cm in greatest dimension

N2b   Metastasis in multiple ipsilateral lymph nodes, none more than 6 cm in greatest dimension

N2c   Metastasis in bilateral or contralateral lymph nodes, none more than 6 cm in greatest dimension

N3   Metastasis in a lymph node, more than 6 cm in greatest dimension

Distant Metastasis (M)

M0   No distant metastasis

M1   Distant metastasis

ANATOMIC STAGE/PROGNOSTIC GROUPS

Stage 0	Tis	N0	M0
Stage I	T1	N0	M0
Stage II	T2	N0	M0
Stage III	T3	N0	M0
	T1	N1	M0
	T2	N1	M0
	T3	N1	M0
Stage IVA	T4a	N0	M0
	T4a	N1	M0
	T1	N2	M0
	T2	N2	M0
	T3	N2	M0
	T4a	N2	M0
Stage IVB	T4b	Any N	M0
	Any T	N3	M0
Stage IVC	Any T	Any N	M1

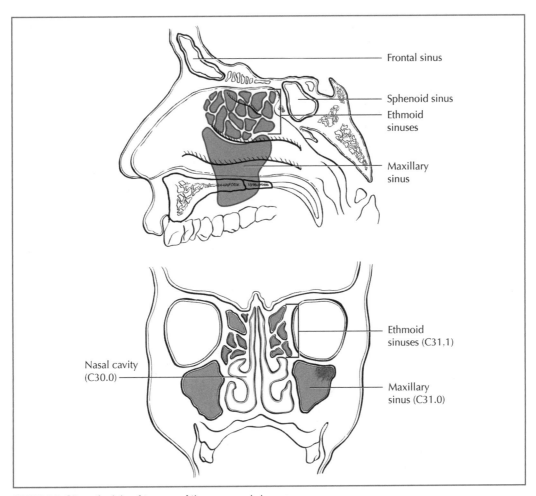

FIGURE 6.1. *Sites of origin of tumors of the paranasal sinuses.*

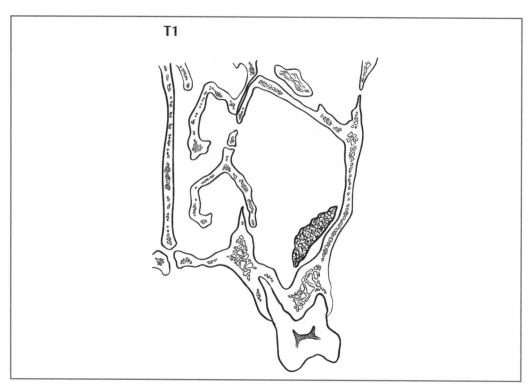

FIGURE 6.2. *T1 in the maxillary sinus is limited to the maxillary sinus mucosa with no erosion or destruction of bone.*

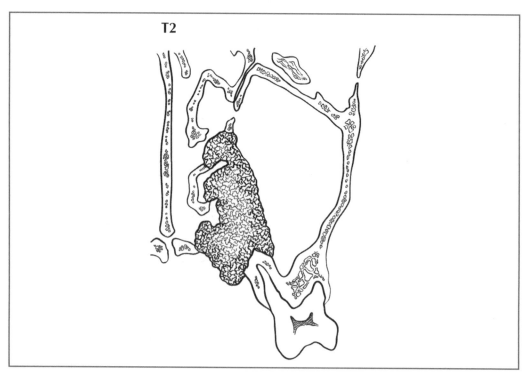

FIGURE 6.3. *T2 in the maxillary sinus causes bone erosion or destruction including extension into the hard palate and/ or middle nasal meatus with the exception of extension to posterior wall of maxillary sinus and pterygoid plates.*

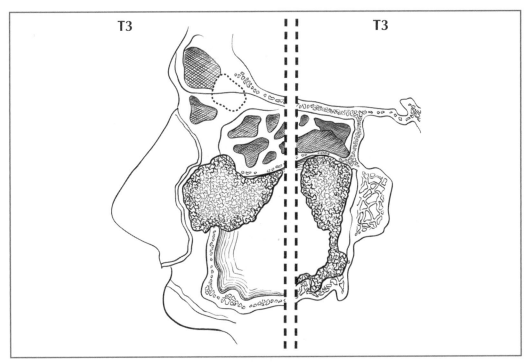

FIGURE 6.4. *Two views of T3 in the maxillary sinus. Tumor invades any of the following: bone of the posterior wall of maxillary sinus, subcutaneous tissues, floor or medial wall of orbit, pterygoid fossa, ethmoid sinuses.*

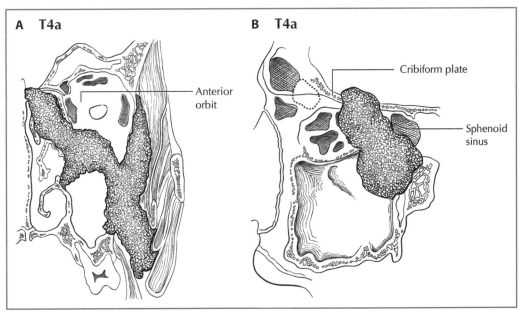

FIGURE 6.5. *(A) T4a in the maxillary sinus is defined as moderately advanced local disease, showing tumor invasion of anterior orbital contents. (B) T4a in the maxillary sinus is defined as moderately advanced local disease, showing tumor invasion of sphenoid sinus and cribriform plate.*

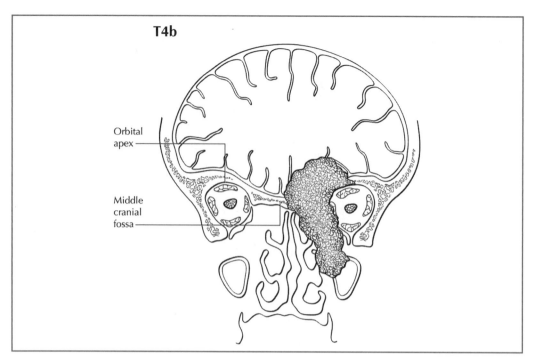

FIGURE 6.6. *Coronal view of T4b in the maxillary sinus, very advanced local disease, shows tumor invading orbital apex.*

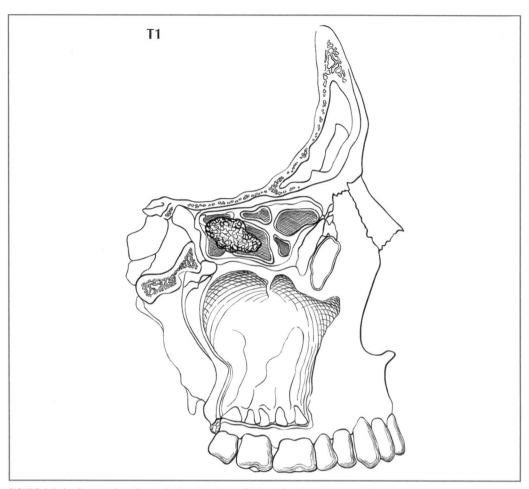

FIGURE 6.7. *In the nasal cavity and ethmoid sinus, T1 is defined as tumor restricted to any one subsite, with or without bony invasion.*

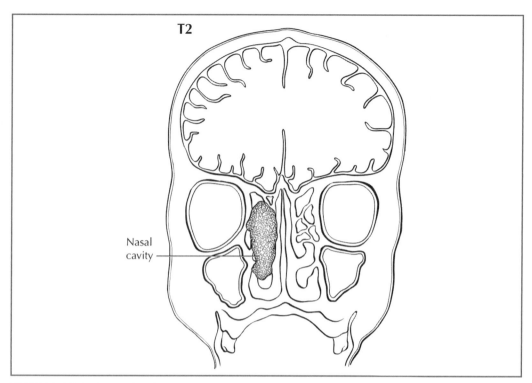

FIGURE 6.8. *T2 in the nasal cavity and ethmoid sinus is defined as invading two subsites in a single region or extending to involve an adjacent region within the nasoethmoidal complex, here the nasal cavity, with or without bony invasion.*

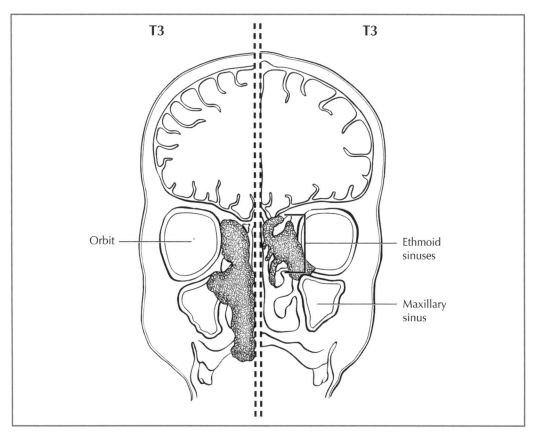

FIGURE 6.9. *Two views of T3 in the nasal cavity and ethmoid sinus showing tumor invading maxillary sinus and palate (left) and extending to the floor of the orbit (right).*

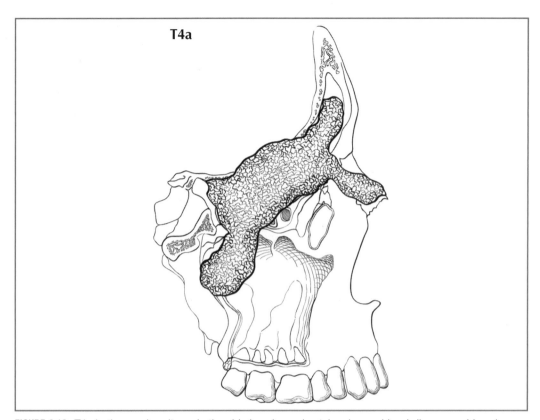

FIGURE 6.10. *T4a in the nasal cavity and ethmoid sinus is moderately advanced local disease and invades any of the following: anterior orbital contents, skin of nose or cheek, minimal extension to anterior cranial fossa, pterygoid plates, sphenoid or frontal sinuses.*

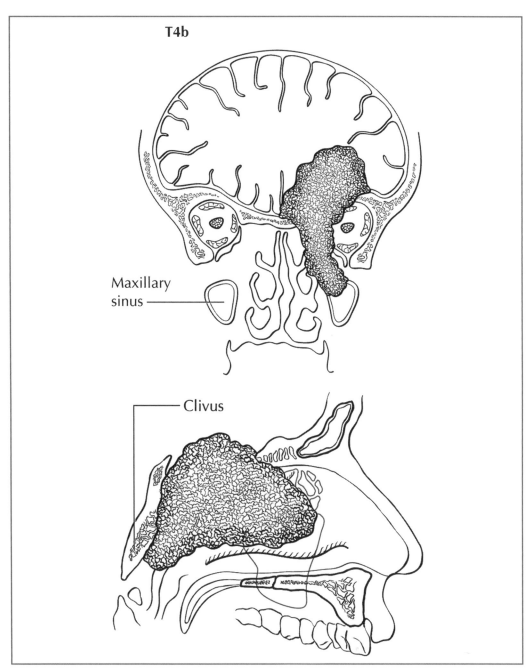

T4b

Maxillary sinus

Clivus

FIGURE 6.11. *Two views of T4b in the nasal cavity and ethmoid sinus. This is very advanced local disease, and the coronal view on the left shows invasion in the orbital apex and brain. On the right, tumor invades the clivus.*

Major Salivary Glands

(Parotid, submandibular, and sublingual)

7

SUMMARY OF CHANGES

- T4 lesions have been divided into T4a (moderately advanced local disease) and T4b (very advanced local disease), leading to the stratification of Stage IV into Stage IVA (moderately advanced local/regional disease), Stage IVB (very advanced local/regional disease), and Stage IVC (distant metastatic disease)

ICD-O-3 TOPOGRAPHY CODES

C07.9	Parotid gland
C08.0	Submandibular gland
C08.1	Sublingual gland
C08.8	Overlapping lesion of major salivary glands
C08.9	Major salivary gland, NOS

ICD-O-3 HISTOLOGY CODE RANGES

8000–8576, 8940–8950, 8980–8982

ANATOMY

Primary Site. The major salivary glands include the parotid, submandibular, and sublingual glands (Figure 7.1). Tumors arising in minor salivary glands (mucus-secreting glands in the lining membrane of the upper aerodigestive tract) are staged according to the anatomic site of origin (e.g., oral cavity, sinuses, etc.).

Primary tumors of the parotid constitute the largest proportion of salivary gland tumors. Sublingual primary cancers are rare and may be difficult to distinguish with certainty from minor salivary gland primary tumors of the anterior floor of the mouth.

Regional Lymph Nodes. Regional lymphatic spread from salivary gland cancer is less common than from head and neck mucosal squamous cancers and varies according to the histology and size of the primary tumor. Most nodal metastases will be clinically apparent on initial evaluation.

Low-grade tumors rarely metastasize to regional nodes, whereas the risk of regional spread is substantially higher from high-grade cancers. Regional dissemination tends to be orderly, progressing from intraglandular to adjacent (periparotid, submandibular) nodes, then to upper and midjugular nodes, apex of the posterior triangle (level Va) nodes, and occasionally to retropharyngeal nodes. Bilateral lymphatic spread is rare.

For pathologic reporting (pN), histologic examination of a selective neck dissection will ordinarily include six or more lymph nodes and a radical or modified radical neck dissection will ordinarily include ten or more lymph nodes. Negative pathologic evaluation of a lesser number of nodes still mandates a pN0 designation.

Distant Metastases. Distant spread is most frequently to the lungs.

DEFINITIONS OF TNM

Primary Tumor (T)

TX	Primary tumor cannot be assessed
T0	No evidence of primary tumor
T1	Tumor 2 cm or less in greatest dimension without extraparenchymal extension* (Figure 7.2)
T2	Tumor more than 2 cm but not more than 4 cm in greatest dimension without extraparenchymal extension* (Figure 7.3)
T3	Tumor more than 4 cm and/or tumor having extraparenchymal extension* (Figure 7.4A, B)
T4a	Moderately advanced disease
	Tumor invades skin, mandible, ear canal, and/or facial nerve (Figure 7.5A, B, C, D)
T4b	Very advanced disease
	Tumor invades skull base and/or pterygoid plates and/or encases carotid artery (Figure 7.6A, B)

*Note: Extraparenchymal extension is clinical or macroscopic evidence of invasion of soft tissues. Microscopic evidence alone does not constitute extraparenchymal extension for classification purposes.

Regional Lymph Nodes (N) (See Part II Head and Neck Figures II.1–II.4)

NX	Regional lymph nodes cannot be assessed
N0	No regional lymph node metastasis
N1	Metastasis in a single ipsilateral lymph node, 3 cm or less in greatest dimension
N2	Metastasis in a single ipsilateral lymph node, more than 3 cm but not more than 6 cm in greatest dimension, or in multiple ipsilateral lymph nodes, none more than 6 cm in greatest dimension, or in bilateral or contralateral lymph nodes, none more than 6 cm in greatest dimension
N2a	Metastasis in a single ipsilateral lymph node, more than 3 cm but not more than 6 cm in greatest dimension
N2b	Metastasis in multiple ipsilateral lymph nodes, none more than 6 cm in greatest dimension
N2c	Metastasis in bilateral or contralateral lymph nodes, none more than 6 cm in greatest dimension
N3	Metastasis in a lymph node, more than 6 cm in greatest dimension

Distant Metastasis (M)

M0   No distant metastasis

M1   Distant metastasis

ANATOMIC STAGE/PROGNOSTIC GROUPS

Stage I	T1	N0	M0
Stage II	T2	N0	M0
Stage III	T3	N0	M0
	T1	N1	M0
	T2	N1	M0
	T3	N1	M0
Stage IVA	T4a	N0	M0
	T4a	N1	M0
	T1	N2	M0
	T2	N2	M0
	T3	N2	M0
	T4a	N2	M0
Stage IVB	T4b	Any N	M0
	Any T	N3	M0
Stage IVC	Any T	Any N	M1

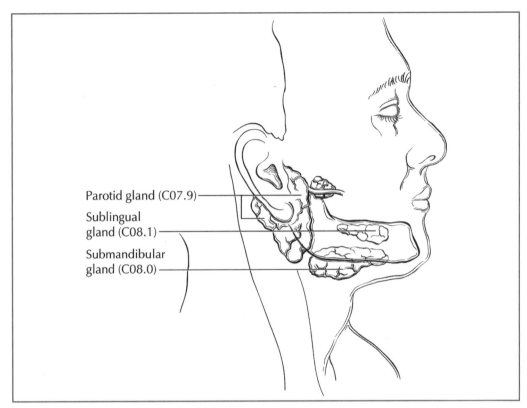

FIGURE 7.1. *Major salivary glands include the parotid, submandibular, and sublingual glands.*

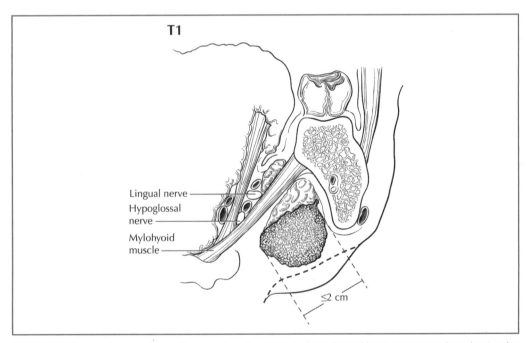

FIGURE 7.2. *T1 is defined as tumor 2 cm or less in greatest dimension without extraparenchymal extension (a coronal section with tumor of the submandibular gland is shown).*

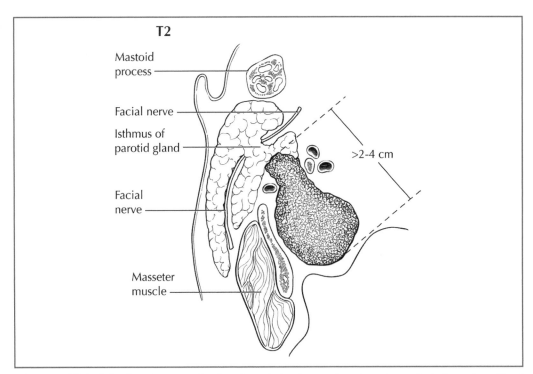

FIGURE 7.3. *T2 is defined as tumor greater than 2 cm but not more than 4 cm in greatest dimension without extraparenchymal extension (an axial section with tumor of the deep lobe of the parotid gland is shown).*

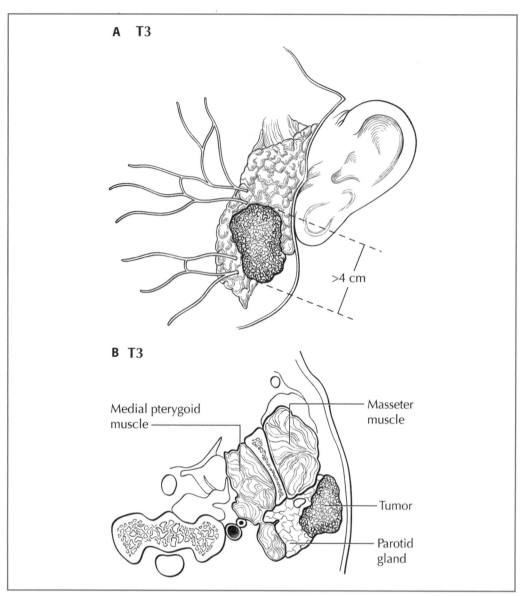

A T3

>4 cm

B T3

Medial pterygoid muscle

Masseter muscle

Tumor

Parotid gland

FIGURE 7.4. (A) T3 is defined as tumor greater than 4 cm and/or tumor having extraparenchymal extension (a tumor of the superficial lobe of the parotid gland is shown). (B) Cross-sectional diagram of T3 tumor with extraparenchymal extension from the parotid gland.

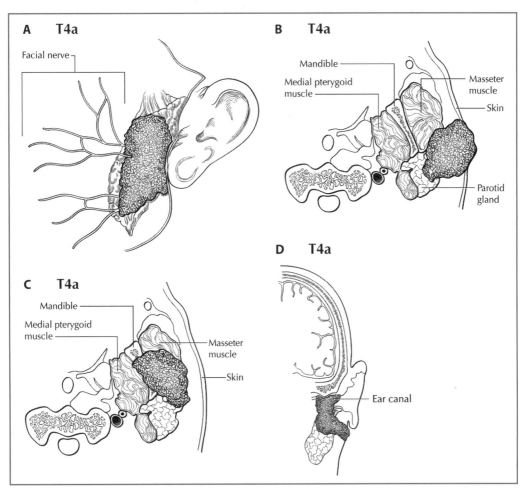

FIGURE 7.5. *(A) T4a is defined as moderately advanced disease, tumor invading skin, mandible, ear canal, and/ or facial nerve (as illustrated here). (B) Cross-sectional diagram of T4a tumor invading skin. (C) Cross-sectional diagram of T4a tumor invading mandible. (D) Coronal section of T4a tumor invading ear canal.*

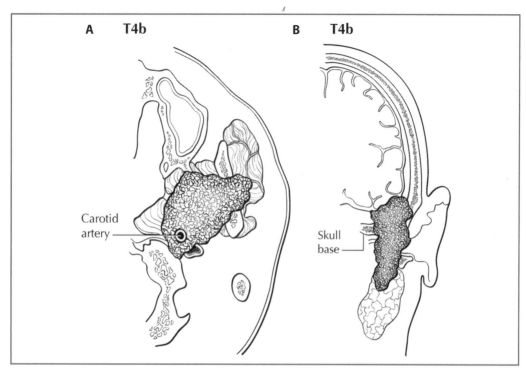

FIGURE 7.6. *(A) T4b is defined as very advanced disease, tumor invading skull base and/or pterygoid plates and/or encases carotid artery. In this cross-sectional diagram, the tumor encases the carotid artery. (B) Coronal section of T4b tumor invading skull base.*

PROGNOSTIC FACTORS (SITE-SPECIFIC FACTORS) *(Recommended for Collection)*	
Required for staging	None
Clinically significant	Size of lymph nodes
	Extracapsular extension from lymph nodes for head and neck
	Head and neck lymph nodes levels I–III
	Head and neck lymph nodes levels IV–V
	Head and neck lymph nodes levels VI–VII
	Other lymph nodes group
	Clinical location of cervical nodes
	Extracapsular spread (ECS) clinical
	Extracapsular spread (ECS) pathologic

Thyroid

8

ICD-O-3 TOPOGRAPHY CODE

C73.9   Thyroid gland

ICD-O-3 HISTOLOGY CODE RANGES

8000–8576, 8940–8950, 8980–8981

ANATOMY

Primary Site. The thyroid gland ordinarily is composed of a right and a left lobe lying adjacent and lateral to the upper trachea and esophagus. An isthmus connects the two lobes, and in some cases a pyramidal lobe is present extending cephalad anterior to the thyroid cartilage (Figure 8.1).

Regional Lymph Nodes. Regional lymph node spread from thyroid cancer is common but of less prognostic significance in patients with well-differentiated tumors (papillary, follicular) than in medullary cancers. The adverse prognostic influence of lymph node metastasis in patients with differentiated carcinomas is observed, only in the older age group. The first echelon of nodal metastasis consists of the paralaryngeal, paratracheal, and prelaryngeal (Delphian) nodes adjacent to the thyroid gland in the central compartment of the neck generally described as Level VI. Metastases secondarily involve the mid- and lower jugular, the supraclavicular, and (much less commonly) the upper deep jugular and spinal accessory lymph nodes. Lymph node metastasis to submandibular and submental lymph nodes is very rare. Upper mediastinal (Level VII) nodal spread occurs frequently both anteriorly and posteriorly. Retropharyngeal nodal metastasis may be seen, usually in the presence of extensive lateral cervical metastasis. Bilateral nodal spread is common. The components of the N category are described as follows: first echelon (central compartment/Level VI), or N1a, and lateral cervical and/or superior mediastinal or N1b. The lymph node metastasis should also be described according to the level of the neck that is involved. Nodal metastases from medullary thyroid cancer carry a much more ominous prognosis, although they follow a similar pattern of spread.

For pN, histologic examination of a selective neck dissection will ordinarily include six or more lymph nodes, whereas histologic examination of a radical or a modified radical comprehensive neck dissection will ordinarily include ten or more lymph nodes. Negative pathologic evaluation of a lesser number of nodes still mandates a pN0 designation.

Metastatic Sites. Distant spread occurs by hematogenous routes – for example to lungs and bones – but many other sites may be involved.

DEFINITIONS OF TNM

Primary Tumor (T)

Note: All categories may be subdivided: (s) solitary tumor and (m) multifocal tumor (the largest determines the classification).

TX	Primary tumor cannot be assessed
T0	No evidence of primary tumor
T1	Tumor 2 cm or less in greatest dimension limited to the thyroid (Figure 8.2)
T1a	Tumor 1 cm or less, limited to the thyroid
T1b	Tumor more than 1 cm but not more than 2 cm in greatest dimension, limited to the thyroid
T2	Tumor more than 2 cm but not more than 4 cm in greatest dimension limited to the thyroid (Figure 8.3)
T3	Tumor more than 4 cm in greatest dimension limited to the thyroid or any tumor with minimal extrathyroid extension (e.g., extension to sternothyroid muscle or perithyroid soft tissues) (Figure 8.4)
T4a	Moderately advanced disease
	Tumor of any size extending beyond the thyroid capsule to invade subcutaneous soft tissues, larynx, trachea, esophagus, or recurrent laryngeal nerve (Figure 8.5A, B)
T4b	Very advanced disease
	Tumor invades prevertebral fascia or encases carotid artery or mediastinal vessels (Figure 8.6)

All anaplastic carcinomas are considered T4 tumors

T4a	Intrathyroidal anaplastic carcinoma
T4b	Anaplastic carcinoma with gross extrathyroid extension

Regional Lymph Nodes (N)

Regional lymph nodes are the central compartment, lateral cervical, and upper mediastinal lymph nodes.

NX	Regional lymph nodes cannot be assessed
N0	No regional lymph node metastasis
N1	Regional lymph node metastasis
N1a	Metastasis to Level VI (pretracheal, paratracheal, and prelaryngeal/Delphian lymph nodes) (Figure 8.7)
N1b	Metastasis to unilateral, bilateral, or contralateral cervical (Levels I, II, III, IV, or V) or retropharyngeal or superior mediastinal lymph nodes (Level VII) (Figure 8.8)

Distant Metastasis (M)

M0	No distant metastasis
M1	Distant metastasis

ANATOMIC STAGE/PROGNOSTIC GROUPS

Separate stage groupings are recommended for papillary or follicular (differentiated), medullary, and anaplastic (undifferentiated) carcinoma

Papillary or Follicular (differentiated)

UNDER 45 YEARS

Stage I	Any T	Any N	M0
Stage II	Any T	Any N	M1

45 YEARS AND OLDER

Stage I	T1	N0	M0
Stage II	T2	N0	M0
Stage III	T3	N0	M0
	T1	N1a	M0
	T2	N1a	M0
	T3	N1a	M0
Stage IVA	T4a	N0	M0
	T4a	N1a	M0
	T1	N1b	M0
	T2	N1b	M0
	T3	N1b	M0
	T4a	N1b	M0
Stage IVB	T4b	Any N	M0
Stage IVC	Any T	Any N	M1

Medullary Carcinoma (all age groups)

Stage I	T1	N0	M0
Stage II	T2	N0	M0
	T3	N0	M0
Stage III	T1	N1a	M0
	T2	N1a	M0
	T3	N1a	M0
Stage IVA	T4a	N0	M0
	T4a	N1a	M0
	T1	N1b	M0
	T2	N1b	M0
	T3	N1b	M0
	T4a	N1b	M0
Stage IVB	T4b	Any N	M0
Stage IVC	Any T	Any N	M1

Anaplastic Carcinoma

All anaplastic carcinomas are considered Stage IV

Stage IVA	T4a	Any N	M0
Stage IVB	T4b	Any N	M0
Stage IVC	Any T	Any N	M1

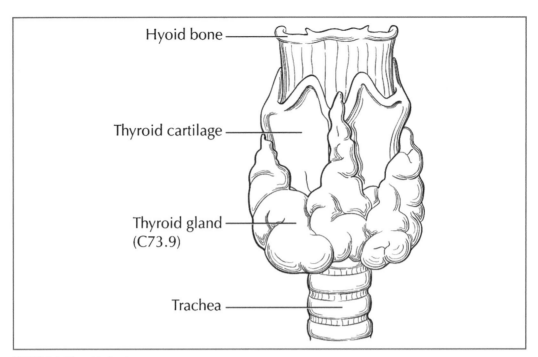

FIGURE 8.1. *Thyroid gland.*

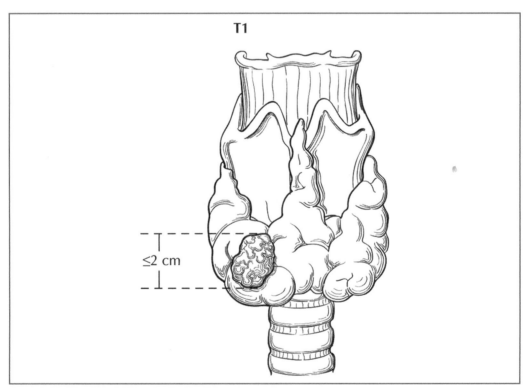

FIGURE 8.2. *T1 is defined as tumor 2 cm or less in greatest dimension limited to the thyroid. T1a is defined as tumor 1 cm or less, limited to the thyroid. T1b is defined as tumor more than 1 cm but not more than 2 cm in greatest dimension, limited to the thyroid.*

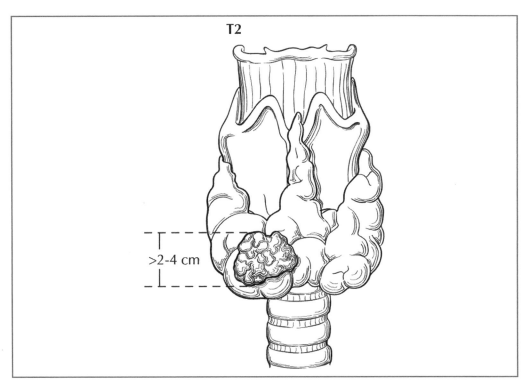

FIGURE 8.3. *T2 is defined as tumor more than 2 cm but not more than 4 cm in greatest dimension limited to the thyroid.*

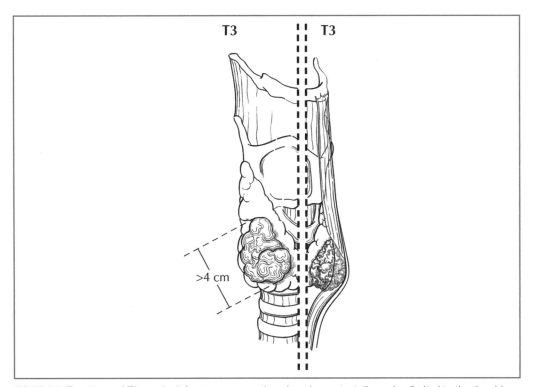

FIGURE 8.4. *Two views of T3: on the left, a tumor more than 4 cm in greatest dimension limited to the thyroid; on the right, a tumor with minimal extrathyroid extension (to either sternothyroid muscle or perithyroid soft tissues).*

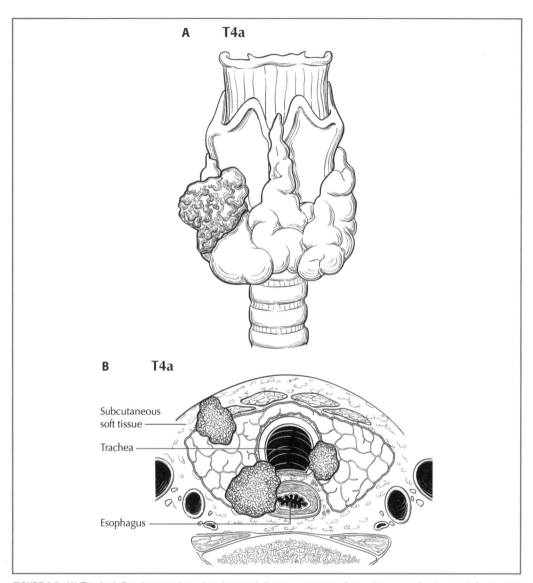

A T4a

B T4a

Subcutaneous
soft tissue

Trachea

Esophagus

FIGURE 8.5. *(A) T4a is defined as moderately advanced disease, a tumor of any size extending beyond the thyroid capsule to invade subcutaneous soft tissues, larynx, trachea, esophagus, or recurrent laryngeal nerve. (B) Cross-sectional diagram of three different parameters of T4a: tumor invading subcutaneous soft tissues; tumor invading trachea; tumor invading esophagus.*

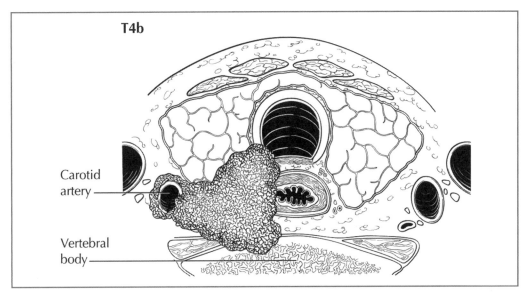

FIGURE 8.6. *T4b is defined as very advanced disease, tumor invading prevertebral fascia or encases carotid artery or mediastinal vessels. Cross-sectional diagram of two different parameters of T4b: tumor encases carotid artery; tumor invades vertebral body.*

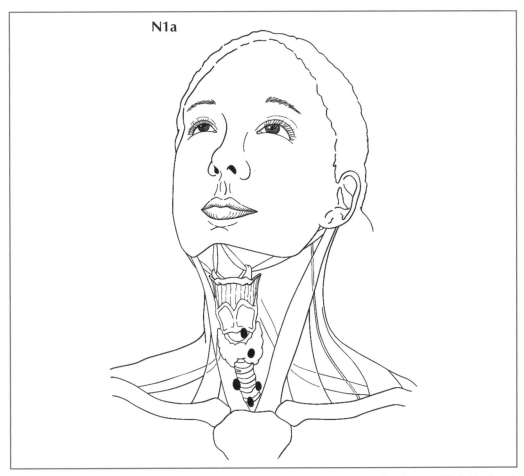

FIGURE 8.7. *N1a is defined as metastasis to Level VI (pretracheal, paratracheal, and prelaryngeal/Delphian lymph nodes).*

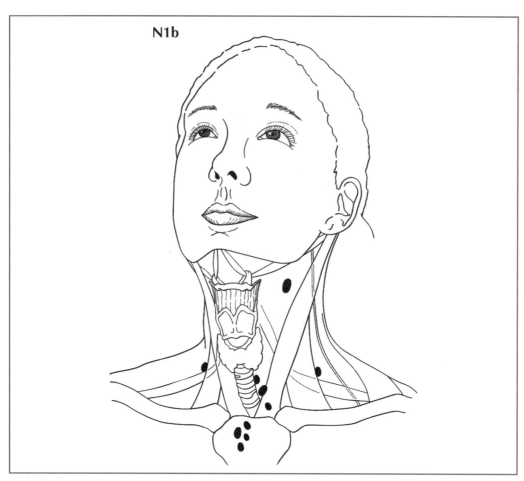

FIGURE 8.8. *N1b is defined as metastasis to unilateral, bilateral, or contralateral cervical (Levels I, II, III, IV, or V) or retropharyngeal or superior mediastinal lymph nodes (Level VII).*

PROGNOSTIC FACTORS (SITE-SPECIFIC FACTORS)
(Recommended for Collection)

Required for staging	None
Clinically significant	Extrathyroid extension
	Histology

Mucosal Melanoma of the Head and Neck

9

ICD-O-3 TOPOGRAPHY CODES

For a complete description of codes, refer to the appropriate anatomic site chapter based on the location of the mucosal melanoma (see Chapters 3–Chapters 6)

Additionally, mucosal melanomas are staged for the following topography codes; however, no staging exists for nonmucosal melanoma in the same anatomic site:

C14.0   Pharynx, NOS
C14.2   Waldeyer's ring
C14.8   Overlapping lesion of lip, oral cavity and pharynx

The following topography codes are excluded:

C07.9   Parotid gland
C08.0   Submandibular gland
C08.1   Sublingual gland
C08.8   Overlapping lesion of major
        salivary glands
C08.9   Major salivary glands, NOS
C30.1   Middle ear
C73.9   Thyroid

ICD-O-3 HISTOLOGY CODE RANGES

8720–8790

ANATOMY

Mucosal melanomas occur throughout the mucosa of the upper aerodigestive tract. For a description of anatomy, refer to the appropriate anatomic site chapter based on the location of the mucosal melanoma.

C.C. Compton et al. (eds.), *AJCC Cancer Staging Atlas: A Companion to the Seventh Editions of the AJCC Cancer Staging Manual and Handbook*, DOI 10.1007/978-1-4614-2080-4_9,
© 2012 American Joint Committee on Cancer

DEFINITIONS OF TNM

Primary Tumor

T3   Mucosal disease (Figure 9.1)

T4a   Moderately advanced disease

      Tumor involving deep soft tissue, cartilage, bone, or overlying skin (Figure 9.2A)

T4b   Very advanced disease

      Tumor involving brain, dura, skull base, lower cranial nerves (IX, X, XI, XII), masticator space, carotid artery, prevertebral space, or mediastinal structures (Figure 9.2B)

Regional Lymph Nodes (See Part II Head and Neck Figures II.1–II.4)

NX   Regional lymph nodes cannot be assessed

N0   No regional lymph node metastases

N1   Regional lymph node metastases present

Distant Metastasis

M0   No distant metastasis

M1   Distant metastasis present

ANATOMIC STAGE/PROGNOSTIC GROUPS

Stage III	T3	N0	M0
Stage IVA	T4a	N0	M0
	T3–T4a	N1	M0
Stage IVB	T4b	Any N	M0
Stage IVC	Any T	Any N	M1

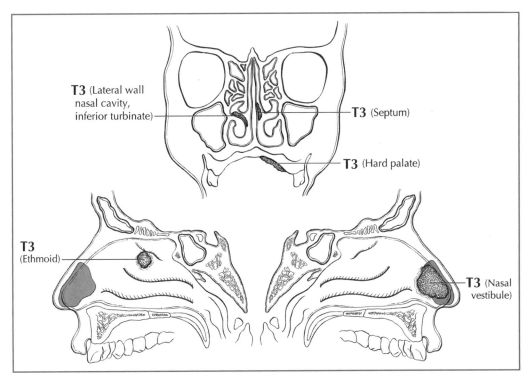

FIGURE 9.1. *T3 is defined as mucosal disease. Involvement of the lateral wall nasal cavity, inferior turbinate is illustrated, as well as septum, hard palate, ethmoid, and nasal vestibule.*

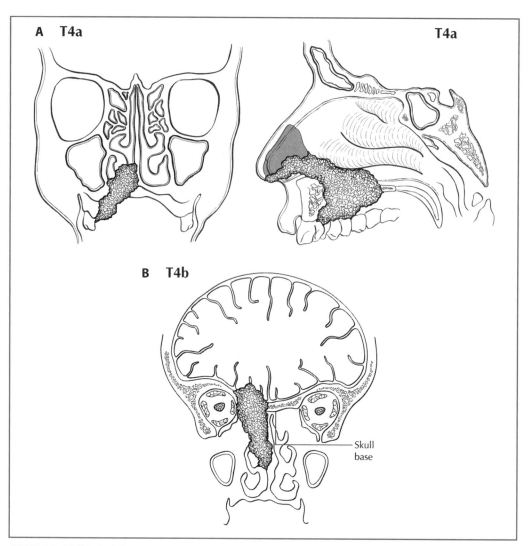

FIGURE 9.2. (A) T4a is defined as moderately advanced disease, with tumor involving deep soft tissue, cartilage, bone, or overlying skin. (B) T4b is defined as very advanced disease, with tumor involving the brain as illustrated, or also involving dura, lower cranial nerves (IX, X, XI, XII), masticator space, carotid artery, prevertebral space, or mediastinal structures.

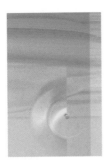

PART III
Digestive System

Esophagus and Esophagogastric Junction

(Nonmucosal cancers are not included)

10

SUMMARY OF CHANGES

- Tumor location is simplified, and esophagogastric junction and proximal 5 cm of stomach are included
- Tis is redefined and T4 is subclassified
- Regional lymph nodes are redefined. N is subclassified according to the number of regional lymph nodes containing metastasis
- M is redefined
- Separate stage groupings for squamous cell carcinoma and adenocarcinoma
- Stage groupings are reassigned using T, N, M, and G classifications

---

ICD-O-3 TOPOGRAPHY CODES

C15.0	Cervical esophagus
C15.1	Thoracic esophagus
C15.2	Abdominal esophagus
C15.3	Upper third of esophagus
C15.4	Middle third of esophagus
C15.5	Lower third of esophagus
C15.8	Overlapping lesion of esophagus
C15.9	Esophagus, NOS
C16.0	Cardia, esophagogastric junction
C16.1	Fundus of stomach, proximal 5 cm only*
C16.2	Body of stomach, proximal 5 cm only*

*Note: If gastric tumor extends to or above esophagogastric junction.

ICD-O-3 HISTOLOGY CODE RANGES

8000–8576, 8940–8950, 8980–8981 (C15 only) 8000–8152, 8154–8231, 8243–8245, 8247–8248, 8250–8576, 8940–8950, 8980–8981 (C16 only)

ANATOMY

Primary Site. The location of the primary tumor is defined by the position of the upper end of the cancer in the esophagus. This is best expressed as the distance from the incisors to the proximal edge of the tumor and conventionally by its location within broad regions of the esophagus. ICD coding recognizes three anatomic compartments traversed by the esophagus: cervical, thoracic, and

---

C.C. Compton et al. (eds.), *AJCC Cancer Staging Atlas: A Companion to the Seventh Editions of the AJCC Cancer Staging Manual and Handbook*, DOI 10.1007/978-1-4614-2080-4_10,
© 2012 American Joint Committee on Cancer

abdominal. It also arbitrarily divides the esophagus into equal thirds: upper, middle, and lower. However, clinical importance of primary site of esophageal cancer is less related to its position in the esophagus than to its relation to adjacent structures (Figure 10.1).

Cervical Esophagus. Anatomically, the cervical esophagus lies in the neck, bordered superiorly by the hypopharynx and inferiorly by the thoracic inlet, which lies at the level of the sternal notch. It is subtended by the trachea, carotid sheaths, and vertebrae. Although length of the esophagus differs somewhat with body habitus, gender, and age, typical endoscopic measurements for the cervical esophagus measured from the incisors are from 15 to <20 cm (Figure 10.1). If esophagoscopy is not available, location can be assessed by computed tomography (CT). If thickening of the esophageal wall begins above the sternal notch, the location is cervical.

Upper Thoracic Esophagus. The upper thoracic esophagus is bordered superiorly by the thoracic inlet and inferiorly by the lower border of the azygos vein. Anterolaterally, it is surrounded by the trachea, arch vessels, and great veins, and posteriorly by the vertebrae. Typical endoscopic measurements from the incisors are from 20 to <25 cm (Figure 10.1). CT location of an upper thoracic cancer is esophageal wall thickening that begins between the sternal notch and the azygos vein.

Middle Thoracic Esophagus. The middle thoracic esophagus is bordered superiorly by the lower border of the azygos vein and inferiorly by the inferior pulmonary veins. It is sandwiched between the pulmonary hilum anteriorly, descending thoracic aorta on the left, and vertebrae posteriorly; on the right, it lies freely on the pleura. Typical endoscopic measurements from the incisors are from 25 to <30 cm (Figure 10.1). CT location is wall thickening that begins between the azygos vein and the inferior pulmonary vein.

Lower Thoracic Esophagus/Esophagogastric Junction. The lower thoracic esophagus is bordered superiorly by the inferior pulmonary veins and inferiorly by the stomach. Because it is the end of the esophagus, it includes the esophagogastric junction (EGJ). It is bordered anteriorly by the pericardium, posteriorly by vertebrae, and on the left by the descending thoracic aorta. It normally passes through the diaphragm to reach the stomach, but there is a variable intra-abdominal portion, and because of hiatal hernia, this portion may be absent. Typical endoscopic measurements from the incisors are from 30 to 40 cm (Figure 10.1). CT location is wall thickening that begins below the inferior pulmonary vein. The abdominal esophagus is included in the lower thoracic esophagus.

The arbitrary 10-cm segment encompassing the distal 5 cm of the esophagus and proximal 5 cm of the stomach, with the EGJ in the middle, is an area of contention. Cancers arising in this segment have been variably staged as esophageal or gastric tumors, depending on orientation of the treating physician. In this edition, cancers whose epicenter is in the lower thoracic esophagus, EGJ, or within the proximal 5 cm of the stomach (cardia) that extend into the EGJ or esophagus (Siewert III) are stage grouped similar to adenocarcinoma of the esophagus. Although Siewert and colleagues subtype EGJ cancers (types I, II, III), not only do their data support a single-stage grouping scheme across this area, but also they demonstrate that prognosis depends on cancer classification (T, N, M, G) and not Siewert type. All other cancers with an epicenter in the stomach greater than 5 cm distal to the EGJ, or those within 5 cm of the EGJ but not extending into the EGJ or esophagus, are stage grouped using the gastric (non-EGJ) cancer staging system (see Chap. 11).

Esophageal Wall. The esophageal wall has three layers: mucosa, submucosa, and muscularis propria (Figure 10.2). The mucosa is composed of epithelium, lamina propria, and muscularis mucosae. A basement membrane isolates the mucosa from the rest of the esophageal wall. In the columnar-lined esophagus the muscularis mucosae may be a two-layered structure. The mucosal division can be classified as m1 (epithelium), m2 (lamina propria), or m3 (muscularis mucosae). The submucosa has no landmarks, but some divide it into inner (sm1), middle (sm2), and outer thirds (sm3). The muscularis propria has inner circular and outer longitudinal muscle layers. There is no serosa; rather, adventitia (periesophageal connective tissue) lies directly on the muscularis propria.

Adjacent Structures. In close proximity to the esophagus lie pleura-peritoneum, pericardium, and diaphragm. Cancers invading these structures may be resectable (T4a). Aorta, carotid vessels, azygos vein, trachea, left main bronchus, and vertebral body also are in close proximity, but cancers invading these structures are usually unresectable (T4b).

Lymphatics. Esophageal lymphatic drainage is intramural and longitudinal (Figure 10.2). Although a lymphatic network is concentrated in the submucosa, lymphatic channels are present in the lamina propria, an arrangement that permits lymphatic metastases early in the course of the disease from superficial cancers that are otherwise confined to the mucosa. Lymphatic drainage of the muscularis propria is more limited, but lymphatic channels pierce this layer to drain into regional lymphatic channels and lymph nodes in the periesophageal fat. Up to 43% of autopsy dissections demonstrate direct drainage from the submucosal plexus into the thoracic duct, which facilitates systemic metastases. The longitudinal nature of the submucosal lymphatic plexus permits lymphatic metastases orthogonal to the depth of tumor invasion. Implications of the longitudinal nature of lymphatic drainage are that the anatomic site of the cancer and the nodes to which lymphatics drain from that site may not be the same.

Regional lymph nodes extend from periesophageal cervical nodes to celiac nodes (Figures 10.3A–C). For radiotherapy, fields of treatment may not be constrained within this definition of regional node.

The data demonstrate that the number of regional lymph nodes containing metastases (positive nodes) is the most important prognostic factor. In classifying N, the data support convenient coarse groupings of the number of positive nodes (0, 1–2, 3–6, 7 or more). These have been designated N1 (1–2), N2 (3–6), and N3 (7 or more). Nevertheless, there are no sharp cut-points; rather, each additional positive node increases risk. Clinical determination of positive lymph node number is possible and correlated with survival. Thus, the staging recommendations apply to both clinical and pathologic staging. The data do not support lymph node ratio (number positive divided by number sampled) as a useful measure of lymph node burden. The number of sampled nodes, the denominator of the ratio, is highly variable, distorting the magnitude of lymph node burden.

Data demonstrate that in general, the more lymph nodes resected, the better the survival. This may be due to either improved N classification or a therapeutic effect of lymphadenectomy. On the basis of worldwide data, it was found that optimum lymphadenectomy depends on T classification: For pT1, approximately ten nodes must be resected to maximize survival; for pT2, 20 nodes and for pT3 or pT4, 30 nodes or more. On the basis of different data and analysis methods that focus on maximizing sensitivity, others have suggested that an adequate lymphadenectomy requires resecting 12–22 nodes. Thus, one should resect as many regional lymph nodes as possible, balancing the extent of lymph node resection with morbidity of radical lymphadenectomy.

Distant Metastatic Sites. Sites of distant metastases are those that are not in direct continuity with the esophagus and include nonregional lymph nodes (M1). The previous M1a and M1b subclassification has not been found useful.

NONANATOMIC TUMOR CHARACTERISTICS

This staging of cancer of the esophagus is based on cancers arising from its epithelium, squamous cell carcinoma, and adenocarcinoma. Nonmucosal cancers arising in the wall should be classified according to their cell of origin.

Highest histologic grade on biopsy or resection specimen is the required data for stage grouping. Because the data indicate that squamous cell carcinoma has a poorer prognosis than adenocarcinoma, if a tumor is of mixed histopathologic type or is not otherwise specified, it shall be recorded as squamous cell carcinoma. If grade is not available, it should be recorded as GX and stage grouped as G1 cancer. G4, undifferentiated cancers, should be recorded as such and stage grouped similar to G3 squamous cell carcinoma.

DEFINITIONS OF TNM

Primary Tumor (T)*

TX	Primary tumor cannot be assessed
T0	No evidence of primary tumor
Tis	High-grade dysplasia** (Figure 10.4)
T1	Tumor invades lamina propria, muscularis mucosae, or submucosa
T1a	Tumor invades lamina propria or muscularis mucosae (Figure 10.4)
T1b	Tumor invades submucosa (Figure 10.4)
T2	Tumor invades muscularis propria (Figure 10.5)
T3	Tumor invades adventitia (Figure 10.5)
T4	Tumor invades adjacent structures
T4a	Resectable tumor invading pleura, pericardium, or diaphragm (Figure 10.6)
T4b	Unresectable tumor invading other adjacent structures, such as aorta, vertebral body, trachea, etc. (Figure 10.6)

*(1) At least maximal dimension of the tumor must be recorded and (2) multiple tumors require the T(m) suffix.
**High-grade dysplasia includes all noninvasive neoplastic epithelia that was formerly called carcinoma in situ, a diagnosis that is no longer used for columnar mucosae anywhere in the gastrointestinal tract.

Regional Lymph Nodes (N)*

NX	Regional lymph nodes cannot be assessed
N0	No regional lymph node metastasis
N1	Metastasis in 1–2 regional lymph nodes (Figure 10.7)
N2	Metastasis in 3–6 regional lymph nodes (Figure 10.8)
N3	Metastasis in seven or more regional lymph nodes (Figure 10.9)

*Number must be recorded for total number of regional nodes sampled and total number of reported nodes with metastases.

Distant Metastasis (M)

M0	No distant metastasis
M1	Distant metastasis

ANATOMIC STAGE/PROGNOSTIC GROUPS

Squamous Cell Carcinoma*

Stage	T	N	M	Grade	Tumor Location**
0	Tis (HGD)	N0	M0	1, X	Any
IA	T1	N0	M0	1, X	Any
IB	T1	N0	M0	2–3	Any
	T2–3	N0	M0	1, X	Lower, X
IIA	T2–3	N0	M0	1, X	Upper, middle
	T2–3	N0	M0	2–3	Lower, X
IIB	T2–3	N0	M0	2–3	Upper, middle
	T1–2	N1	M0	Any	Any
IIIA	T1–2	N2	M0	Any	Any
	T3	N1	M0	Any	Any
	T4a	N0	M0	Any	Any
IIIB	T3	N2	M0	Any	Any
IIIC	T4a	N1–2	M0	Any	Any
	T4b	Any	M0	Any	Any
	Any	N3	M0	Any	Any
IV	Any	Any	M1	Any	Any

*Or mixed histology including a squamous component or NOS.
**Location of the primary cancer site is defined by the position of the upper (proximal) edge of the tumor in the esophagus.

Adenocarcinoma

Stage	T	N	M	Grade
0	Tis (HGD)	N0	M0	1, X
IA	T1	N0	M0	1–2, X
IB	T1	N0	M0	3
	T2	N0	M0	1–2, X
IIA	T2	N0	M0	3
IIB	T3	N0	M0	Any
	T1–2	N1	M0	Any
IIIA	T1–2	N2	M0	Any
	T3	N1	M0	Any
	T4a	N0	M0	Any
IIIB	T3	N2	M0	Any
IIIC	T4a	N1–2	M0	Any
	T4b	Any	M0	Any
	Any	N3	M0	Any
IV	Any	Any	M1	Any

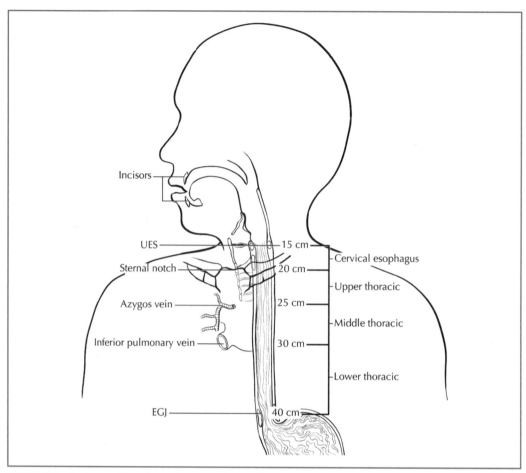

FIGURE 10.1. *Anatomy of esophageal cancer primary site, including anatomic features defining the region (left) and typical endoscopic measurements of each region measured from the incisors (right). Exact measurements are dependent on body size and height.*

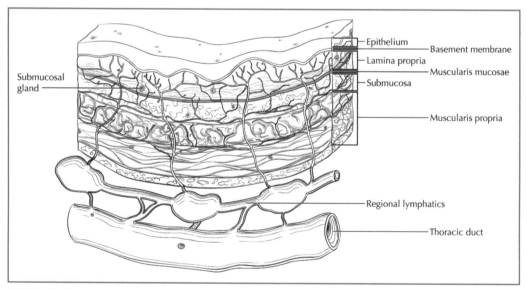

FIGURE 10.2. *Esophageal wall.*

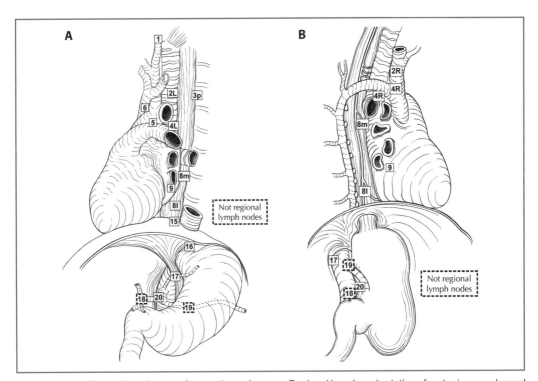

FIGURE 10.3. *(A–C) Lymph node maps for esophageal cancer. Regional lymph node stations for staging esophageal cancer, from different views. 1, Supraclavicular nodes; above suprasternal notch and clavicles. 2R, Right upper paratracheal nodes; between intersection of caudal margin of innominate artery with trachea and the apex of the lung. 2L, Left upper paratracheal nodes; between the top of aortic arch and apex of the lung. 3p, Posterior mediastinal nodes; upper paraesophageal nodes, above tracheal bifurcation. 4R, Right lower paratracheal nodes; between intersection of caudal margin of innominate artery with trachea and cephalic border of azygos vein. 4L, Left lower paratracheal nodes; between top of aortic arch and carina. 5, Aortopulmonary nodes; subaortic and para-aortic nodes lateral to the ligamentum arteriosum. 6, Anterior mediastinal nodes; anterior to ascending aorta or innominate artery. 7, Subcarinal nodes; caudal to the carina of the trachea. 8m, Middle paraesophageal lymph nodes; from the tracheal bifurcation to the caudal margin of the inferior pulmonary vein. 8l, Lower paraesophageal lymph nodes; from the caudal margin of the inferior pulmonary vein to the esophagogastric junction. 9, Pulmonary ligament nodes; within the inferior pulmonary ligament. 10R, Right tracheobronchial nodes; from cephalic border of azygos vein to origin of RUL bronchus. 10L, Left tracheobronchial nodes; between carina and LUL bronchus. 15, Diaphragmatic nodes; lying on the dome of the diaphragm and adjacent to or behind its crura. 16, Paracardial nodes; immediately adjacent to the gastroesophageal junction. 17, Left gastric nodes; along the course of the left gastric artery. 18, Common hepatic nodes; along the course of the common hepatic artery. 19, Splenic nodes; along the course of the splenic artery. 20, Celiac nodes; at the base of the celiac artery. Stations 18 and 19 are not considered regional lymph nodes.*

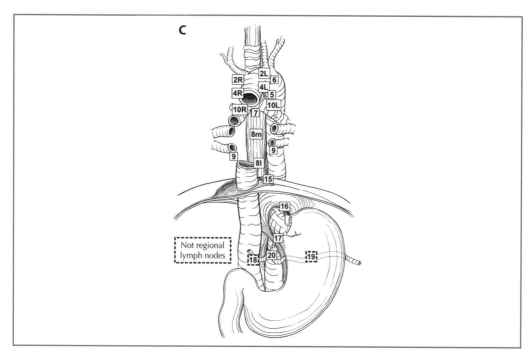

FIGURE 10.3. *(continued) (A–C) Lymph node maps for esophageal cancer. Regional lymph node stations for staging esophageal cancer, from different views. 1, Supraclavicular nodes; above suprasternal notch and clavicles. 2R, Right upper paratracheal nodes; between intersection of caudal margin of innominate artery with trachea and the apex of the lung. 2L, Left upper paratracheal nodes; between the top of aortic arch and apex of the lung. 3p, Posterior mediastinal nodes; upper paraesophageal nodes, above tracheal bifurcation. 4R, Right lower paratracheal nodes; between intersection of caudal margin of innominate artery with trachea and cephalic border of azygos vein. 4L, Left lower paratracheal nodes; between top of aortic arch and carina. 5, Aortopulmonary nodes; subaortic and para-aortic nodes lateral to the ligamentum arteriosum. 6, Anterior mediastinal nodes; anterior to ascending aorta or innominate artery. 7, Subcarinal nodes; caudal to the carina of the trachea. 8m, Middle paraesophageal lymph nodes; from the tracheal bifurcation to the caudal margin of the inferior pulmonary vein. 8l, Lower paraesophageal lymph nodes; from the caudal margin of the inferior pulmonary vein to the esophagogastric junction. 9, Pulmonary ligament nodes; within the inferior pulmonary ligament. 10R, Right tracheobronchial nodes; from cephalic border of azygos vein to origin of RUL bronchus. 10L, Left tracheobronchial nodes; between carina and LUL bronchus. 15, Diaphragmatic nodes; lying on the dome of the diaphragm and adjacent to or behind its crura. 16, Paracardial nodes; immediately adjacent to the gastroesophageal junction. 17, Left gastric nodes; along the course of the left gastric artery. 18, Common hepatic nodes; along the course of the common hepatic artery. 19, Splenic nodes; along the course of the splenic artery. 20, Celiac nodes; at the base of the celiac artery. Stations 18 and 19 are not considered regional lymph nodes.*

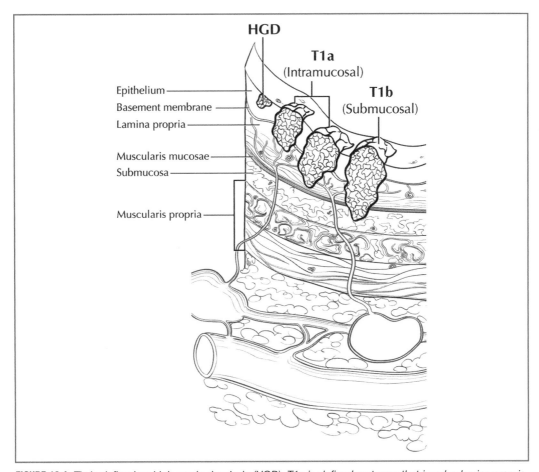

FIGURE 10.4. *Tis is defined as high-grade dysplasia (HGD). T1a is defined as tumor that invades lamina propria. T1b is defined as tumor that invades submucosa.*

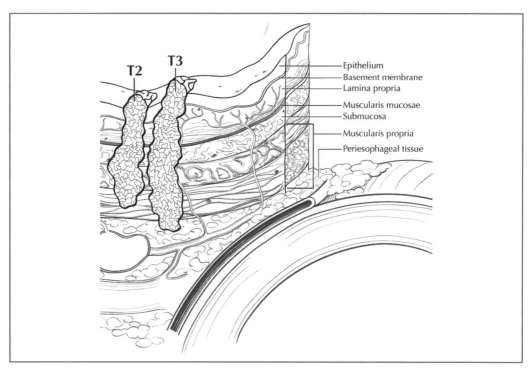

FIGURE 10.5. *T2 is defined as tumor that invades muscularis propria. T3 is defined as tumor that invades adventitia.*

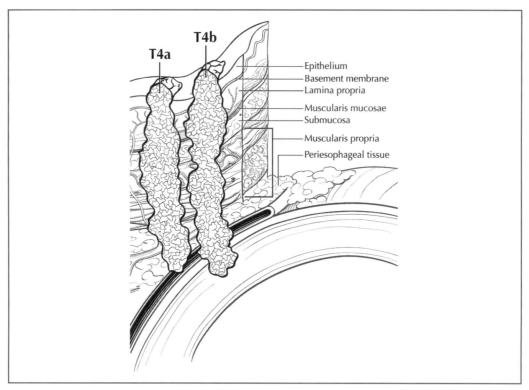

FIGURE 10.6. *T4 is defined as tumor that invades adjacent structures. T4a is defined as resectable tumor that invades pleura, pericardium or diaphragm. T4b is defined as unresectable tumor that invades other adjacent structures, such as aorta, vertebral body, trachea, etc.*

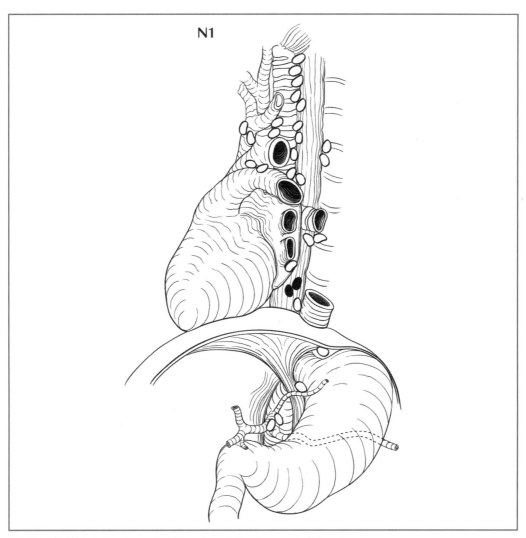

FIGURE 10.7. *N1 is defined as regional lymph node involvement in 1–2 nodes.*

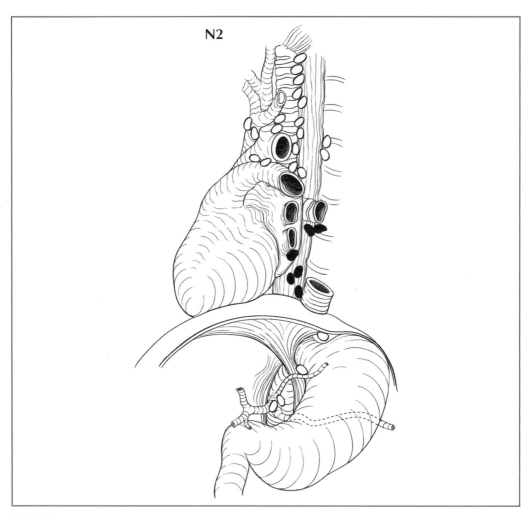

FIGURE 10.8. *N2 is defined as regional lymph node involvement in 3–6 nodes.*

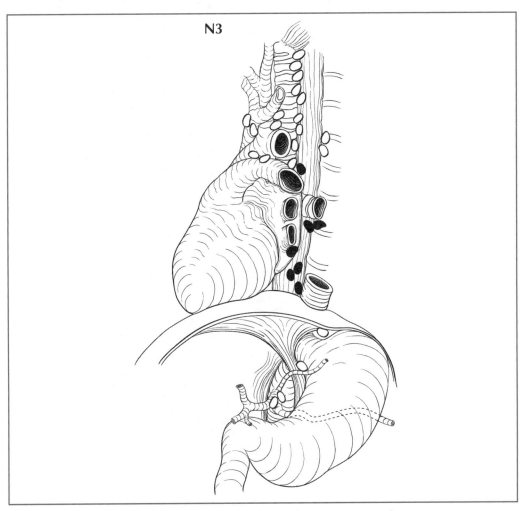

FIGURE 10.9. *N3 is defined as regional lymph node involvement in seven or more nodes.*

PROGNOSTIC FACTORS (SITE-SPECIFIC FACTORS)
(Recommended for Collection)

Squamous Cell Carcinoma

Required for staging	Location – based on the position of the upper (proximal) edge of the tumor in the esophagus (upper or middle – cancers above lower border of inferior pulmonary vein; lower – below inferior pulmonary vein)
	Grade
Clinically significant	Distance to proximal edge of tumor from incisors
	Distance to distal edge of tumor from incisors
	Number of regional nodes with extracapsular tumor

Adenocarcinoma

Required for staging	Grade
Clinically significant	Distance to proximal edge of tumor from incisors
	Distance to distal edge of tumor from incisors
	Number of regional nodes with extracapsular tumor

Stomach

(Lymphomas, sarcomas, and carcinoid tumors [low-grade neuroendocrine tumors] are not included)

11

SUMMARY OF CHANGES

- Tumors arising at the esophagogastric junction, or arising in the stomach ≤5 cm from the esophagogastric junction and crossing the esophagogastric junction are staged using the TNM system for esophageal adenocarcinoma (see Chap. 10)
- T categories have been modified to harmonize with T categories of the esophagus and small and large intestine

  - T1 lesions have been subdivided into T1a and T1b
  - T2 is defined as a tumor that invades the muscularis propria
  - T3 is defined as a tumor that invades the subserosal connective tissue
  - T4 is defined as a tumor that invades the serosa (visceral peritoneum) or adjacent structures

- N categories have been modified, with N1 = 1–2 positive lymph nodes, N2 = 3–6 positive lymph nodes, N3 = 7 or more positive lymph nodes
- Positive peritoneal cytology is classified as M1
- Stage groupings have been changed

ICD-O-3 TOPOGRAPHY CODES

C16.1   Fundus of stomach*
C16.2   Body of stomach*
C16.3   Gastric antrum
C16.4   Pylorus
C16.5   Lesser curvature of stomach, NOS
C16.6   Greater curvature of stomach, NOS
C16.8   Overlapping lesion of stomach
C16.9   Stomach, NOS
Note: See first statement in Summary of Changes.

ICD-O-3 HISTOLOGY CODE RANGES

8000–8152, 8154–8231, 8243–8245, 8247–8248, 8250–8576, 8940–8950, 8980–8990

ANATOMY

Primary Site. The stomach is the first division of the abdominal portion of the alimentary tract, beginning at the esophagogastric junction and extending to the pylorus (Figure 11.1). The proximal stomach is located immediately below the diaphragm and is termed the cardia. The remaining portions are the fundus and body of the stomach, and the distal portion of the stomach is known as the antrum. The pylorus is a muscular ring that controls the flow of food content from the stomach into the first portion of the duodenum. The medial and lateral curvatures of the stomach are known as the lesser and greater curvatures, respectively. Histologically, the wall of the stomach has five layers: mucosal, submucosal, muscular, subserosal, and serosal.

The arbitrary 10-cm segment encompassing the distal 5 cm of the esophagus and proximal 5 cm of the stomach (cardia), with the EGJ in the middle, is an area of contention. Cancers arising in this segment have been variably staged as esophageal or gastric tumors, depending on orientation of the treating physician. In this edition, cancers whose midpoint is in the lower thoracic esophagus, EGJ, or within the proximal 5 cm of the stomach (cardia) that extend into the EGJ or esophagus (Siewert III) are staged as adenocarcinoma of the esophagus (see Chap. 10). All other cancers with a midpoint in the stomach lying more than 5 cm distal to the EGJ, or those within 5 cm of the EGJ but not extending into the EGJ or esophagus, are staged using the gastric (non-EGJ) cancer staging system (Figure 11.2).

Staging of primary gastric adenocarcinoma is dependent on the depth of penetration of the primary tumor. The T1 designation has been subdivided into T1a (invasion of the lamina propria or muscularis mucosae) and T1b (invasion of the submucosa). T2 designation has been changed to invasion of the muscularis propria, and T3 to invasion of the subserosal connective tissue without invasion of adjacent structures or the serosa (visceral peritoneum). T4 tumors penetrate the serosa (T4a) or invade adjacent structures (T4b). These T categories have been changed to harmonize with those of other gastrointestinal sites.

Regional Lymph Nodes. Several groups of regional lymph nodes drain the wall of the stomach. These perigastric nodes are found along the lesser and greater curvatures. Other major nodal groups follow the main arterial and venous vessels from the aorta and the portal circulation. Adequate nodal dissection of these regional nodal areas is important to ensure appropriate designation of the pN determination. Although it is suggested that at least 16 regional nodes be assessed pathologically, a pN0 determination may be assigned on the basis of the actual number of nodes evaluated microscopically.

Involvement of other intra-abdominal lymph nodes, such as the hepatoduodenal, retropancreatic, mesenteric, and para-aortic, is classified as distant metastasis. The specific nodal areas are as follows (Figure 11.3A, B):

Greater Curvature of Stomach. Greater curvature, greater omental, gastroduodenal, gastroepiploic, pyloric, and pancreaticoduodenal

Pancreatic and Splenic Area. Pancreaticolienal, peripancreatic, splenic

Lesser Curvature of Stomach. Lesser curvature, lesser omental, left gastric, cardioesophageal, common hepatic, celiac, and hepatoduodenal

Distant Nodal Groups. Retropancreatic, para-aortic, portal, retroperitoneal, mesenteric

Metastatic Sites. The most common metastatic distribution is to the liver, peritoneal surfaces, and nonregional or distant lymph nodes. Central nervous system and pulmonary metastases occur but are less frequent. With large, bulky lesions, direct extension may occur to the liver, transverse colon, pancreas, or undersurface of the diaphragm. Positive peritoneal cytology is classified as metastatic disease.

PROGNOSTIC FEATURES

Treatment is a major prognostic factor for gastric cancer. Patients who are not resected have a poor prognosis, with survival ranging from 3 to 11 months. Depth of invasion into the gastric wall (T) correlates with reduced survival, but regional lymphatic spread is probably the most powerful prognostic factor. For those patients undergoing complete resection, the factors that affect prognosis include the location of the tumor in the stomach, histologic grade, and lymphovascular invasion. The prognosis for proximal gastric cancer is less favorable than for distal lesions. Asian race, female sex, and younger age are predictive of a better outcome, while high preoperative serum levels for tumor markers CEA and CA 19–9 have been associated with a less favorable outcome.

DEFINITIONS OF TNM

Primary Tumor (T)

TX	Primary tumor cannot be assessed
T0	No evidence of primary tumor
Tis	Carcinoma in situ: intraepithelial tumor without invasion of the lamina propria
T1	Tumor invades lamina propria, muscularis mucosae, or submucosa
T1a	Tumor invades lamina propria or muscularis mucosae (Figure 11.4)
T1b	Tumor invades submucosa (Figure 11.4)
T2	Tumor invades muscularis propria* (Figure 11.4)
T3	Tumor penetrates subserosal connective tissue without invasion of visceral peritoneum or adjacent structures**,*** (Figure 11.4, Figure 11.5A, B)
T4	Tumor invades serosa (visceral peritoneum) or adjacent structures**,***
T4a	Tumor invades serosa (visceral peritoneum) (Figure 11.6A, B, Figure 11.7)
T4b	Tumor invades adjacent structures (Figure 11.7)

*Note: A tumor may penetrate the muscularis propria with extension into the gastrocolic or gastrohepatic ligaments, or into the greater or lesser omentum, without perforation of the visceral peritoneum covering these structures. In this case, the tumor is classified T3. If there is perforation of the visceral peritoneum covering the gastric ligaments or the omentum, the tumor should be classified T4.

**The adjacent structures of the stomach include the spleen, transverse colon, liver, diaphragm, pancreas, abdominal wall, adrenal gland, kidney, small intestine, and retroperitoneum.

***Intramural extension to the duodenum or esophagus is classified by the depth of the greatest invasion in any of these sites, including the stomach.

Regional Lymph Nodes (N)

NX	Regional lymph node(s) cannot be assessed
N0	No regional lymph node metastasis*
N1	Metastasis in 1–2 regional lymph nodes (Figure 11.8)
N2	Metastasis in 3–6 regional lymph nodes (Figure 11.9)
N3	Metastasis in seven or more regional lymph nodes (Figure 11.10)
N3a	Metastasis in 7–15 regional lymph nodes
N3b	Metastasis in 16 or more regional lymph nodes

*Note: A designation of pN0 should be used if all examined lymph nodes are negative, regardless of the total number removed and examined.

Distant Metastasis (M)

M0	No distant metastasis
M1	Distant metastasis (Figure 11.11)

ANATOMIC STAGE/PROGNOSTIC GROUPS

Stage 0	Tis	N0	M0
Stage IA	T1	N0	M0
Stage IB	T2	N0	M0
	T1	N1	M0
Stage IIA	T3	N0	M0
	T2	N1	M0
	T1	N2	M0
Stage IIB	T4a	N0	M0
	T3	N1	M0
	T2	N2	M0
	T1	N3	M0
Stage IIIA	T4a	N1	M0
	T3	N2	M0
	T2	N3	M0
Stage IIIB	T4b	N0	M0
	T4b	N1	M0
	T4a	N2	M0
	T3	N3	M0
Stage IIIC	T4b	N2	M0
	T4b	N3	M0
	T4a	N3	M0
Stage IV	Any T	Any N	M1

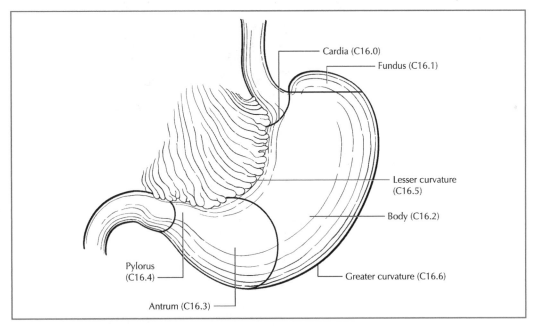

FIGURE 11.1. *Anatomical subsites of the stomach.*

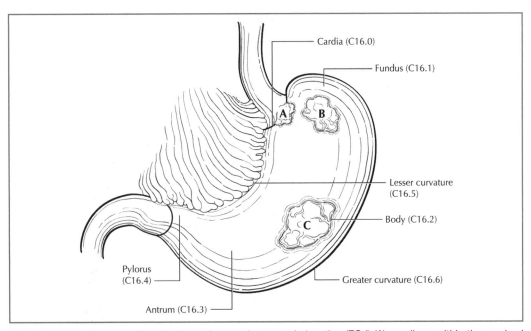

FIGURE 11.2. *Carcinomas with midpoint at the esophagogastric junction (EGJ) (A), cardia or within the proximal five centimeters of the stomach and extending into the EGJ or esophagus are staged as esophageal cancers (see Chap. 10). Carcinomas with a midpoint within 5 cm of the EGJ but not extending into the EGJ or esophagus (B) and those a midpoint lying more than 5 cm distal to the EGJ (C) are staged as gastric cancers.*

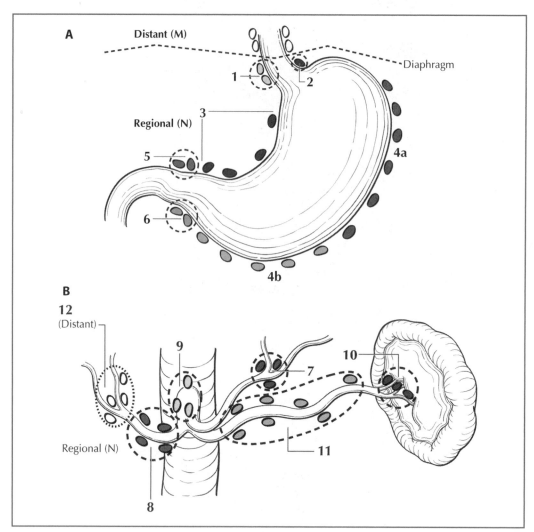

FIGURE 11.3. (A) Regional lymph nodes of the stomach. 1: right paracardial nodes; 2: left paracardial nodes; 3: perigastric nodes of the lesser curvature; 4a, 4b: perigastric nodes along the greater curvature; 5: suprapyloric nodes; 6: infrapyloric nodes. Involvement of nodes above the diaphragm is defined as distant metastasis. (B) Other lymph node groups of the stomach. 7: left gastric nodes; 8: nodes along the common hepatic artery; 9: nodes along the celiac artery; 10: splenic hilum nodes; 11: nodes along the splenic artery. Involvement of hepatoduodenal lymph nodes (12) is regarded as distant metastatic disease.

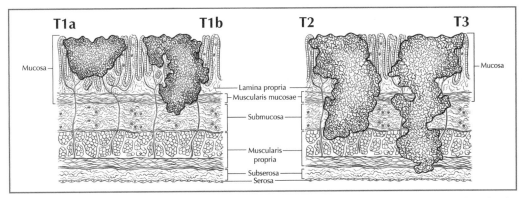

FIGURE 11.4. *T1a is defined as tumor that invades the lamina propria. T1b is defined as tumor that invades the submucosa. T2 is defined as tumor that invades muscularis propria whereas T3 is defined as tumor that extends through muscularis propria into subserosal tissue.*

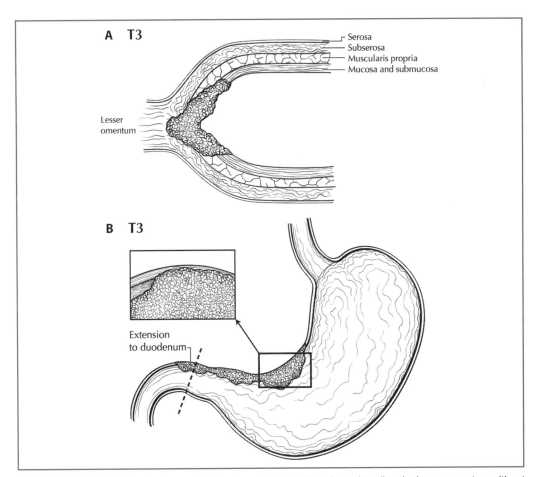

FIGURE 11.5. *(A) T3 is defined as tumor that invades subserosa, here shown invading the lesser omentum without involvement of serosa (visceral peritoneum). (B) Distal extension to duodenum does not affect the T category.*

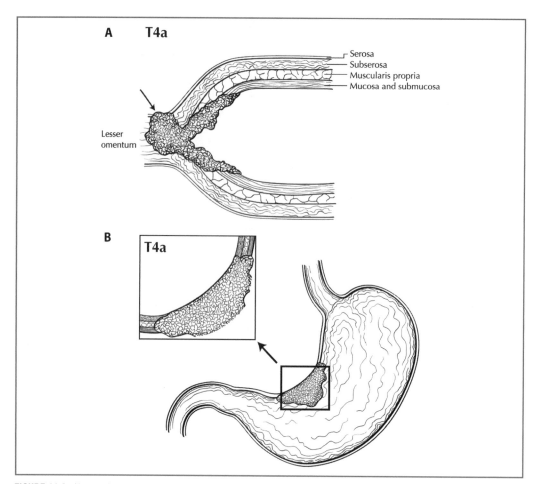

FIGURE 11.6. *(A and B) T4a is defined as tumor that penetrates the serosa (visceral peritoneum) without invasion of adjacent structures.*

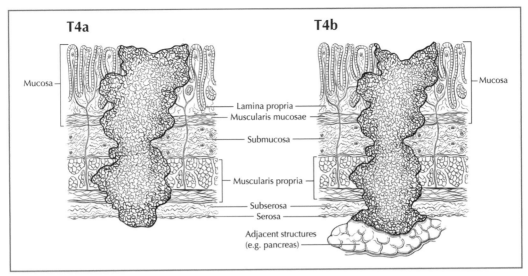

FIGURE 11.7. *T4a is defined as tumor that penetrates the serosa (visceral peritoneum) without invasion of adjacent structures whereas T4b is defined as tumor that radially invades adjacent structures, shown here invading the pancreas.*

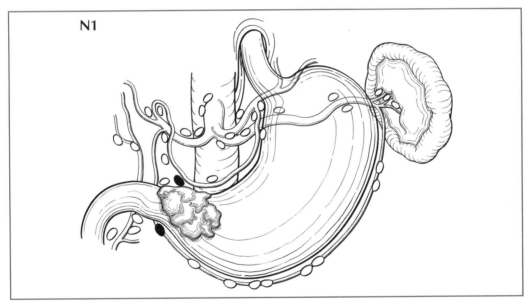

FIGURE 11.8. *N1 is defined as metastasis in 1 to 2 regional lymph nodes.*

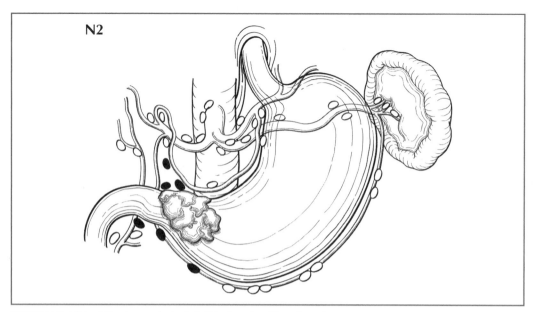

FIGURE 11.9. *N2 is defined as metastasis in 3 to 6 regional lymph nodes.*

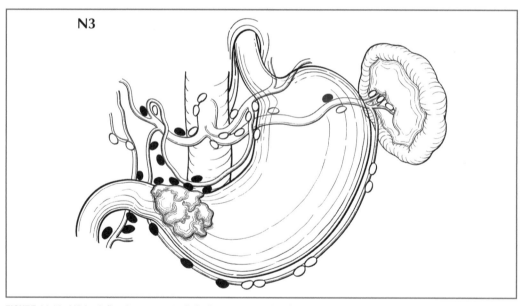

FIGURE 11.10. *N3 is defined as metastasis in 7 or more regional lymph nodes. N3a is defined as 7 to 15 involved lymph nodes whereas N3b is defined as 16 or more involved nodes.*

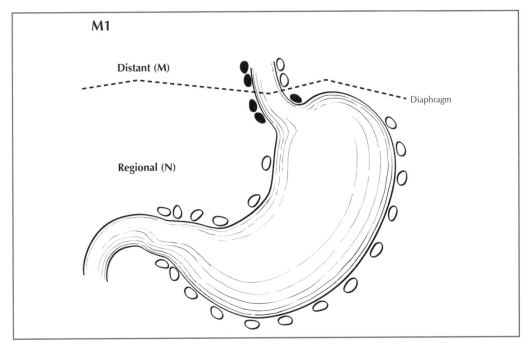

FIGURE 11.11. *Involvement of lymph nodes above the diaphragm is defined as distant metastasis or M1.*

PROGNOSTIC FACTORS (SITE-SPECIFIC FACTORS)	
(Recommended for Collection)	
Required for staging	None
Clinically significant	Tumor location
	Serum carcinoembryonic antigen
	Serum CA19.9

Small Intestine

(Lymphomas, carcinoid tumors, and visceral sarcomas are not included)

12

ICD-O-3 TOPOGRAPHY CODES

C17.0   Duodenum
C17.1   Jejunum
C17.2   Ileum
C17.8   Overlapping lesion of small intestine
C17.9   Small intestine, NOS

ICD-O-3 HISTOLOGY CODE RANGES

8000–8152, 8154–8231, 8243–8245, 8247–8248, 8250–8576, 8940–8950, 8980–8981

ANATOMY

Primary Site. This classification applies to carcinomas arising in the duodenum, jejunum, and ileum (Figure 12.1). It does not apply to carcinomas arising in the ileocecal valve or to carcinomas that may arise in Meckel's diverticulum. Carcinomas arising in the ampulla of Vater are staged according to the system described in Chap. 23.

Duodenum. About 25 cm in length, the duodenum extends from the pyloric sphincter of the stomach to the jejunum. It is usually divided anatomically into four parts, with the common bile duct and pancreatic duct opening into the second part at the ampulla of Vater.

Jejunum and Ileum. The jejunum (8 ft in length) and ileum (12 ft in length) extend from the junction with the duodenum proximally to the ileocecal valve distally. The division point between the jejunum and the ileum is arbitrary. As a general rule, the jejunum includes the proximal 40% and the ileum includes the distal 60% of the small intestine, exclusive of the duodenum.

General. The jejunal and ileal portions of the small intestine are supported by a fold of the peritoneum containing the blood supply and the regional lymph nodes, the mesentery. The shortest segment, the duodenum, has no real mesentery and is covered only by peritoneum anteriorly. The wall of all parts of the small intestine has five layers: mucosal, submucosal, muscular, subserosal, and serosal. A very thin layer of smooth muscle cells, the muscularis mucosae, separates the mucosa from the submucosa. The small intestine is entirely ensheathed by peritoneum, except for a narrow strip of bowel that is attached to the mesentery and that part of the duodenum that is located retro-peritoneally.

Regional Lymph Nodes. For pN, histologic examination of a regional lymphadenectomy speci-men will ordinarily include a representative number of lymph nodes distributed along the mesen-teric vessels extending to the base of the mesentery. Histologic examination of a regional lymphadenectomy specimen will ordinarily include six or more lymph nodes. If the lymph nodes are negative, but the number ordinarily examined is not met, pN0 should be assigned. The number of lymph nodes sampled and the number of involved lymph nodes should be recorded.

Duodenum (Figure 12.2)
Duodenal
Hepatic
Pancreaticoduodenal
Infrapyloric
Gastroduodenal
Pyloric
Superior mesenteric
Pericholedochal
Regional lymph nodes, NOS

Ileum and Jejunum (Figure 12.3)
Cecal (terminal ileum only)
Ileocolic (terminal ileum only)
Superior mesenteric
Mesenteric, NOS
Regional lymph nodes, NOS

Metastatic Sites. Cancers of the small intestine can metastasize to most organs, especially the liver, or to the peritoneal surfaces. Involvement of regional lymph nodes and invasion of adjacent structures are most common. Involvement of the celiac nodes is considered M1 disease for carcino-mas of the duodenum, jejunum, and ileum. The presence of distant metastases and the presence of residual disease (R) have the most influence on survival.

PROGNOSTIC FEATURES

The anatomic extent of the tumor is the strongest indicator of outcome when the tumor can be resected. Prognosis after incomplete removal or for those patients who do not undergo cancer-directed surgery is poor. The presence of Crohn's disease and patients' age greater than 75 years are also associated with poorer outcome.

The pathologic extent of tumor, in terms of the depth of invasion through the bowel wall, is a significant prognostic factor, as is regional lymphatic spread. Histologic grade has not emerged as a significant predictor of outcome in multivariate analysis. There are insufficient data to assess the impact of other more sophisticated pathologic factors and serum tumor markers, but it is logical to believe that the effect of those factors would be similar to that observed with colorectal cancer.

DEFINITIONS OF TNM

Primary Tumor (T)

TX   Primary tumor cannot be assessed

T0   No evidence of primary tumor

Tis   Carcinoma in situ

T1a   Tumor invades lamina propria (Figure 12.4)

T1b   Tumor invades submucosa* (Figure 12.4)

T2   Tumor invades muscularis propria (Figure 12.5)

T3   Tumor invades through the muscularis propria into the subserosa or into the nonperitonealized perimuscular tissue (mesentery or retroperitoneum) with extension 2 cm or less* (Figures 12.6)

T4   Tumor perforates the visceral peritoneum or directly invades other organs or structures (includes other loops of small intestine, mesentery, or retroperitoneum more than 2 cm, and abdominal wall by way of serosa; for duodenum only, invasion of pancreas or bile duct) (Figures 12.6, 12.7, 12.8, and 12.9)

*Note: The nonperitonealized perimuscular tissue is, for jejunum and ileum, part of the mesentery and, for duodenum in areas where serosa is lacking, part of the interface with the pancreas.

Regional Lymph Nodes (N)

NX   Regional lymph nodes cannot be assessed

N0   No regional lymph node metastasis

N1   Metastasis in 1–3 regional lymph nodes (Figure 12.10A, B, C)

N2   Metastasis in four or more regional lymph nodes (Figure 12.11A, B, C)

Distant Metastasis (M)

M0   No distant metastasis

M1   Distant metastasis (Figure 12.12)

ANATOMIC STAGE/PROGNOSTIC GROUPS

Stage	T	N	M
Stage 0	Tis	N0	M0
Stage I	T1	N0	M0
	T2	N0	M0
Stage IIA	T3	N0	M0
Stage IIB	T4	N0	M0
Stage IIIA	Any T	N1	M0
Stage IIIB	Any T	N2	M0
Stage IV	Any T	Any N	M1

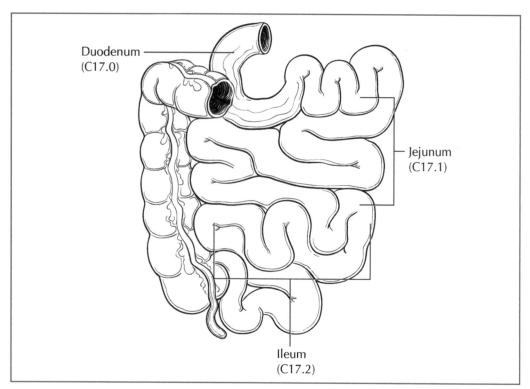

FIGURE 12.1. *Anatomical sites of the small intestine.*

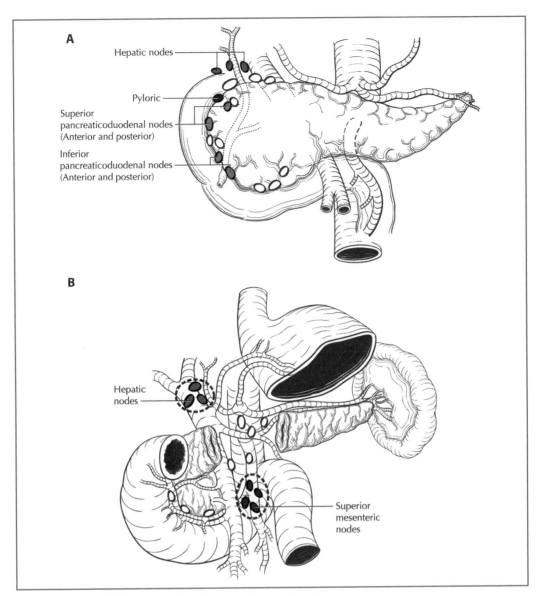

A

Hepatic nodes

Pyloric

Superior
pancreaticoduodenal nodes
(Anterior and posterior)

Inferior
pancreaticoduodenal nodes
(Anterior and posterior)

B

Hepatic
nodes

Superior
mesenteric
nodes

FIGURE 12.2. *(A and B) The regional lymph nodes of the duodenum.*

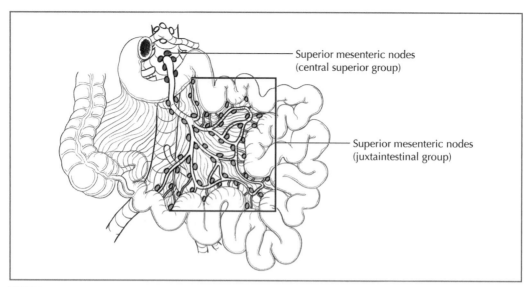

FIGURE 12.3. *The regional lymph nodes of the ileum and jejunum.*

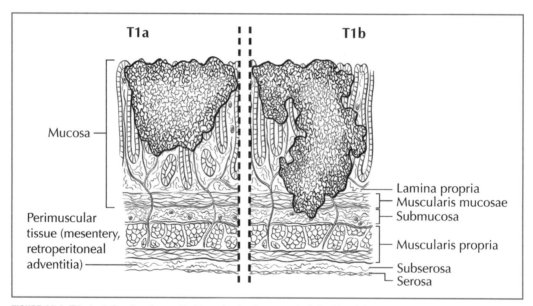

FIGURE 12.4. *T1a is defined as tumor that invades lamina propria (left side of figure) and T1b is defined as tumor that invades submucosa (right side of figure).*

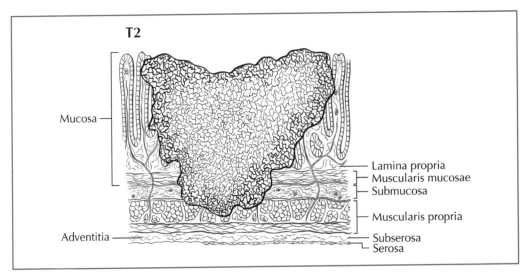

FIGURE 12.5. *T2 is defined as tumor that invades muscularis propria.*

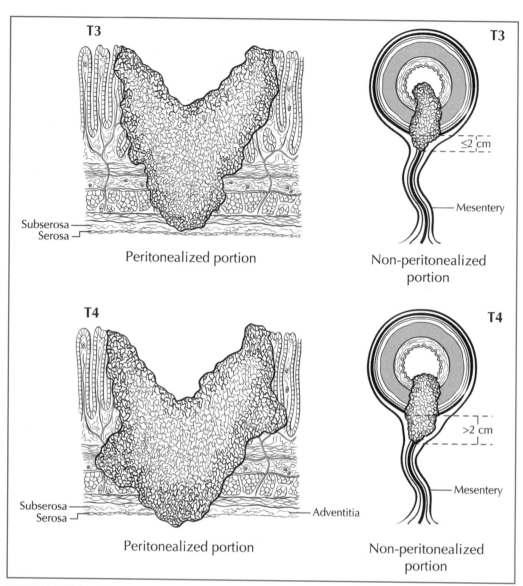

FIGURE 12.6. *T3 is defined as tumor that invades through the muscularis propria into the subserosa, whereas T4 is defined as tumor that perforates (penetrates) the visceral peritoneum. T3 is defined as tumor that invades into the nonperitonealized perimuscular tissue (mesentery or retroperitoneum) with extension 2 cm or less, whereas T4 is defined as tumor that directly invades other organs or structures (includes mesentery, or retroperitoneum) more than 2 cm.*

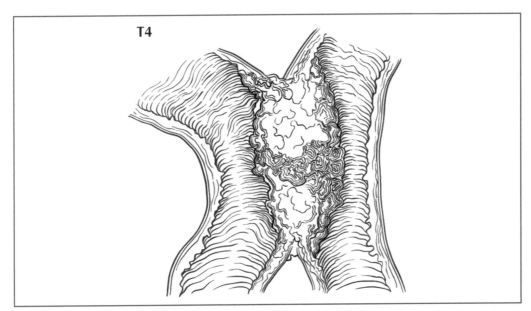

FIGURE 12.7. *T4 is defined as tumor that directly invades other organs or structures, including other loops of small intestine.*

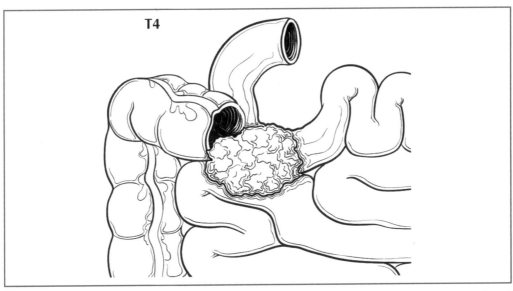

FIGURE 12.8. *T4 is defined as tumor that directly invades other organs or structures, including other loops of small intestine.*

T4 (duodenum only)

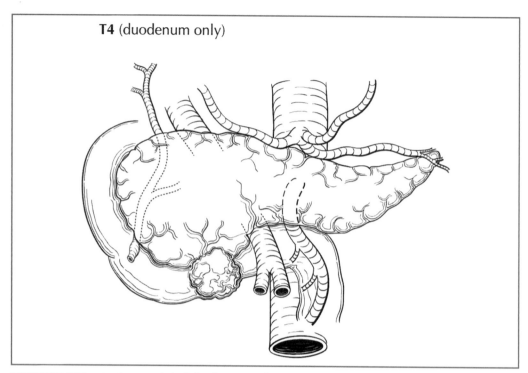

FIGURE 12.9. *T4 for duodenum only is defined as tumor that invades the pancreas.*

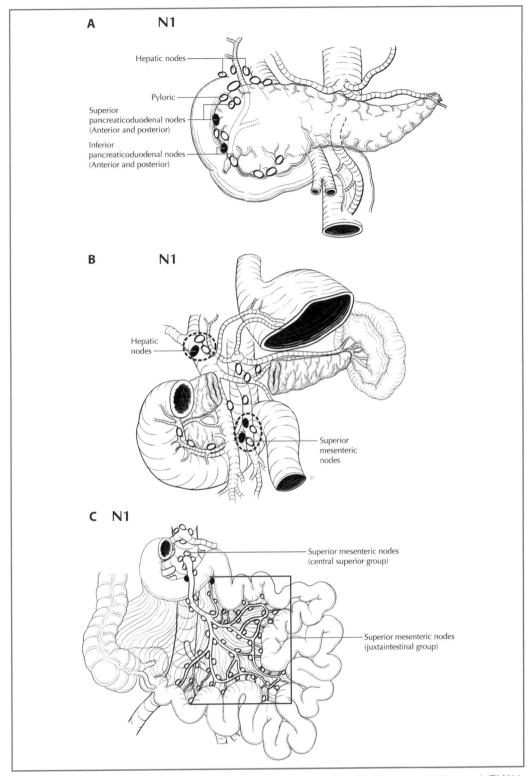

FIGURE 12.10. *(A) N1 is defined as metastasis in 1 to 3 regional lymph nodes. The duodenum is illustrated. (B) N1 is defined as metastasis in 1 to 3 regional lymph nodes. The duodenum is illustrated. (C) N1 is defined as metastasis in 1 to 3 regional lymph nodes. The jejunum and ileum are illustrated.*

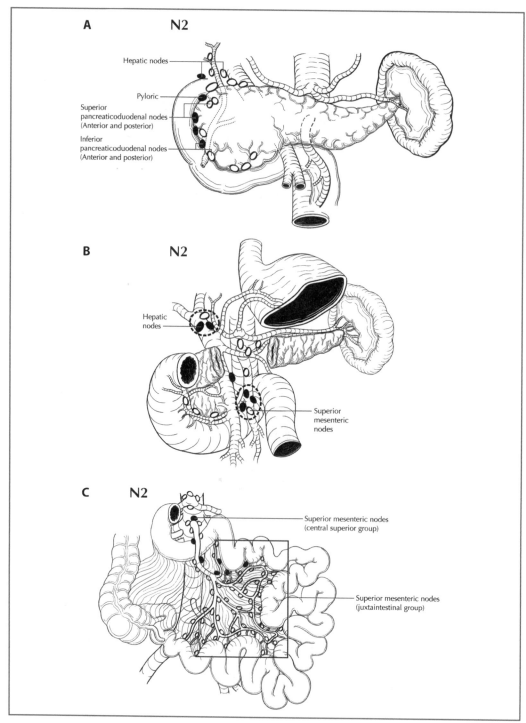

FIGURE 12.11. *(A) N2 is defined as metastasis in four or more regional lymph nodes. The duodenum is illustrated. (B) N2 is defined as metastasis in four or more regional lymph nodes. The duodenum is illustrated. (C) N2 is defined as metastasis in four or more regional lymph nodes. The jejunum and ileum are illustrated.*

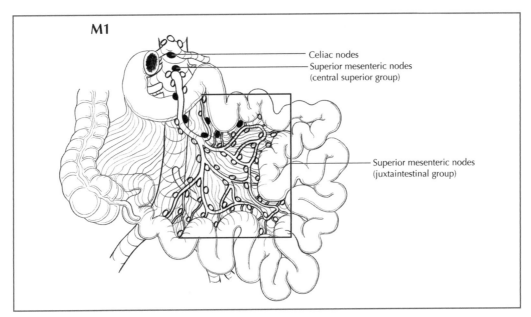

FIGURE 12.12. *Involvement of the celiac nodes is considered M1 disease.*

PROGNOSTIC FACTORS (SITE-SPECIFIC FACTORS)	
(Recommended for Collection)	
Required for staging	None
Clinically significant	Presurgical carcinoembryonic antigen (CEA)
	Microsatellite instability (MSI)
	Presence of Crohn's disease

Appendix

(Carcinomas and carcinoid tumors of the appendix are included, but separately categorized)

13

SUMMARY OF CHANGES

Appendiceal Carcinomas

- In the seventh edition, appendiceal carcinomas are separately classified. In the sixth edition, appendiceal carcinomas were classified according to the definitions for colorectal tumors
- Appendiceal carcinomas are now separated into mucinous and nonmucinous types. Histologic grading is considered of particular importance for mucinous tumors. This is reflected in the staging considerations for metastatic tumors. The change is based on published data and analysis of NCDB data
- In the seventh edition, the T4 category is divided into T4a and T4b as in the colon and is reflected in the subdivision of Stage II
- M1 is divided into M1a and M1b where pseudomyxoma peritonei, M1a, is separated from nonperitoneal metastasis, M1b
- Regional lymph node metastasis is unchanged from the sixth edition, in contrast to the subdivision of N for colorectal tumors, as there are no data justifying such a division for the appendiceal tumors. Therefore, Stage III for the appendix is unchanged from the sixth edition
- In the seventh edition, Stage IV is subdivided on the basis of N, M, and G status, unlike colorectal carcinomas
- Clinically significant prognostic factors are identified for collection in cancer registries including pretreatment CEA and CA 19.9, the number of tumor deposits in the mesentery, and where available, the presence of microsatellite instability and 18q loss of heterozygosity

Appendiceal Carcinoids

- A new classification is added for carcinoid tumors that were not classified previously by TNM. This is a new classification. There are substantial differences between the classification schemas of appendiceal carcinomas and carcinoids and between appendiceal carcinoids and other well-differentiated gastrointestinal neuroendocrine tumors (carcinoids) (see chapters of the digestive system for staging of other gastrointestinal carcinoids)
- Serum chromogranin A is identified as a significant prognostic factor

---

ICD-O-3 TOPOGRAPHY CODE

C18.1   Appendix

ICD-O-3 HISTOLOGY CODE RANGES

8000–8576, 8940–8950, 8980–8981

ANATOMY

Primary Site. The appendix is a tubular structure that arises from the base of the cecum (Figure 13.1). Its length varies but is about 10 mm. It is connected to the ileal mesentery by the mesoappendix, through which its blood supply passes from the ileocolic artery.

Regional Lymph Nodes. Lymphatic drainage passes into the ileocolic chain of lymph nodes (Figure 13.2).

Metastatic Sites. Mucinous adenocarcinomas commonly spread along the peritoneal surfaces even in the absence of lymph node metastasis. The pattern of spread of nonmucinous adenocarcinomas, in contrast, resembles cecal (colonic) tumors. Appendiceal carcinoids also tend to spread, like cecal tumors, to regional lymph nodes and the liver. Goblet cell carcinoids appear to have a predilection for metastasis to ovary.

PROGNOSTIC FEATURES

Carcinoma. Appendiceal mucinous carcinomas that spread to the peritoneum have a much better prognosis than nonmucinous tumors. Mucus that has spread beyond the right lower quadrant is a poor prognostic factor as is the presence of epithelial cells in the peritoneal cavity outside the appendix. Poor prognosis in pseudomyxoma peritonei is associated with high histological grade and/or invasion deep to the peritoneal surface. Debulking of peritoneal mucus can prolong survival, particularly in low-grade tumors. Cytological and DNA flow cytometry studies on aspirated mucus in pseudomyxoma peritonei cases are not helpful for prognostic purposes.

Carcinoid. There is controversy about the prognostic significance of mesoappendiceal invasion by a carcinoid. Tumor size appears to be the dominant local criterion for aggressive behavior. Neural invasion is commonly seen in appendiceal carcinoids and does not appear to have prognostic significance. Tubular carcinoids are typically indolent. Goblet cell carcinoids are considered more aggressive than are other appendiceal carcinoids and are classified according to the criteria for appendiceal carcinomas (see previous discussion). They tend to grow in a concentric manner along the longitudinal axis of the appendix without appearing as an easily measurable tumor mass and may even extend imperceptively into the cecum. Therefore, the line of resection is very important in assessing residual tumor. The carcinoid syndrome is typically associated with carcinoids that are metastatic to the liver. An elevated level of serum chromogranin A is considered a poor prognostic indicator for patients with metastatic carcinoid.

DEFINITIONS OF TNM

CARCINOMA

Primary Tumor (T)

TX	Primary tumor cannot be assessed
T0	No evidence of primary tumor
Tis	Carcinoma in situ: intraepithelial or invasion of lamina propria*
T1	Tumor invades submucosa (Figure 13.3)
T2	Tumor invades muscularis propria (Figure 13.4)
T3	Tumor invades through muscularis propria into subserosa or into mesoappendix (Figure 13.5)
T4	Tumor penetrates visceral peritoneum, including mucinous peritoneal tumor within the right lower quadrant and/or directly invades other organs or structures**,***
T4a	Tumor penetrates visceral peritoneum, including mucinous peritoneal tumor within the right lower quadrant (Figure 13.6)
T4b	Tumor directly invades other organs or structures (Figure 13.7)

*Tis includes cancer cells confined within the glandular basement membrane (intraepithelial) or lamina propria (intramucosal) with no extension through muscularis mucosae into submucosa.

**Direct invasion in T4 includes invasion of other segments of the colorectum by way of the serosa, e.g., invasion of ileum.

***Tumor that is adherent to other organs or structures, grossly, is classified cT4b. However, if no tumor is present in the adhesion, microscopically, the classification should be pT1-3 depending on the anatomical depth of wall invasion.

Regional Lymph Nodes (N)

NX	Regional lymph nodes cannot be assessed
N0	No regional lymph node metastasis
N1	Metastasis in 1–3 regional lymph nodes (Figure 13.8)
N2	Metastasis in four or more regional lymph nodes (Figure 13.9)

Note: A satellite peritumoral nodule or tumor deposit (TD) in the periappendiceal adipose tissue of a primary carcinoma without histologic evidence of residual lymph node in the nodule may represent discontinuous spread (T3), venous invasion with extravascular spread (T3, V1/2), or a totally replaced lymph node (N1/2). Replaced nodes should be counted as positive nodes while discontinuous spread or venous invasion should be counted in the site-specific factor TD.

Distant Metastasis (M)

M0	No distant metastasis
M1	Distant metastasis
M1a	Intraperitoneal metastasis beyond the right lower quadrant, including pseudomyxoma peritonei (Figure 13.10)
M1b	Nonperitoneal metastasis (Figure 13.11)

pTNM Pathologic Classification. The pT, pN, and pM categories correspond to the T, N, and M categories.

pN0. Histological examination of a regional lymphadenectomy specimen will ordinarily include 12 or more lymph nodes. If the lymph nodes are negative, but the number ordinarily examined is not met, classify as pN0.

Primary Tumor (T)

TX	Primary tumor cannot be assessed
T0	No evidence of primary tumor
T1	Tumor 2 cm or less in greatest dimension (Figure 13.12)
T1a	Tumor 1 cm or less in greatest dimension
T1b	Tumor more than 1 cm but not more than 2 cm
T2	Tumor more than 2 cm but not more than 4 cm or with extension to the cecum (Figures 13.13 and 13.14)
T3	Tumor more than 4 cm or with extension to the ileum (Figures 13.15 and 13.16)
T4	Tumor directly invades other adjacent organs or structures, e.g., abdominal wall and skeletal muscle* (Figure 13.17)

Note: Tumor that is adherent to other organs or structures, grossly, is classified cT4. However, if no tumor is present in the adhesion, microscopically, the classification should be classified pT1-3 depending on the anatomical depth of wall invasion. *Penetration of the mesoappendix does not seem to be as important a prognostic factor as the size of the primary tumor and is not separately categorized.

Regional Lymph Nodes (N)

NX	Regional lymph nodes cannot be assessed
N0	No regional lymph node metastasis
N1	Regional lymph node metastasis (Figure 13.18)

Distant Metastasis (M)

M0	No distant metastasis
M1	Distant metastasis

pTNM Pathologic Classification. The pT, pN, and pM categories correspond to the T, N, and M categories except that pM0 does not exist as a category.

pN0. Histological examination of a regional lymphadenectomy specimen will ordinarily include 12 or more lymph nodes. If the lymph nodes are negative, but the number ordinarily examined is not met, classify as pN0.

ANATOMIC STAGE/PROGNOSTIC GROUPS

Carcinoma

Stage 0	Tis	N0	M0
Stage I	T1	N0	M0
	T2	N0	M0
Stage IIA	T3	N0	M0
Stage IIB	T4a	N0	M0
Stage IIC	T4b	N0	M0

(continued)

ANATOMIC STAGE/PROGNOSTIC GROUPS (*continued*)

Stage IIIA	T1	N1	M0	
	T2	N1	M0	
Stage IIIB	T3	N1	M0	
	T4	N1	M0	
Stage IIIC	Any T	N2	M0	
Stage IVA	Any T	N0	M1a	G1
Stage IVB	Any T	N0	M1a	G2, 3
	Any T	N1	M1a	Any G
	Any T	N2	M1a	Any G
Stage IVC	Any T	Any N	M1b	Any G

ANATOMIC STAGE/PROGNOSTIC GROUPS

Carcinoid

Stage I	T1	N0	M0
Stage II	T2, T3	N0	M0
Stage III	T4	N0	M0
	Any T	N1	M0
Stage IV	Any T	Any N	M1

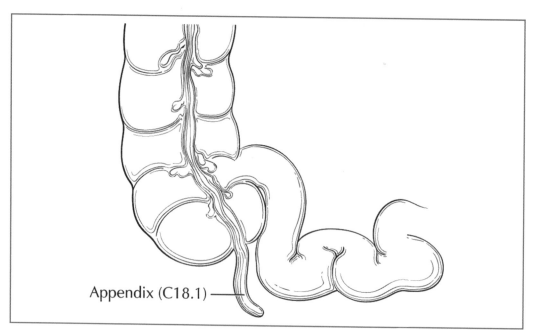

FIGURE 13.1. *Anatomic location of the appendix.*

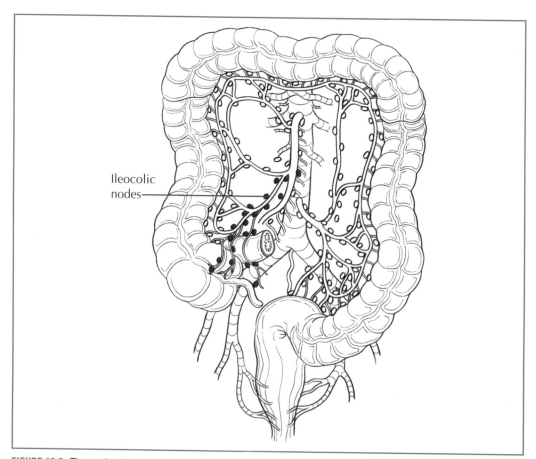

FIGURE 13.2. *The regional lymph nodes of the appendix.*

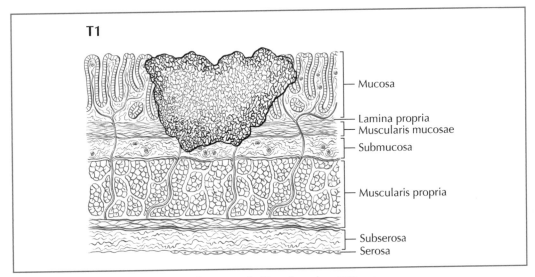

FIGURE 13.3. *For carcinoma T1 is defined as tumor that invades submucosa.*

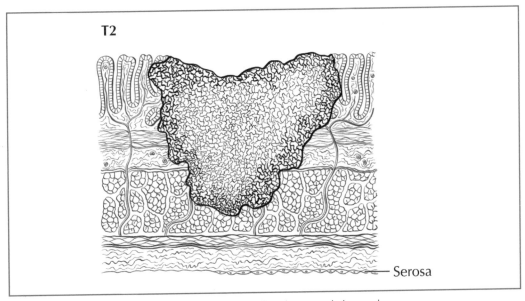

FIGURE 13.4. *For carcinoma T2 is defined as tumor that invades muscularis propria.*

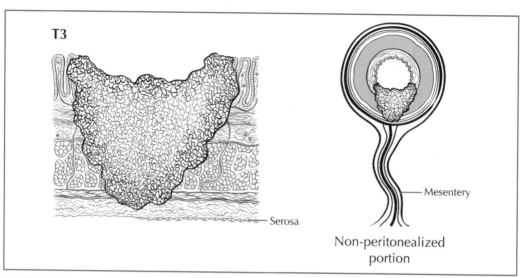

FIGURE 13.5. *For carcinoma T3 is defined as tumor that invades through muscularis propria into subserosa or into mesoappendix.*

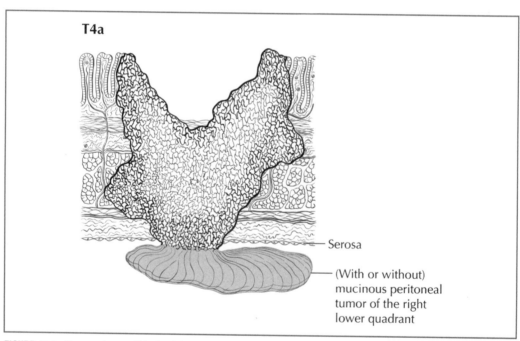

FIGURE 13.6. *For carcinoma T4a is defined as tumor that penetrates visceral peritoneum, including mucinous peritoneal tumor within the right lower quadrant.*

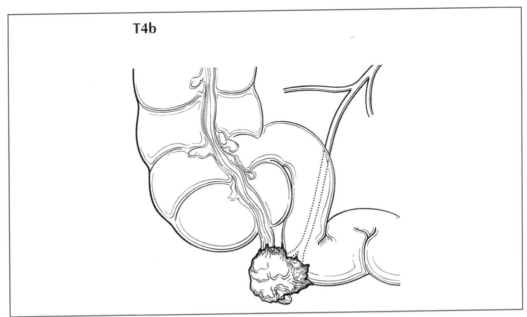

FIGURE 13.7. *For carcinoma T4b is defined as tumor that directly invades other organs or structures.*

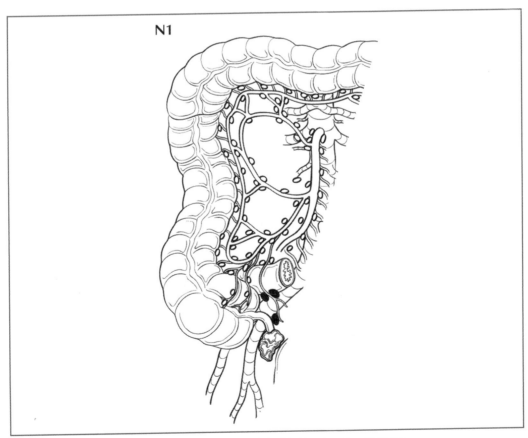

FIGURE 13.8. *For carcinoma N1 is defined as metastasis in 1 to 3 regional lymph nodes.*

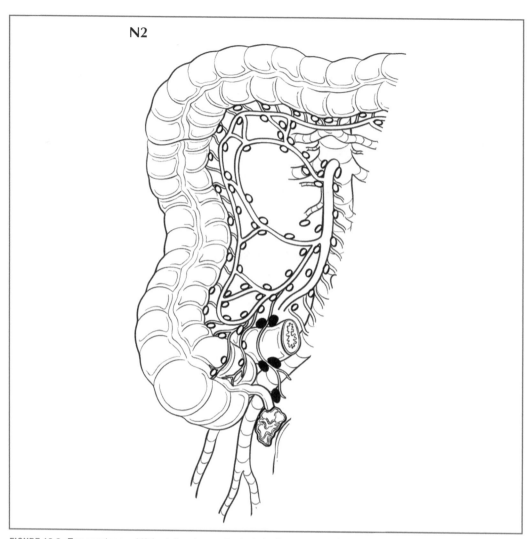

N2

FIGURE 13.9. *For carcinoma N2 is defined as metastasis in 4 or more regional lymph nodes.*

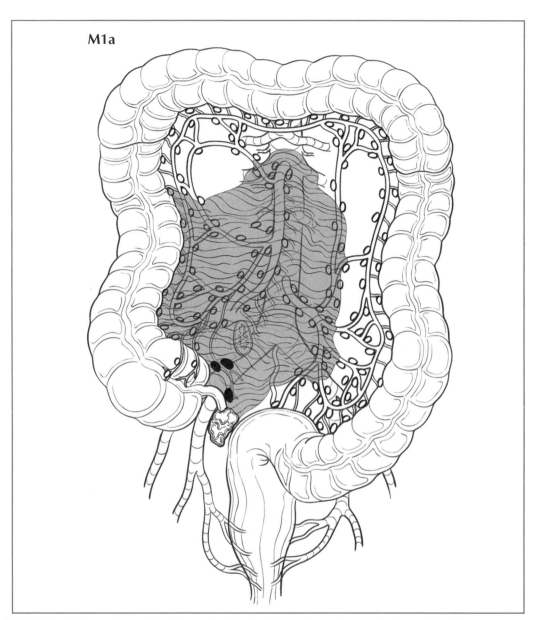

FIGURE 13.10. *For carcinoma M1a disease is defined as intraperitoneal metastasis beyond the right lower quadrant, including pseudomyxoma peritonei. The gray area depicts pseudomyxoma peritonei and is shown with coincident metastatic involvement of 3 regional lymph nodes (N1).*

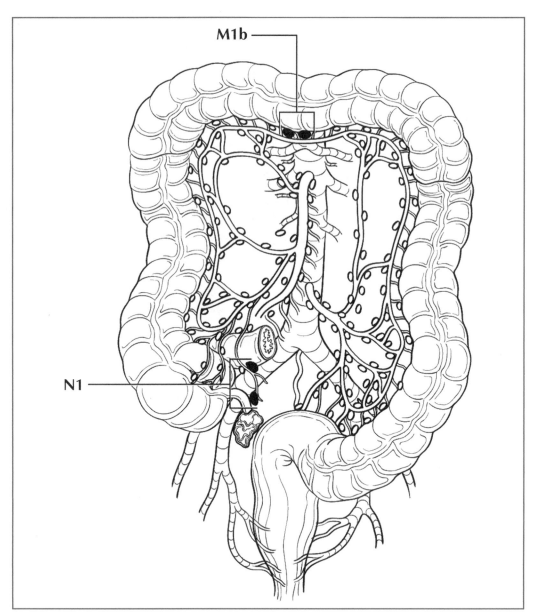

FIGURE 13.11. *For carcinoma M1b disease is defined as nonperitoneal metastasis.*

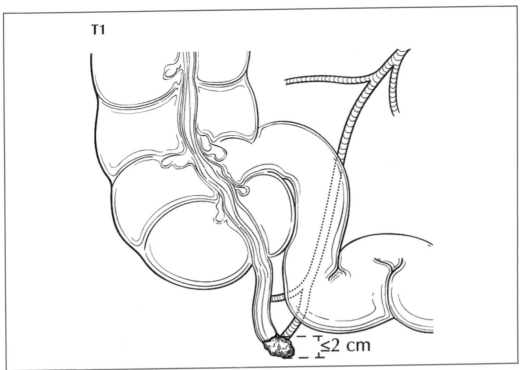

FIGURE 13.12. *For carcinoid T1 is defined as tumor that is 2 cm or less in greatest dimension. T1a is defined as tumor that is 1 cm or less in greatest dimension. T1b is defined as tumor that is more than 1 cm but not greater than 2 cm.*

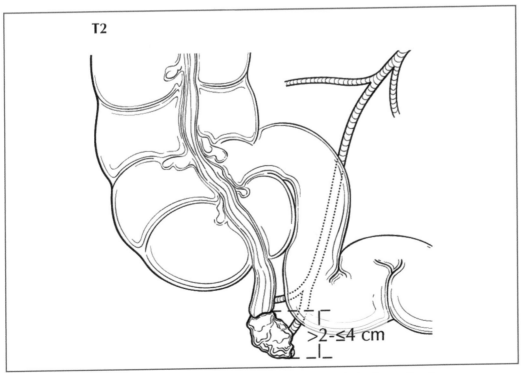

FIGURE 13.13. *For carcinoid T2 is defined as tumor that is more than 2 cm but not more than 4 cm.*

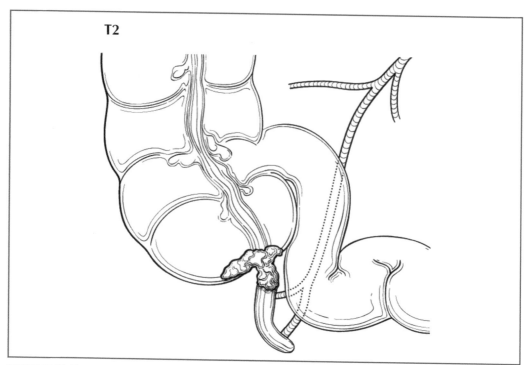

FIGURE 13.14. *For carcinoid T2 is defined as tumor with extension to the cecum.*

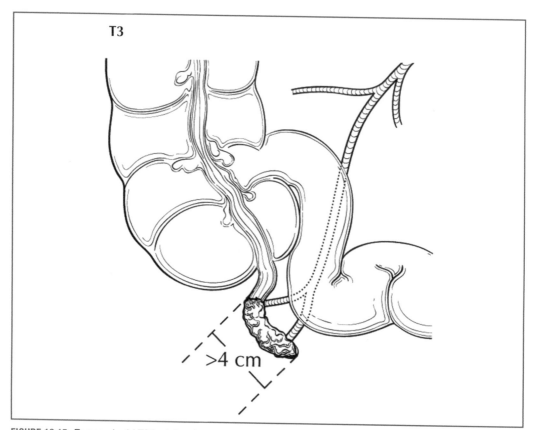

>4 cm

FIGURE 13.15. *For carcinoid T3 is defined as tumor that is more than 4 cm.*

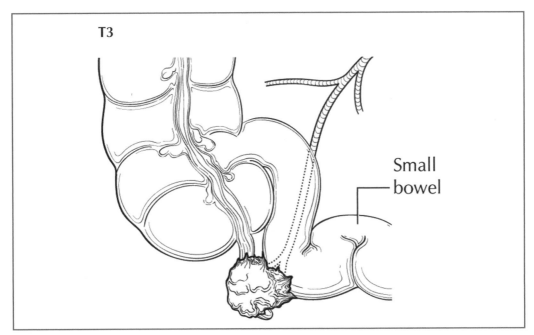

FIGURE 13.16. *For carcinoid T3 is defined as tumor with extension to the ileum.*

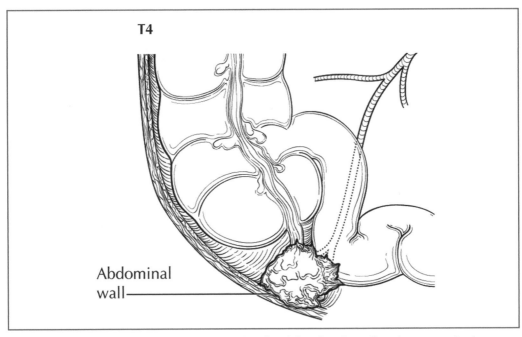

FIGURE 13.17. *For carcinoid T4 is defined as tumor that directly invades other adjacent organs or structures, e.g., abdominal wall and skeletal muscle.*

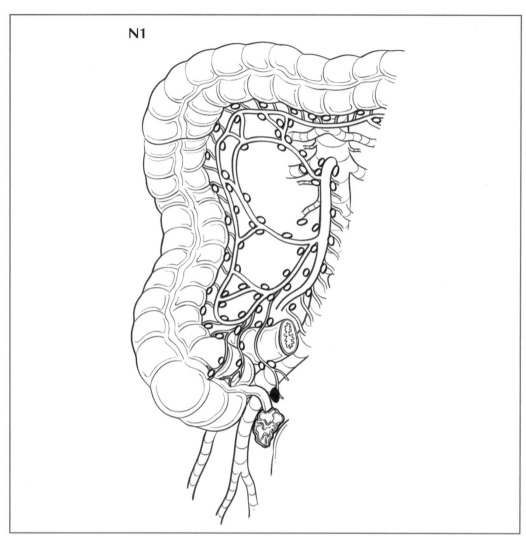

FIGURE 13.18. *For carcinoid N1 is defined as regional lymph node metastasis.*

PROGNOSTIC FACTORS (SITE-SPECIFIC FACTORS)
(Recommended for Collection for Carcinoma)

Required for staging	Grade
Clinically significant	Preoperative/pretreatment carcinoembryonic antigen (CEA)
	Preoperative/pretreatment CA 19-9
	Tumor deposits (TD)
	Microsatellite instability (MSI)
	18q Loss of Heterozygosity (LOH)

PROGNOSTIC FACTORS (SITE-SPECIFIC FACTORS)
(Recommended for Collection for Carcinoid)

Required for staging	None
Clinically significant	Serum chromogranin A

Colon and Rectum

(Sarcomas, lymphomas, and carcinoid tumors of the large intestine are not included)

14

SUMMARY OF CHANGES

- In the sixth edition, Stage II was subdivided into IIA and IIB on the basis of whether the primary tumor was T3N0 or T4N0, respectively, and Stage III was subdivided into IIIA (T1-2N1M0), IIIB (T3-4N1M0), or IIIC (any TN2M0). In the seventh edition, further substaging of Stage II and III has been accomplished, based on survival and relapse data that was not available for the prior edition
- Expanded data sets have shown differential prognosis within T4 lesions based on extent of disease. Accordingly T4 lesions are subdivided as T4a (Tumor penetrates the surface of the visceral peritoneum) and as T4b. (Tumor directly invades or is histologically adherent to other organs or structures)
- The potential importance of satellite tumor deposits is now defined by the new site-specific factor Tumor Deposits (TD) that describes their texture and number. T1-2 lesions that lack regional lymph node metastasis but have tumor deposit(s) will be classified in addition as N1c
- The number of nodes involved with metastasis influences prognosis within both N1 and N2 groups. Accordingly N1 will be subdivided as N1a (metastasis in 1 regional node) and N1b (metastasis in 2–3 nodes), and N2 will be subdivided as N2a (metastasis in 4–6 nodes) and N2b (metastasis in 7 or more nodes)
- Stage Group II is subdivided into IIA (T3N0), IIB (T4aN0) and IIC (T4bN0)
- Stage Group III:

  - A category of N1 lesions, T4bN1, that was formerly classified as IIIB was found to have outcomes more akin to IIIC and has been reclassified from IIIB to IIIC
  - Similarly, several categories of N2 lesions formerly classified as IIIC have outcomes more akin to other stage groups; therefore, T1N2a has been reclassified as IIIA and T1N2b, T2N2a-b, and T3N2a have all been reclassified as IIIB

- M1 has been subdivided into M1a for single metastatic site vs. M1b for multiple metastatic sites

---

ICD-O-3 TOPOGRAPHY CODES

C18.0	Cecum
C18.2	Ascending colon
C18.3	Hepatic flexure of colon
C18.4	Transverse colon
C18.5	Splenic flexure of colon
C18.6	Descending colon
C18.7	Sigmoid colon
C18.8	Overlapping lesion of colon
C18.9	Colon, NOS
C19.9	Rectosigmoid junction
C20.9	Rectum, NOS

C.C. Compton et al. (eds.), *AJCC Cancer Staging Atlas: A Companion to the Seventh Editions of the AJCC Cancer Staging Manual and Handbook*, DOI 10.1007/978-1-4614-2080-4_14, © 2012 American Joint Committee on Cancer

ICD-O-3 HISTOLOGY CODE RANGES

8000–8152, 8154–8231, 8243–8245, 8247–8248, 8250–8576, 8940–8950, 8980–8981

ANATOMY

The divisions of the colon and rectum are as follows (Figures 14.1 and 14.2, respectively):

Cecum
Ascending colon
Hepatic flexure
Transverse colon
Splenic flexure
Descending colon
Sigmoid colon
Rectosigmoid junction
Rectum

Primary Site. The large intestine (colorectum) extends from the terminal ileum to the anal canal. Excluding the rectum and vermiform appendix, the colon is divided into four parts: the right or ascending colon, the middle or transverse colon, the left or descending colon, and the sigmoid colon. The sigmoid colon is continuous with the rectum which terminates at the anal canal.

The cecum is a large, blind pouch that arises from the proximal segment of the right colon. It measures 6–9 cm in length and is covered with a visceral peritoneum (serosa). The ascending colon measures 15–20 cm in length. The posterior surface of the ascending (and descending) colon lacks peritoneum and thus is in direct contact with the retroperitoneum. In contrast, the anterior and lateral surfaces of the ascending (and descending) colon have serosa and are intraperitoneal. The hepatic flexure connects the ascending colon with the transverse colon, passing just inferior to the liver and anterior to the duodenum.

The transverse colon is entirely intraperitoneal, supported on a mesentery that is attached to the pancreas. Anteriorly, its serosa is continuous with the gastrocolic ligament. The splenic flexure connects the transverse colon to the descending colon, passing inferior to the spleen and anterior to the tail of the pancreas. As noted above, the posterior aspect of the descending colon lacks serosa and is in direct contact with the retroperitoneum, whereas the lateral and anterior surfaces have serosa and are intraperitoneal. The descending colon measures 10–15 cm in length. The colon becomes completely intraperitoneal once again at the sigmoid colon, where the mesentery develops at the medial border of the left posterior major psoas muscle and extends to the rectum. The transition from sigmoid colon to rectum is marked by the fusion of the taenia of the sigmoid colon to the circumferential longitudinal muscle of the rectum. This occurs roughly 12–15 cm from the dentate line.

Approximately 12 cm in length, the rectum extends from the fusion of the taenia to the puborectalis ring. The rectum is covered by peritoneum in front and on both sides in its upper third and only on the anterior wall in its middle third. The peritoneum is reflected laterally from the rectum to form the perirectal fossa and, anteriorly, the uterine or rectovesical fold. There is no peritoneal covering in the lower third, which is often known as the rectal ampulla.

The anal canal, which measures 3–5 cm in length, extends from the superior border of the puborectalis sling to the anal verge. The superior border of the puborectalis sling is the proximal portion of the palpable anorectal ring on digital rectal examination and is approximately 1–2 cm proximal to the dentate line.

Regional Lymph Nodes. Regional nodes are located (1) along the course of the major vessels supplying the colon and rectum, (2) along the vascular arcades of the marginal artery, and (3) adjacent to the colon – that is, located along the mesocolic border of the colon. Specifically, the regional lymph nodes are the pericolic and perirectal nodes and those found along the ileocolic, right colic, middle colic, left colic, inferior mesenteric artery, superior rectal (hemorrhoidal), and internal iliac arteries (Figure 14.3).

In the assessment of pN, the number of lymph nodes sampled should be recorded. The number of nodes examined from an operative specimen has been reported to be associated with improved survival, possibly because of increased accuracy in staging. It is important to obtain at least 10–14 lymph nodes in radical colon and rectum resections in patients without neoadjuvant therapy, but in cases in which tumor is resected for palliation or in patients who have received preoperative radiation, fewer lymph nodes may be removed or present. In all cases, however, it is essential that the total number of regional lymph nodes recovered from the resection specimen be described since that number is prognostically important. A pN0 determination is assigned when these nodes are histologically negative, even though fewer than the recommended number of nodes has been analyzed. However, when fewer than the number of nodes recommended by the College of American Pathologists (CAP) have been found, it is important that the pathologist report the degree of diligence of their efforts to find lymph nodes in the specimen.

The regional lymph nodes for each segment of the large bowel are designated as follows:

Segment	Regional Lymph Nodes
Cecum	Pericolic, anterior cecal, posterior cecal, ileocolic, right colic
Ascending colon	Pericolic, ileocolic, right colic, middle colic
Hepatic flexure	Pericolic, middle colic, right colic
Transverse colon	Pericolic, middle colic
Splenic flexure	Pericolic, middle colic, left colic, inferior mesenteric
Descending colon	Pericolic, left colic, inferior mesenteric, sigmoid
Sigmoid colon	Pericolic, inferior mesenteric, superior rectal (hemorrhoidal), sigmoidal, sigmoid mesenteric
Rectosigmoid	Pericolic, perirectal, left colic, sigmoid mesenteric, sigmoidal, inferior mesenteric, superior rectal (hemorrhoidal), middle rectal (hemorrhoidal)
Rectum	Perirectal, sigmoid mesenteric, inferior mesenteric, lateral sacral, presacral, internal iliac, sacral promontory, superior rectal (hemorrhoidal), middle rectal (hemorrhoidal), inferior rectal (hemorrhoidal)

Metastatic Sites. Although carcinomas of the colon and rectum can metastasize to almost any organ, the liver and lungs are most commonly affected. Seeding of other segments of the colon, small intestine, or peritoneum also can occur.

Tumor Deposits. Discrete foci of tumor found in the pericolic or perirectal fat or in adjacent mesentery (mesocolic fat) away from the leading edge of the tumor and showing no evidence of residual lymph node tissue but within the lymph drainage area of the primary carcinoma are considered to be peritumoral deposits or satellite nodules, and their number should be recorded in the site-specific Prognostic Markers on the staging form as Tumor Deposits (TD) (Figure 14.4). Such tumor deposits may represent discontinuous spread, venous invasion with extravascular spread (V1/2), or a totally replaced lymph node (N1/2). If tumor deposits are observed in lesions that would otherwise be classified as T1 or T2, then the primary tumor classification is not changed, but the nodule is recorded in the TD category and as a N1c positive node.

PROGNOSTIC FEATURES

Seven new prognostic factors that are clinically significant are included for collection, in addition to the prior notation of serum CEA levels. The new site-specific factors include: tumor deposits (TD, the number of satellite tumor deposits discontinuous from the leading edge of the carcinoma and that lack evidence of residual lymph node); a tumor regression grade that enables the pathologic response to neoadjuvant therapy to be graded, the circumferential resection margin (CRM, measured in mm from the edge of tumor to the nearest dissected margin of the surgical resection); microsatellite instability (MSI), an important but controversial prognostic factor especially for colon cancer; and perineural invasion (PN, histologic evidence of invasion of regional nerves) that may have a similar prognosis as lymphovascular invasion. KRAS mutation status will also be collected since recent analyses indicate that mutation in KRAS is associated with lack of response to treatment with monoclonal antibodies directed against the epidermal growth factor receptor (EGFR) in patients with metastatic colorectal carcinoma. The 18q LOH assay has been validated, and there is work to qualify this as a prognostic marker that would suggest the need for adjuvant therapy in stage II colon cancer.

Tumor Regression Grade. The pathologic response to preoperative adjuvant treatment should be recorded according to the CAP guidelines for recording the tumor regression grade (see CAP Protocol for the examination of Specimens from Patients with Carcinomas of the Colon and Rectum) because neoadjuvant chemoradiation in rectal cancer is often associated with significant tumor response and down-staging. Although the data are not definitive, complete eradication of the tumor, as detected by pathologic examination of the resected specimen, may be associated with a better prognosis and, conversely, failure of the tumor to respond to neoadjuvant treatment appears to be an adverse prognostic factor. Therefore, specimens from patients receiving neoadjuvant chemoradiation should be thoroughly examined at the primary tumor site, in regional nodes and for peritumoral satellite nodules or deposits in the remainder of the specimen. The degree of tumor response may correlate with prognosis. Those patients with minimal or no residual disease after therapy may have a better prognosis than gross residual disease. Whereas a number of different grading systems for tumor regression have been advocated, a four-point tumor regression grade will be used to assess response that is similar to that of Ryan et al. except that the complete absence of viable tumor will be recorded as a Grade 0.

Circumferential Resection Margins. It is essential that accurate pathologic evaluation of the CRM adjacent to the deepest point of tumor invasion be performed. The CRM is the surgically dissected nonperitonealized surface of the specimen. It corresponds to any aspect of the colorectum that is not covered by a serosal layer of mesothelial cells and must be dissected from the retroperitoneum or subperitoneum in order to remove the viscus. In contradistinction, serosalized surfaces of the colorectum are not dissected; they are naturally occurring anatomic structures and are not pathologic surgical margins. The circumferential surface of surgical resection specimens of ascending colon, descending colon, or upper rectum is only partially peritonealized, and the demarcation between the peritonealized surface and the nonperitonealized surface (corresponding to the CRM) of such specimens is not always easily appreciated on pathologic examination. Therefore, the surgeon is encouraged to mark the peritoneal reflection and/or the area of deepest tumor penetration adjacent to a nonperitonealized surface with a clip or suture so that the pathologist may accurately identify and evaluate the CRM.

For mid and distal rectal cancers (subperitoneal location), the entire surface of the resection specimen corresponds to a CRM (anterior, posterior, medial, lateral). For proximal rectal or retroperitoneal colon cancers (ascending, descending, possibly cecum), surgically dissected margins will include those that lie in a retroperitoneal or subperitoneal location as described above (Figure 14.5). For segments of the colon that are entirely covered by a visceral peritoneum (transverse, sigmoid, possibly cecum), the only specimen margin that is surgically dissected is the mesenteric margin, unless the cancer is adherent to or invading an adjacent organ or structure. Therefore, for cancers of the cecum, transverse or sigmoid colon that extends to the cut edge of the mesentery, assignment of a positive CRM is appropriate.

For rectal cancer, the quality of the surgical technique is likely a key factor in the success of surgical outcomes relative to local recurrence and possibly long-term survival. Numerous nonrandomized studies have demonstrated that total mesorectal excision (TME) with adequate surgical clearance around the penetrating edge of the tumor decreases the rate of local relapse. The TME technique entails precise sharp dissection within the areolar plane of loose connective tissue outside (lateral to) the visceral mesorectal fascia in order to remove the rectum. With this approach, all mesorectal soft tissues encasing the rectum, which includes the mesentery and all regional nodes, are removed intact. Thus, the circumferential surface (CRM) of TME resection specimens is the mesorectal or Waldeyer's fascia. Rectal resection performed by less precise techniques may be associated with incomplete excision of the mesorectum. It is critical that the analysis of the surgical specimen follows the CAP guidelines that refer to examination of the TME specimen. In addition, it is essential that the distance between the closest leading edge of the tumor and the CRM (known as the surgical clearance) be measured pathologically and recorded in mm in the CRM field on the staging form. A margin of greater than 1 mm is required with TME to be considered a negative margin because surgical clearance of 1 mm or less is associated with a significantly increased risk of local recurrence and should be classified as positive (Figure 14.5).

Residual Tumor (R). The completeness of resection is largely dependent on the status of the CRM, although the designation is global and would include the transverse margins and other disease observed but not removed at surgery. The resection (R) codes should be given for each procedure:

- R0—Complete tumor resection with all margins histologically negative
- R1—Incomplete tumor resection with microscopic surgical resection margin involvement (margins grossly uninvolved)
- R2—Incomplete tumor resection with gross residual tumor that was not resected (primary tumor, regional nodes, macroscopic margin involvement)

Isolated Tumor Cells and Molecular Node Involvement. As technology progresses and sentinel node biopsy or other procedures may become feasible in colon and rectal surgery, the issue of interpretation of very small amounts of detected tumor in regional lymph nodes will continue to be classified as pN0, and the universal terminology for these isolated tumor cells (ITC) will follow the terminology referenced in Chap. 1. The prognostic significance of ITCs, defined as single malignant cells or a few tumor cells in microclusters, identified in regional lymph nodes that otherwise would be considered to be negative is still unclear. Therefore, ITC identified the collection of data on ITC that may be generated by pathologists who use special immunohistochemical stains or molecular analysis procedures to identify ITC in nodes that might otherwise be considered negative for metastasis by standard hematoxylin and eosin (H&E). It should be noted that isolated tumor cells identified on H&E stains alone are also classified as ITC and are annotated in the same fashion as ITC seen on immunohistochemical stains (i.e., pN0(i+); "i" = "isolated tumor cells").

KRAS. Analysis of multiple recent clinical trials has shown that the presence of a mutation in either codon 12 or 13 of KRAS (abnormal or "mutated" KRAS) is strongly associated with a lack of response to treatment with anti-EGFR antibodies in patients with metastatic colorectal carcinoma. It is recommended that patients with advanced colorectal carcinoma be tested for the presence of mutations in KRAS if treatment will include an anti-EGFR antibody. Where the status of KRAS is known, it should be recorded as a site-specific factor as either Normal (Wild Type) or Abnormal (Mutated).

Anatomic Boundary. The boundary between the rectum and anal canal most often has been equated with the dentate line, which is identified pathologically. However, with advances in sphincter-preservation surgery, defining the boundary between the rectum and the anus as the anorectal ring, which corresponds to the proximal border of the puborectalis muscle palpable on digital rectal examination, is more appropriate.

TNM Stage of Disease. Since publication of the sixth edition, new prognostic data with regard to survival and disease relapse justifies further substaging of both Stages II and III by anatomic criteria. Differential prognosis has been shown for patients with T4 lesions based on the extent of disease in SEER analyses for both rectal cancer and colon cancer. Accordingly, for the seventh edition of AJCC, T4 lesions have been subdivided as T4a (tumor penetrates to the surface of the visceral peritoneum) and T4b (tumor directly invades or is adherent to other organs or structures). In addition, the number of nodes involved by metastasis has been shown to influence prognosis within both N1 and N2 groups, in separate analyses of SEER. For the SEER analyses, both relative and observed survival are listed by TN category of disease (relative survival is survival corrected by age-related comorbidity; see Chap. 2 for more information). Also the total number of nodes examined has an important impact on survival in colon and rectal cancer. The impact of increased nodes examined in the resected specimen is clearly associated with better outcome in colon cancer for all combinations of T and N whereas the association holds in T1–T3 lesions in rectal cancer but appears to be less important in T4a and T4b lesions, perhaps because of the greater use of preoperative radiation or concurrent chemoradiation of the smaller number of patients in the rectal carcinoma subgroups.

Stage Group II has been further subdivided into IIA (T3N0), IIB (T4aN0), and IIC (T4bN0), based on differential survival prognosis. These differences are shown in the SEER analyses for both rectal cancer and colon cancer.

Within Stage III, a number of changes have been made based on differential prognosis found in the rectal cancer pooled analyses, the SEER rectal and colon cancer analyses, and the NCDB colon cancer analysis. A category of N1 tumors has prognosis more akin to IIIC (T4bN1) and has been shifted from Stage IIIB to IIIC. In addition, several categories of N2 tumors have prognosis more akin to IIIA (the T1N2a group) or IIIB (the T1N2b, T2N2a-b, and T3N2a groups) and have been shifted out of Stage IIIC accordingly.

Independent Prognostic Factors and Molecular Markers. In addition to the TNM, independent prognostic factors that are generally used in patient management and are well supported in the literature include residual disease, histologic type, histologic grade, serum carcinoembryonic antigen and cytokine levels, extramural venous invasion, and submucosal vascular invasion by carcinomas arising in adenomas. Small cell carcinomas, signet ring cell carcinomas, and undifferentiated carcinomas have a less favorable outcome than other histologic types. In contrast, medullary carcinoma is more favorable prognostically. Submucosal vascular invasion by carcinomas arising in adenomas is associated with a greater risk of regional lymph node involvement. Lymphatic, venous, and perineural invasion also have been shown to have a less favorable outcome. A number of these independent prognostic factors are currently being evaluated in nomograms that also include TNM stage of disease.

In the future, the intratumoral expression of specific molecules, e.g., Deleted in Colorectal Cancer (DCC) or 18q loss of heterozygosity (LOH), p27^{Kip1}, DNA microsatellite instability, KRAS mutation, or thymidylate synthase, may be proven to be associated either with prognosis or response to therapy that is independent of TNM stage group or histologic grade. Currently, these molecular markers are not part of the staging system, but it is recommended that they be recorded if available and especially if studied within the context of a clinical trial. Furthermore, it is now clear that there is interaction between the T and N designations that is likely to rely on the expression of specific molecules within the cancer. Thus, by the time of the next edition of TNM staging it may be possible to add molecular profiling information to the TNM information to enhance the precision of predicting prognosis or even response to therapy. Finally, it is important to consider that other factors such as age, gender, race/ethnicity are important factors that affect response to therapy and disease outcome. Although these factors are not included in the TNM Summary or Working Stages at this time, several groups are studying the interaction of these clinicopathological factors with TNM and other prognostic factors in various nomograms such as those at http://www.nomograms.org. In order to determine the optimal way to integrate these various clinical, pathologic, and molecular factors with TNM, collection of the appropriate information prior to the next edition must be carried out.

DEFINITIONS OF TNM

The same classification is used for both clinical and pathologic staging.

Primary Tumor (T)

TX	Primary tumor cannot be assessed
T0	No evidence of primary tumor
Tis	Carcinoma in situ: intraepithelial or invasion of lamina propria*
T1	Tumor invades submucosa (Figure 14.6)
T2	Tumor invades muscularis propria (Figure 14.7)
T3	Tumor invades through the muscularis propria into pericolorectal tissues (Figure 14.8)
T4a	Tumor penetrates to the surface of the visceral peritoneum** (Figure 14.9A, B)
T4b	Tumor directly invades or is adherent to other organs or structures**,*** (Figure 14.9C, D)

*Note: Tis includes cancer cells confined within the glandular basement membrane (intraepithelial) or mucosal lamina propria (intramucosal) with no extension through the muscularis mucosae into the submucosa.

**Note: Direct invasion in T4 includes invasion of other organs or other segments of the colorectum as a result of direct extension through the serosa, as confirmed on microscopic examination (for example, invasion of the sigmoid colon by a carcinoma of the cecum) or, for cancers in a retroperitoneal or subperitoneal location, direct invasion of other organs or structures by virtue of extension beyond the muscularis propria (i.e., respectively, a tumor on the posterior wall of the descending colon invading the left kidney or lateral abdominal wall; or a mid or distal rectal cancer with invasion of prostate, seminal vesicles, cervix, or vagina).

***Note: Tumor that is adherent to other organs or structures, grossly, is classified cT4b. However, if no tumor is present in the adhesion, microscopically, the classification should be pT1-4a depending on the anatomical depth of wall invasion. The V and L classifications should be used to identify the presence or absence of vascular or lymphatic invasion whereas the PN site-specific factor should be used for perineural invasion.

Regional Lymph Nodes (N)

NX	Regional lymph nodes cannot be assessed
N0	No regional lymph node metastasis
N1	Metastasis in 1–3 regional lymph nodes
N1a	Metastasis in one regional lymph node (Figure 14.10)

N1b	Metastasis in 2–3 regional lymph nodes (Figure 14.10)
N1c	Tumor deposit(s) in the subserosa, mesentery, or nonperitonealized pericolic or perirectal tissues without regional nodal metastasis
N2	Metastasis in four or more regional lymph nodes
N2a	Metastasis in 4–6 regional lymph nodes (Figure 14.11A)
N2b	Metastasis in seven or more regional lymph nodes (Figure 14.11A, B)

Note: A satellite peritumoral nodule in the pericolorectal adipose tissue of a primary carcinoma without histologic evidence of residual lymph node in the nodule may represent discontinuous spread, venous invasion with extravascular spread (V1/2), or a totally replaced lymph node (N1/2). Replaced nodes should be counted separately as positive nodes in the N category, whereas discontinuous spread or venous invasion should be classified and counted in the Site-Specific Factor category Tumor Deposits (TD).

Distant Metastasis (M)

M0	No distant metastasis
M1	Distant metastasis
M1a	Metastasis confined to one organ or site (e.g., liver, lung, ovary, nonregional node) (Figure 14.12)
M1b	Metastases in more than one organ/site or the peritoneum

ANATOMIC STAGE/PROGNOSTIC GROUPS

Stage	T	N	M	Dukes*	MAC*
0	Tis	N0	M0	–	–
I	T1	N0	M0	A	A
	T2	N0	M0	A	B1
IIA	T3	N0	M0	B	B2
IIB	T4a	N0	M0	B	B2
IIC	T4b	N0	M0	B	B3
IIIA	T1–T2	N1/N1c	M0	C	C1
	T1	N2a	M0	C	C1
IIIB	T3–T4a	N1/N1c	M0	C	C2
	T2–T3	N2a	M0	C	C1/C2
	T1–T2	N2b	M0	C	C1
IIIC	T4a	N2a	M0	C	C2
	T3–T4a	N2b	M0	C	C2
	T4b	N1–N2	M0	C	C3
IVA	Any T	Any N	M1a	–	–
IVB	Any T	Any N	M1b	–	–

Note: cTNM is the clinical classification, pTNM is the pathologic classification. The y prefix is used for those cancers that are classified after neoadjuvant pretreatment (e.g., ypTNM). Patients who have a complete pathologic response are ypT0N0cM0 that may be similar to Stage Group 0 or I. The r prefix is to be used for those cancers that have recurred after a disease-free interval (rTNM).
*Dukes B is a composite of better (T3 N0 M0) and worse (T4 N0 M0) prognostic groups, as is Dukes C (Any TN1 M0 and Any T N2 M0). MAC is the modified Astler-Coller classification.

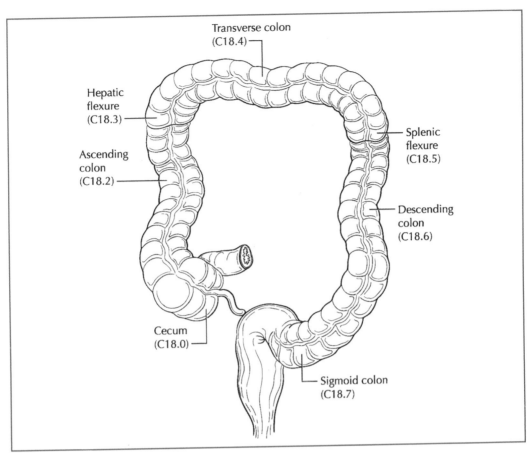

FIGURE 14.1. *Anatomic subsites of the colon.*

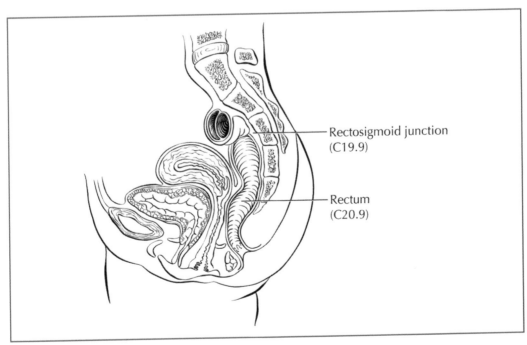

FIGURE 14.2. *Anatomic subsites of the rectum.*

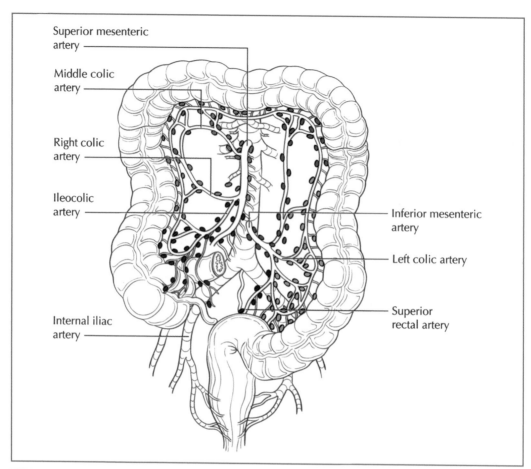

Superior mesenteric artery

Middle colic artery

Right colic artery

Ileocolic artery

Internal iliac artery

Inferior mesenteric artery

Left colic artery

Superior rectal artery

FIGURE 14.3. *The regional lymph nodes of the colon and rectum are colored by anatomic location, e.g., dark brown – right colon and cecum; blue – hepatic flexure to mid transverse colon; red – splenic flexure, left colon and sigmoid colon.*

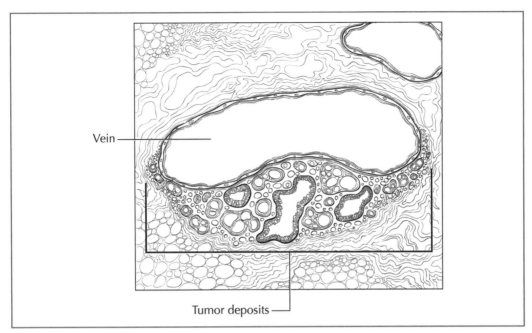

FIGURE 14.4. *Tumor deposit. Discrete foci of tumor found in the pericolic or perirectal fat or in adjacent mesentery (mesocolic fat) away from the leading edge of the tumor and showing no evidence of residual lymph node tissue but within the lymph drainage area of the primary carcinoma are considered to be peritumoral deposits or satellite nodules, and their number should be recorded in the site-specific Prognostic Markers on the staging form as Tumor Deposits (TD).*

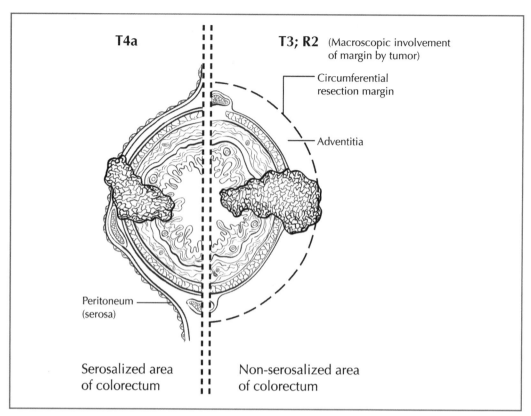

FIGURE 14.5. *Circumferential resection margin. T4a (left side) has perforated the visceral peritoneum. In contrast, T3; R2 (right side) shows macroscopic involvement of the circumferential resection margin of a non-peritonealized surface of the colorectum by tumor with gross disease remaining after surgical excision.*

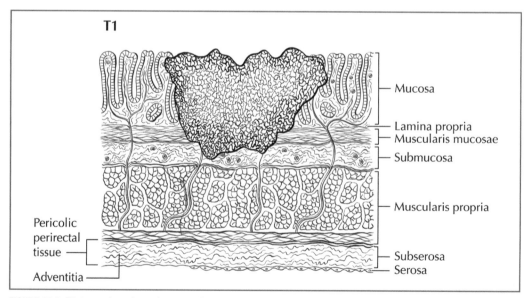

FIGURE 14.6. *T1 tumor invades submucosal.*

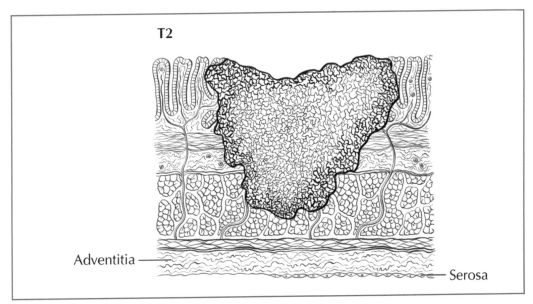

T2

Adventitia

Serosa

FIGURE 14.7. *T2 tumor invades muscularis propria.*

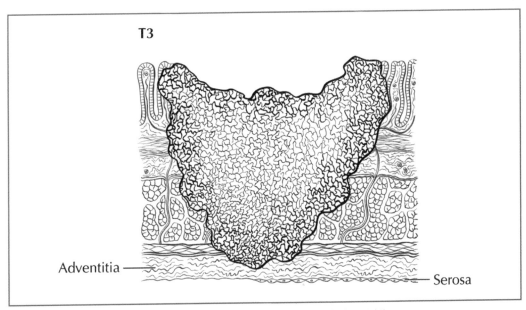

T3

Adventitia

Serosa

FIGURE 14.8. *T3 tumor invades through the muscularis propria into pericolorectal tissues.*

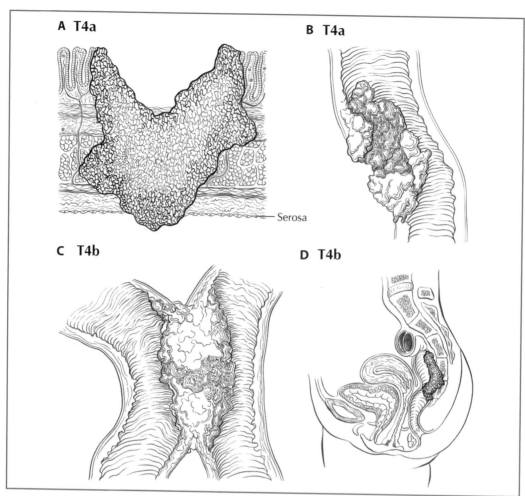

FIGURE 14.9. *(A) T4a tumor penetrates to the surface of the visceral peritoneum. The tumor perforates (penetrates) visceral peritoneum, as illustrated here. (B) T4a tumor perforates visceral peritoneum (shown with gross bowel perforation through the tumor). (C) T4b tumor directly invades or is adherent to other organs or structures, as illustrated here with extension into an adjacent loop of small bowel. (D) T4b tumor directly invades or is adherent to other organs or structures (such as the sacrum shown here).*

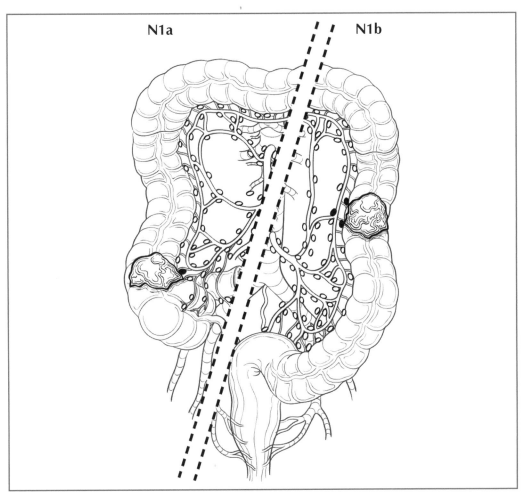

FIGURE 14.10. *N1a is defined as metastasis in one regional lymph node. N1b is defined as metastasis in 2 to 3 regional lymph nodes.*

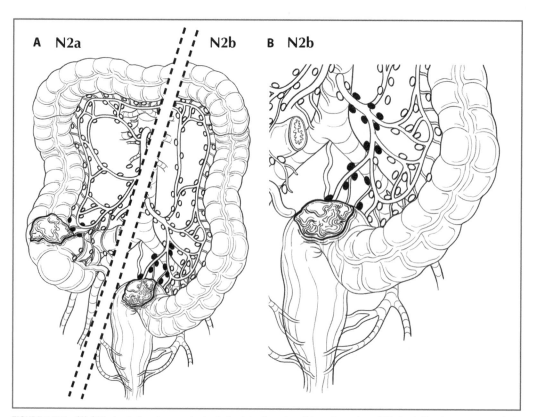

FIGURE 14.11. *(A) N2a is defined as metastasis in 4 to 6 regional lymph nodes. N2b is defined as metastasis in seven or more regional lymph nodes. (B) N2b showing nodal masses in more than 7 regional lymph nodes.*

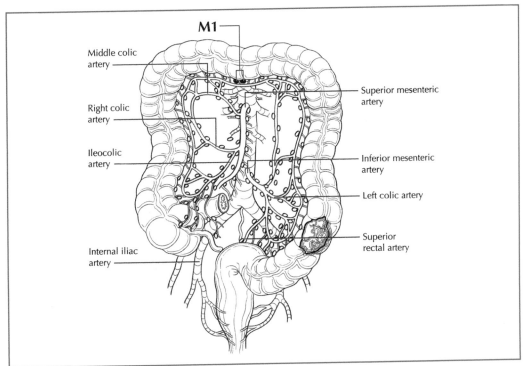

FIGURE 14.12. *M1a disease is defined as distant metastasis confined to one organ or site (e.g., liver, lung, ovary, nonregional node). In this case, involvement is outside the regional nodes of the primary tumor.*

PROGNOSTIC FACTORS (SITE-SPECIFIC FACTORS)
(Recommended for Collection)

Required for staging	None
Clinically significant	Preoperative or pretreatment carcinoembryonic antigen (CEA) (ng/ml)
	Tumor deposits (TD)
	Circumferential resection margin (CRM)
	Perineural invasion (PN)
	Microsatellite instability (MSI)
	Tumor regression grade (with neoadjuvant therapy)
	KRAS gene analysis

Anus

(The classification applies to carcinomas only; melanomas, carcinoid tumors, and sarcomas are not included.)

15

SUMMARY OF CHANGES

- The definitions of TNM and the stage groupings for this chapter have not changed from the sixth edition
- The descriptions of both the boundaries of the anal canal and anal carcinomas have been clarified
- The collection of the reported status of the tumor for the presence of human papilloma virus is included

---

ICD-O-3 TOPOGRAPHY CODES

C21.0   Anus, NOS
C21.1   Anal canal
C21.2   Cloacogenic zone
C21.8   Overlapping lesion of rectum, anus, and anal canal

ICD-O-3 HISTOLOGY CODE RANGES

8000–8152, 8154–8231, 8243–8245, 8250–8576, 8940–8950, 8980–8981

ANATOMY

Primary Site. The anatomic subsites of the anal canal are illustrated in Figure 15.1. The anal canal begins where the rectum enters the puborectalis sling at the apex of the anal sphincter complex (palpable as the anorectal ring on digital rectal examination and approximately 1–2 cm proximal to the dentate line) and ends with the squamous mucosa blending with the perianal skin, which roughly coincides with the palpable intersphincteric groove or the outermost boundary of the internal sphincter muscle. The most proximal aspect of the anal canal is lined by colorectal mucosa in which squamous metaplasia may occur. When involved by metaplasia, this zone also may be referred to as the transformation zone. Immediately proximal to the macroscopically visible dentate line, a narrow zone of transitional mucosa that is similar to urothelium is variably present. The proximal zone of the anal canal that extends from the top of the puborectalis to the dentate line measures approximately 1–2 cm. In the region of the dentate line, anal glands are subjacent to the mucosa, often penetrating through the internal sphincter into the intersphincteric plane. The distal zone of the anal canal extends from the dentate line to the mucocutaneous junction with the perianal skin and is lined by a nonkeratinizing squamous epithelium devoid of epidermal appendages (hair follicles, apocrine glands, and sweat glands).

Determination of the anatomic site of origin of carcinomas that overlap the anorectal junction may be problematic. For staging purposes, such tumors should be classified as rectal cancers if their epicenter is located more than 2 cm proximal to the dentate line or proximal to the anorectal ring on

---

digital examination and as anal canal cancers if their epicenter is 2 cm or less from the dentate line. For rectal cancers that extend beyond the dentate line, as for anal canal cancers, the superficial inguinal lymph nodes are among the regional nodal groups at risk of metastatic spread and included in cN/pN analysis.

Regional Lymph Nodes. Lymphatic drainage and nodal involvement of anal cancers depend on the location of the primary tumor. Tumors above the dentate line spread primarily to the anorectal, perirectal, and internal iliac nodes, whereas tumors below the dentate line spread primarily to the superficial inguinal nodes.

The regional lymph nodes are as follows (Figure 15.2):

Perirectal
    Anorectal
    Perirectal
    Lateral sacral
Internal iliac (hypogastric)
Inguinal
    Superficial

All other nodal groups represent sites of distant metastasis.

Metastatic Sites. Cancers of the anus may metastasize to any organs, but the liver and lungs are the distal organs that are most frequently involved. Involvement of the abdominal cavity is not unusual.

PROGNOSTIC FEATURES

For carcinoma of the anal canal, the 5-year observed survival rates for each of the stage groups are as follows: Stage I, 69.5%; Stage II, 61.8%; Stage IIIA, 45.6%; Stage IIIB, 39.6%; Stage IV, 15.3%.

Notably, within each stage grouping, overall 5-year survival rates for anal canal carcinomas vary significantly according to histologic type. At each stage, survival rates for patients with squamous cell carcinomas are better than that for patients with nonsquamous tumors.

Historically recognized histologic variants of squamous cell carcinoma, such as large cell keratinizing, large cell nonkeratinizing and basaloid subtypes, have no associated prognostic differences. Therefore, the World Health Organization recommends that the generic term *squamous cell carcinoma* be used for all squamous tumors of the anal canal. Nonsquamous histologies of anal canal carcinomas include adenocarcinoma, mucinous adenocarcinoma, small cell carcinoma (high-grade neuroendocrine carcinoma), and undifferentiated carcinoma.

Human papilloma virus (HPV) may be an etiologic agent in anal carcinoma. When the data are reported, it is of value to record the HPV status in the cancer registry.

DEFINITIONS OF TNM

Primary Tumor (T)

TX	Primary tumor cannot be assessed
T0	No evidence of primary tumor
Tis	Carcinoma in situ (Bowen's disease, high-grade squamous intraepithelial lesion (HSIL), anal intraepithelial neoplasia II–III (AIN II–III)
T1	Tumor 2 cm or less in greatest dimension (Figure 15.3)
T2	Tumor more than 2 cm but not more than 5 cm in greatest dimension (Figure 15.4)
T3	Tumor more than 5 cm in greatest dimension (Figure 15.5)
T4	Tumor of any size invades adjacent organ(s), e.g., vagina, urethra, bladder* (Figure 15.6)

*Note: Direct invasion of the rectal wall, perirectal skin, subcutaneous tissue, or the sphincter muscle(s) is not classified as T4.

Regional Lymph Nodes (N)

NX	Regional lymph nodes cannot be assessed
N0	No regional lymph node metastasis
N1	Metastasis in perirectal lymph node(s) (Figure 15.7)
N2	Metastasis in unilateral internal iliac and/or inguinal lymph node(s) (Figure 15.8A, B)
N3	Metastasis in perirectal and inguinal lymph nodes and/or bilateral internal iliac and/or inguinal lymph nodes (Figure 15.9A–C)

Distant Metastasis (M)

M0	No distant metastasis
M1	Distant metastasis

ANATOMIC STAGE/PROGNOSTIC GROUPS

0	Tis	N0	M0
I	T1	N0	M0
II	T2	N0	M0
	T3	N0	M0
IIIA	T1	N1	M0
	T2	N1	M0
	T3	N1	M0
	T4	N0	M0
IIIB	T4	N1	M0
	Any T	N2	M0
	Any T	N3	M0
IV	Any T	Any N	M1

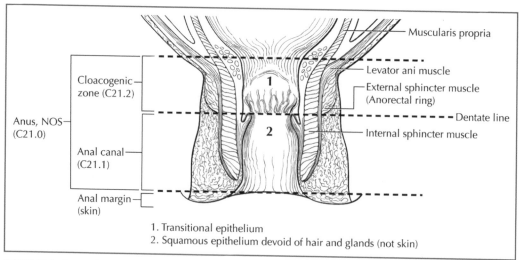

FIGURE 15.1. *Anatomic subsites of the anus. The epithelium in the peri-anal region and the vulvar zone is at risk for squamous carcinomas, along with HPV and other skin infections. While these are of a lower malignant potential, they can be troublesome. In women, there are diseases that give rise to peri-vulvar squamous carcinoma that can be a problem. In men, there may be condylomas in HIV positive disease, and perhaps some HPV positive disease that can morph into squamous cell carcinoma.*

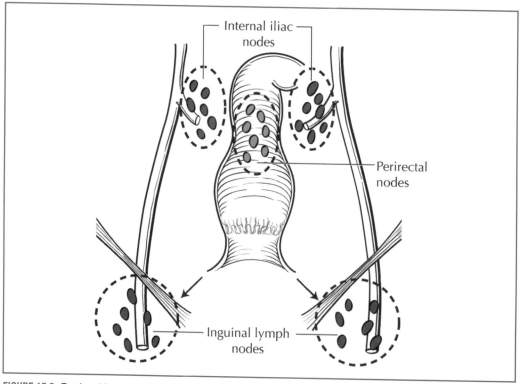

FIGURE 15.2. *Regional lymph nodes of the anus.*

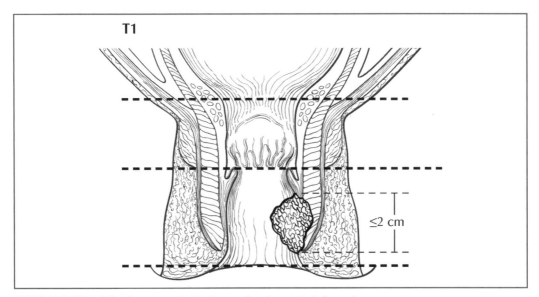

FIGURE 15.3. *T1 is defined as tumor that is 2 cm or less in greatest dimension.*

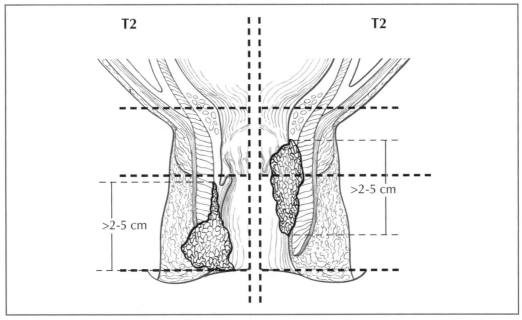

FIGURE 15.4. *Two views of T2 showing tumor that is more than 2 cm but not more than 5 cm in greatest dimension. On the right side of the diagram, the tumor extends above the dentate line.*

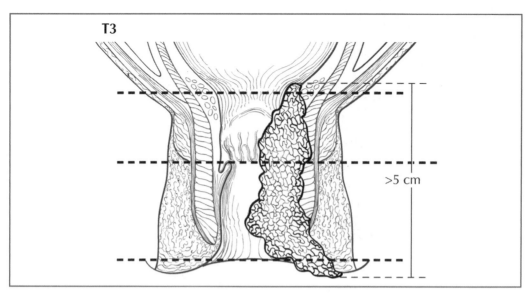

FIGURE 15.5. *T3 is defined as tumor that is more than 5 cm in greatest dimension.*

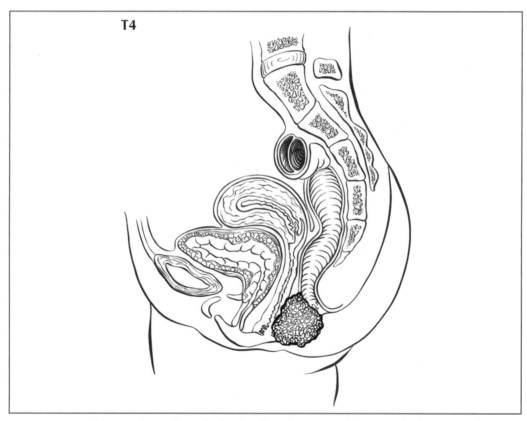

FIGURE 15.6. *T4 is defined as tumor of any size that invades adjacent organ(s), e.g., vagina (as illustrated), urethra, and bladder. Note: Direct invasion of the rectal wall, perirectal skin, subcutaneous tissue, or the sphincter muscle(s) is not classified as T4.*

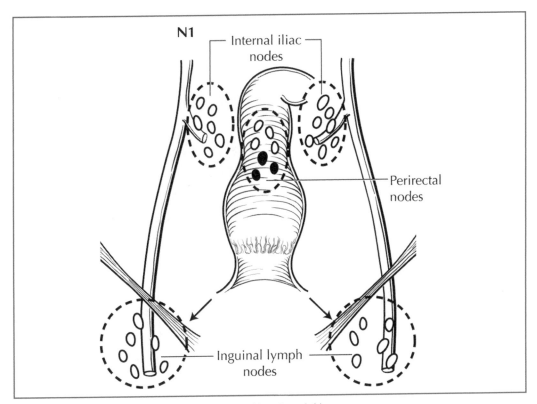

FIGURE 15.7. *N1 is defined as metastasis in perirectal lymph node(s).*

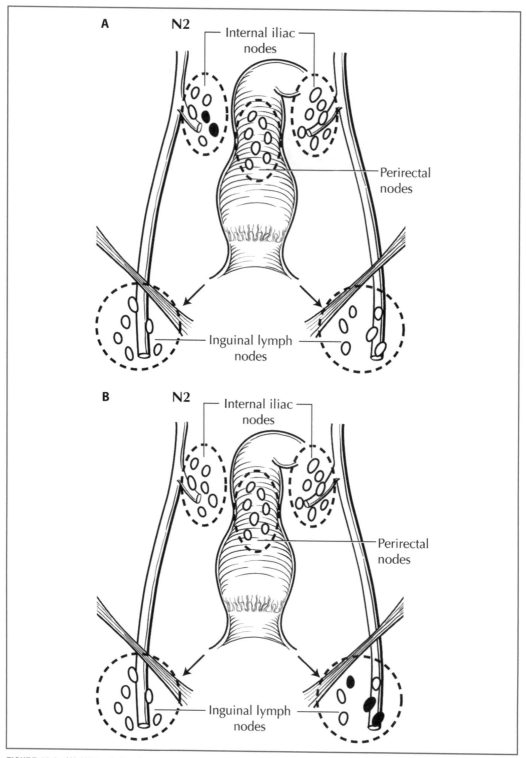

FIGURE 15.8. *(A) N2 is defined as metastasis in unilateral internal iliac. (B) N2 is defined as metastasis in inguinal lymph node(s).*

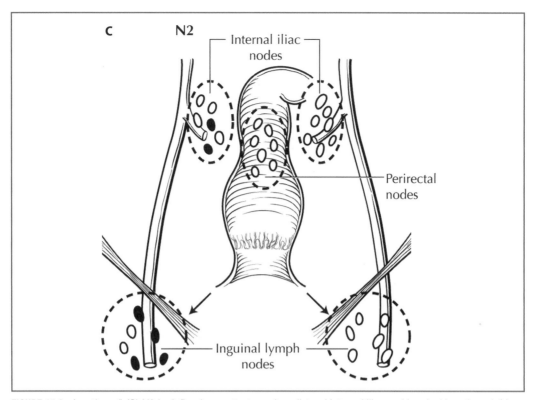

FIGURE 15.8. *(continued) (C) N2 is defined as metastases in unilateral internal iliac and inguinal lymph node(s).*

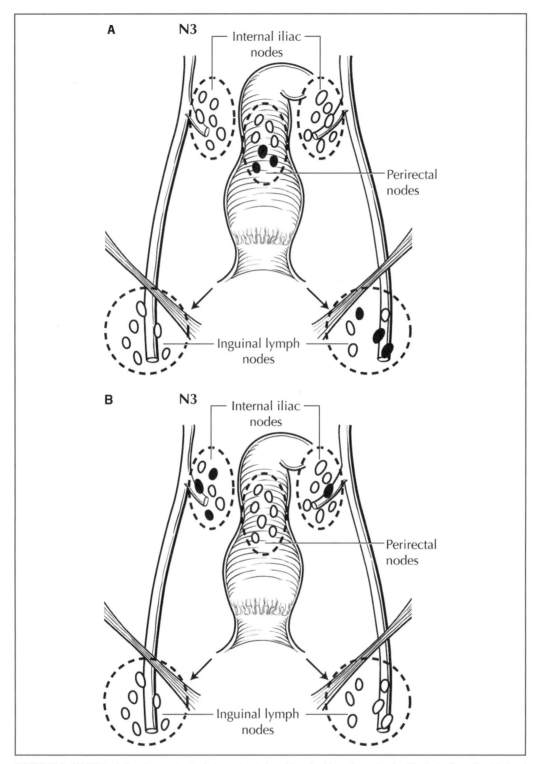

FIGURE 15.9. *(A) N3 is defined as metastasis in perirectal and inguinal lymph nodes (as illustrated) and/or bilateral internal iliac and/or inguinal lymph nodes. (B) N3 is defined as metastases in bilateral internal iliac lymph nodes.*

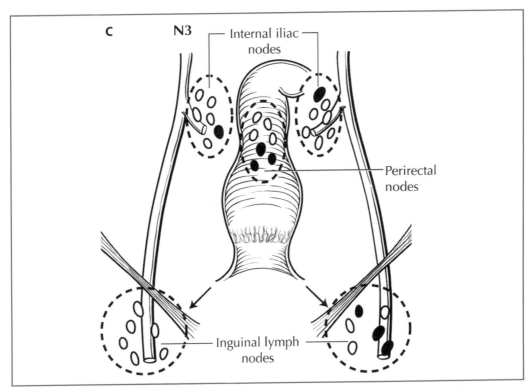

FIGURE 15.9. *(continued) (C) N3 is defined as metastases in bilateral internal iliac and inguinal lymph nodes.*

PROGNOSTIC FACTORS (SITE-SPECIFIC FACTORS)	
(Recommended for Collection)	
Required for staging	None
Clinically significant	HPV Status

Gastrointestinal Stromal Tumor

16

ICD-O-3 TOPOGRAPHY CODES

C15.0–C15.9	Esophagus
C16.0–C16.9	Stomach
C17.0–C17.2, C17.8–C17.9	Small intestine
C18.0–C18.9	Colon
C19.9	Recto-sigmoid junction
C20.9	Rectum
C48.0–C48.8	Retroperi-toneum and Peritoneum

ICD-O-3 HISTOLOGY CODE RANGES

8935, 8936

ANATOMY

Primary Site. GISTs occur throughout the gastrointestinal tract. They are most common in the stomach (60%) and small intestine (jejunum and ileum) (30%) and are relatively rare in the duodenum (5%), rectum (3%), colon (1–2%), and esophagus (<1%). In some cases, they present as disseminated tumors without a known primary site, and a small number of GISTs may be primary in the omentum or mesenteries.

Regional Lymph Nodes. Nodal metastasis is very rare and virtually unheard of in GIST, especially if one adheres to its rigorous histologic verification. Surgeons generally agree that nodal dissection is not indicated for GIST. In the absence of information on regional lymph node status, N0/pN0 is appropriate; NX should not be used.

Metastatic Sites. Metastases include intra-abdominal soft tissue, liver, and distant metastases. Presence of any of these is designated M1. Distant metastases are relatively rare in GISTs, but they are increasingly detected with sophisticated radiological studies. The most common distinct, nonabdominal metastatic sites are bone, soft tissues, and skin, whereas lung metastases are distinctly rare.

C.C. Compton et al. (eds.), *AJCC Cancer Staging Atlas: A Companion to the Seventh Editions of the AJCC Cancer Staging Manual and Handbook*, DOI 10.1007/978-1-4614-2080-4_16, © 2012 American Joint Committee on Cancer

PROGNOSTIC FEATURES

In some cases, patients have survived for a long time after a solitary intra-abdominal GIST metastasis. Tumors with mitotic rates in the lower end of "high mitotic rate" (6–10 mitoses/50 HPFs) may behave better than those with significantly elevated mitotic rates (>10 mitoses/50 HPFs).

There may be differences in behavior between GISTs with different types of KIT and PDGFRA mutations. Because of limitations of the universal application of mutation studies (most importantly, their limited availability), mutations are not considered in this staging system. Further research is needed to examine these and other prognostic factors in detail.

DEFINITIONS OF TNM (FOR GISTS AT ALL SITES)

Primary Tumor (T)

TX	Primary tumor cannot be assessed
T0	No evidence for primary tumor
T1	Tumor 2 cm or less (Figure 16.1)
T2	Tumor more than 2 cm but not more than 5 cm (Figure 16.1)
T3	Tumor more than 5 cm but not more than 10 cm (Figure 16.2)
T4	Tumor more than 10 cm in greatest dimension (Figure 16.2)

Regional Lymph Nodes (N)

N0	No regional lymph node metastasis[*]
N1	Regional lymph node metastasis

[*]If regional node status is unknown, use N0, not NX.
Note: Please refer to the corresponding carcinoma chapter for the relevant nodal groups.

Distant Metastasis (M)

M0	No distant metastasis
M1	Distant metastasis

HISTOPATHOLOGIC GRADE

Grading for GISTs is dependent on mitotic rate
Low mitotic rate: 5 or fewer per 50 HPF
High mitotic rate: over 5 per 50 HPF

ANATOMIC STAGE/PROGNOSTIC GROUPS

Gastric GIST*

Group	T	N	M	Mitotic rate
Stage IA	T1 or T2	N0	M0	Low
Stage IB	T3	N0	M0	Low
Stage II	T1	N0	M0	High
	T2	N0	M0	High
	T4	N0	M0	Low
Stage IIIA	T3	N0	M0	High
Stage IIIB	T4	N0	M0	High
Stage IV	Any T	N1	M0	Any rate
	Any T	Any N	M1	Any rate

Small Intestinal GIST**

Group	T	N	M	Mitotic rate
Stage I	T1 or T2	N0	M0	Low
Stage II	T3	N0	M0	Low
Stage IIIA	T1	N0	M0	High
	T4	N0	M0	Low
Stage IIIB	T2	N0	M0	High
	T3	N0	M0	High
	T4	N0	M0	High
Stage IV	Any T	N1	M0	Any rate
	Any T	Any N	M1	Any rate

*Note: Also to be used for omentum.

**Note: Also to be used for esophagus, colorectal, mesentery, and peritoneum.

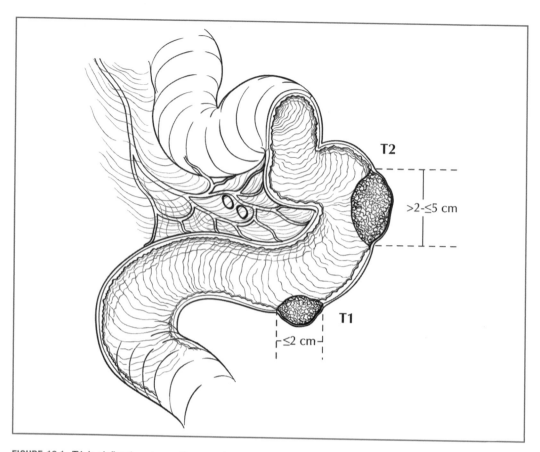

FIGURE 16.1. *T1 is defined as tumor 2 cm or less. T2 is defined as tumor more than 2 cm but not more than 5 cm.*

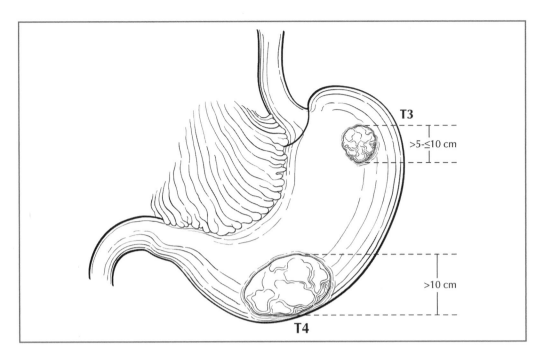

FIGURE 16.2. *T3 is defined as tumor more than 5 cm but not more than 10 cm. T4 is defined as tumor more than 10 cm in greatest dimension.*

<table>
<tr><td colspan="2">PROGNOSTIC FACTORS (SITE-SPECIFIC FACTORS)
(FOR GISTS AT ALL SITES)
(Recommended for Collection)</td></tr>
<tr><td>Required for staging</td><td>Mitotic rate</td></tr>
<tr><td>Clinically significant</td><td>KIT immunohistochemistry
Mutational status of KIT, PDGFRA</td></tr>
</table>

Neuroendocrine Tumors

(Gastric, small bowel, colonic, rectal, and ampulla of vater carcinoid tumors [well-differentiated neuroendocrine tumors and well-differentiated neuroendocrine carcinomas]; carcinoid tumors of the appendix [see Chap. 13] and neuroendocrine tumors of the pancreas [see Chap. 24] are not included.)

SUMMARY OF CHANGES

- This staging system is new for the 7th edition

ICD-O-3 TOPOGRAPHY CODES

C16.0–C16.9	Stomach
C17.0–C17.9	Small intestine
C18.0,	Colon
C18.2–C18.9	(excludes C18.1)
C19.9	Recto-sigmoid junction
C20.9	Rectum
C24.1	Ampulla of Vater

ICD-O-3 HISTOLOGY CODE RANGES

8153, 8240–8242, 8246, 8249

ANATOMY

Primary Site. Neuroendocrine tumors (NETs) can arise from neuroendocrine cells of the entire gastroenteropancreatic system (Figure 17.1), although the small intestine is the commonest overall location (20.7%). The terminal ileal area is the most common location and lesions may be multicentric. The progenitor cell of the majority of gastrointestinal NETs is the enterochromaffin (EC) cell. Gastric NETs arise from the enterochromaffin-like (ECL) cells of the fundic gastric glands. Among 12,259 GEP-NETs in the SEER database, 8.2% were gastric, 5.4% pancreatic, and 20.7% small intestinal (duodenal 19.1%, jejunal 9.2%, ileal 71.7%). The proportion of nonfunctional lesions in GEP-NETs ranges from 10 to 25% depending upon the rigorousness with which criteria of nonfunctionality are applied; some series indicate an incidence as high as 48%.

Regional Lymph Nodes. A rich lymphatic network surrounds the gastrointestinal organs, and NETs exhibit an almost equal affinity for spread via the lymphatic system as well as the bloodstream (Figures 17.2, 17.3A, 17.3B, and 17.4).

Stomach

- *Greater curvature of the stomach.* Greater curvature, greater omental, gastroduodenal, gastroepiploic, pyloric and pancreaticoduodenal nodes
- *Pancreatic and splenic areas.* Pancreaticolienal, peripancreatic, and splenic nodes

---

C.C. Compton et al. (eds.), *AJCC Cancer Staging Atlas: A Companion to the Seventh Editions of the AJCC Cancer Staging Manual and Handbook*, DOI 10.1007/978-1-4614-2080-4_17,
© 2012 American Joint Committee on Cancer

- *Lesser curvature of the stomach.* Lesser curvature, lesser omental, left gastric, cardioesophageal, common hepatic, celiac, and hepatoduodenal nodes
- *"Distant metastasis" nodal groups.* Retropancreatic, para-aortic, portal, retroperitoneal, and mesenteric

Small Intestine

- *Duodenum.* Duodenal, hepatic, pancreaticoduodenal, infrapyloric, gastroduodenal, pyloric, superior mesenteric, and pericholedochal nodes
- *Ileum and jejunum.* Posterior cecal (terminal ileum only), superior mesenteric, and mesenteric NOS nodes
- *"Distant metastasis" nodal groups.* Celiac nodes

Large Intestine

- *Cecum.* Pericolic, anterior cecal, posterior cecal, ileocolic, right colic
- *Ascending colon.* Pericolic, ileocolic, right colic, middle colic
- *Hepatic flexure.* Pericolic, middle colic, right colic
- *Transverse colon.* Pericolic, middle colic
- *Splenic flexure.* Pericolic, middle colic, left colic, inferior mesenteric
- *Descending colon.* Pericolic, left colic, inferior mesenteric, sigmoid
- *Sigmoid colon.* Pericolic, inferior mesenteric, superior rectal (hemorrhoidal), sigmoidal, sigmoid mesenteric
- *Rectosigmoid.* Pericolic, perirectal, left colic, sigmoid mesenteric, sigmoidal, inferior mesenteric, superior rectal (hemorrhoidal), middle rectal (hemorrhoidal)
- *Rectum.* Perirectal, sigmoid mesenteric, inferior mesenteric, lateral sacral presacral, internal iliac, sacral promontory (Gerota's), internal iliac, superior rectal (hemorrhoidal), middle rectal (hemorrhoidal), inferior rectal (hemorrhoidal)

Metastatic Sites. The most common metastatic distribution for GEP-NETs is lymph nodes (89.8%), the liver (44.1%), lung (13.6%), peritoneum (13.6%), and pancreas (6.8%). Local spread to adjacent organs is often characterized by associated extensive fibrosis.

PROGNOSTIC FEATURES

Important determinants of survival in NETs are neuroendocrine cell type, nodal status, and Ki67 index. Negative predictable variables are the presence of clinical symptoms, size of primary tumor, elevated CgA and hormonally active tumor by-products, and a high mitotic index.

Gastric NETs may be subdivided into ECL cell carcinoid type I–III. Type I tumors (approximately 80–90%) originate in a hypergastrinemic milieu (rarely metastasize approximately 1–3%, 5-year survival of approximately 100%). Type II lesions are rare (5–7%), occur in the context of MEN-1 and exhibit a more aggressive neoplastic phenotype (10–30% metastasis, 5-year survival of 60–90%). Type III lesions occur in a normogastrinemic environment and constitute approximately 10–15% of tumors, behave as adenocarcinomas, are usually metastatic (50%), and have a 5-year survival <50%). Little biological information exists regarding the mechanisms responsible for human ECL cell transformation.

The malignancy of gastric NETs types can be further defined by elevation of levels of CCN2, metastasis associated protein 1 – MTA1, and melanoma antigen D2 – MAGE-D2, whose gene and protein expression correlates with invasion and metastatic potential.

Duodenal NETs with a tumor size greater than 2 cm, involvement of the muscularis propria, and presence of mitotic figures have a poor prognosis. The presence of regional lymph node metastases, however, cannot be predicted reliably on the basis of tumor size or depth of invasion, although EUS is of use. In a study including 89 patients with duodenal NETs, the overall 5-year survival was 60%.

Jejunoileal NETs typically present at an advanced stage and have a poor 5-year survival rate (60.5%) compared with other GI NETs. Tumor size is the most predictive factor and spread to regional lymph nodes is common at diagnosis.

Well-differentiated NETs arising in the colon are relatively rare, occurring most commonly in the cecum, although some in this location may represent extension from appendiceal carcinoids. Tumor size is probably an important prognostic indicator, but is less useful for colonic NETs because most are greater than 2 cm and involve the muscularis propria at diagnosis. Overall survival is 33–42%.

Rectal NETs have a low propensity for metastasis and have a favorable prognosis, with overall 5-year survival of 88.3%. Features predictive of poor outcome are tumor size greater than 2 cm and invasion of the muscularis propria.

DEFINITIONS OF TNM

Stomach

Primary Tumor (T)

TX	Primary tumor cannot be assessed
T0	No evidence of primary tumor
Tis	Carcinoma in situ/dysplasia (tumor size less than 0.5 mm), confined to mucosa (Figure 17.5)
T1	Tumor invades lamina propria or submucosa and 1 cm or less in size (Figure 17.6)
T2	Tumor invades muscularis propria or more than 1 cm in size (Figure 17.7)
T3	Tumor penetrates subserosa (Figure 17.8)
T4	Tumor invades visceral peritoneum (serosal) or other organs or adjacent structures (Figure 17.9)
	For any T, add (m) for multiple tumors

Regional Lymph Nodes (N)

NX	Regional lymph nodes cannot be assessed
N0	No regional lymph node metastasis
N1	Regional lymph node metastasis (Figure 17.10)

Distant Metastases (M)

M0	No distant metastases
M1	Distant metastasis

Duodenum/Ampulla/Jejunum/Ileum

Primary Tumor (T)

TX	Primary tumor cannot be assessed
T0	No evidence of primary tumor
T1	Tumor invades lamina propria or submucosa and size 1 cm or less* (small intestinal tumors); tumor 1 cm or less (ampullary tumors) (Figure 17.11)
T2	Tumor invades muscularis propria or size > 1 cm (small intestinal tumors); tumor > 1 cm (ampullary tumors) (Figure 17.12)
T3	Tumor invades through the muscularis propria into subserosal tissue without penetration of overlying serosa (jejunal or ileal tumors) or invades pancreas or retroperitoneum (ampullary or duodenal tumors) or into non-peritonealized tissues (Figure 17.13)
T4	Tumor invades visceral peritoneum (serosa) or invades other organs (Figure 17.14)
	For any T, add (m) for multiple tumors

*Note: Tumor limited to ampulla of Vater for ampullary gangliocytic paraganglioma.

Regional Lymph Nodes (N)

NX	Regional lymph nodes cannot be assessed
N0	No regional lymph node metastasis
N1	Regional lymph node metastasis (Figures 17.15A, B)

Distant Metastases (M)

M0	No distant metastases
M1	Distant metastasis

Colon or Rectum

Primary Tumor (T)

TX	Primary tumor cannot be assessed
T0	No evidence of primary tumor
T1	Tumor invades lamina propria or submucosa and size 2 cm or less
T1a	tumor size less than 1 cm in greatest dimension (Figure 17.16)
T1b	tumor size 1–2 cm in greatest dimension (Figure 17.17)
T2	Tumor invades muscularis propria or size more than 2 cm with invasion of lamina propria or submucosa (Figure 17.18)
T3	Tumor invades through the muscularis propria into the subserosa, or into non-peritonealized pericolic or perirectal tissues (Figure 17.19)
T4	Tumor invades peritoneum or other organs (Figure 17.20)
	For any T, add (m) for multiple tumors

Regional Lymph Nodes (N)

NX	Regional lymph nodes cannot be assessed
N0	No regional lymph node metastasis
N1	Regional lymph node metastasis (Figure 17.21)

Distant Metastases (M)

M0	No distant metastases
M1	Distant metastasis

ANATOMIC STAGE/PROGNOSTIC GROUPS

Stage 0	Tis	N0	M0
Stage I	T1	N0	M0
Stage IIA	T2	N0	M0
Stage IIB	T3	N0	M0
Stage IIIA	T4	N0	M0
Stage IIIB	Any T	N1	M0
Stage IV	Any T	Any N	M1

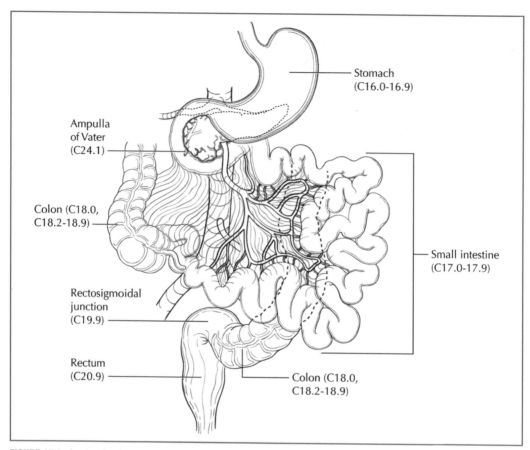

FIGURE 17.1. *Anatomic sites used in the staging of neuroendocrine tumors.*

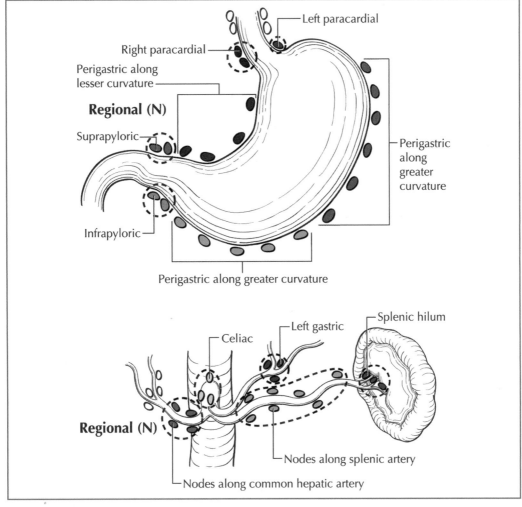

FIGURE 17.2. *The regional lymph nodes of the stomach for neuroendocrine tumors.*

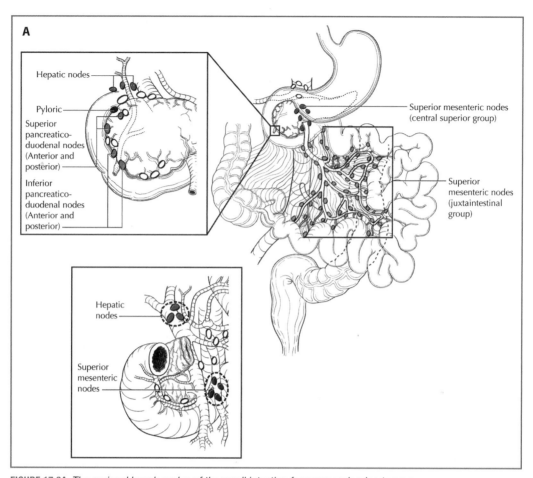

FIGURE 17.3A. *The regional lymph nodes of the small intestine for neuroendocrine tumors.*

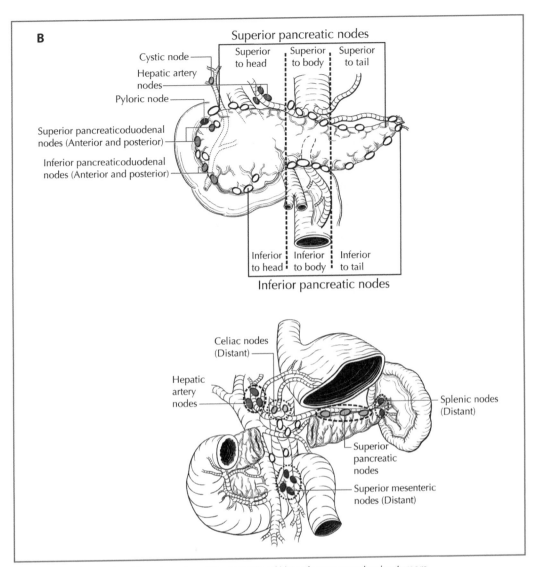

FIGURE 17.3B. *The regional lymph nodes of the ampulla of Vater for neuroendocrine tumors.*

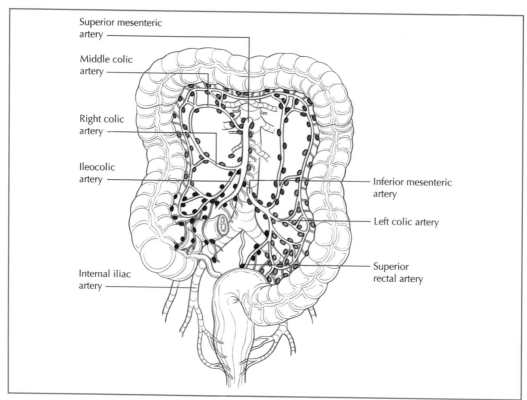

FIGURE 17.4. *The regional lymph nodes of the large intestine for neuroendocrine tumors.*

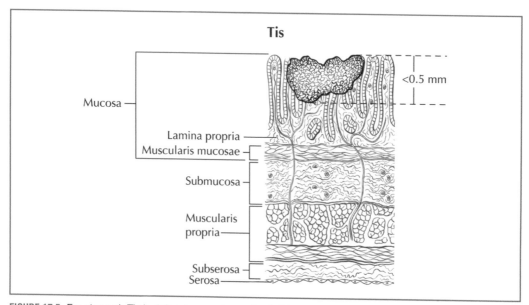

FIGURE 17.5. *For stomach Tis is defined as carcinoma in situ/dysplasia (tumor size less than 0.5 mm), confined to mucosa.*

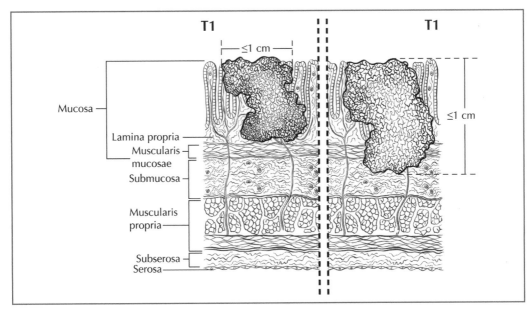

FIGURE 17.6. *For stomach T1 is defined as tumor that invades lamina propria (left side) or submucosa (right side) and 1 cm or less in size.*

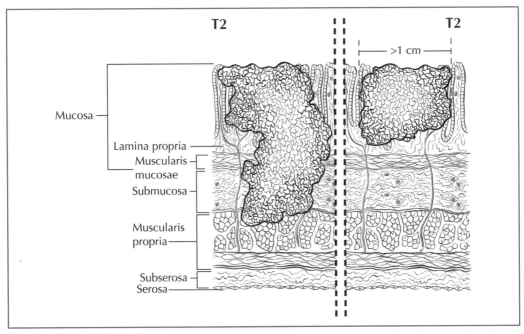

FIGURE 17.7. *For stomach T2 is defined as tumor that invades muscularis propria (left side) or more than 1 cm in size (right side).*

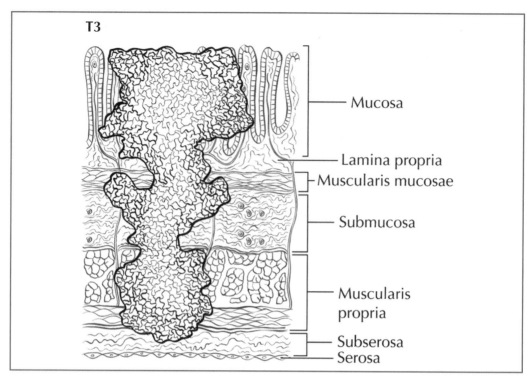

FIGURE 17.8. *For stomach T3 is defined as tumor that penetrates subserosa.*

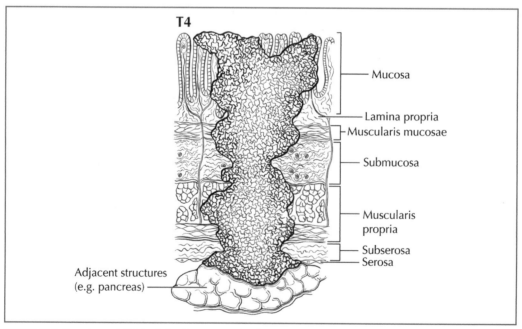

FIGURE 17.9. *For stomach T4 is defined as tumor that invades visceral peritoneum (serosa) or other organs or adjacent structures.*

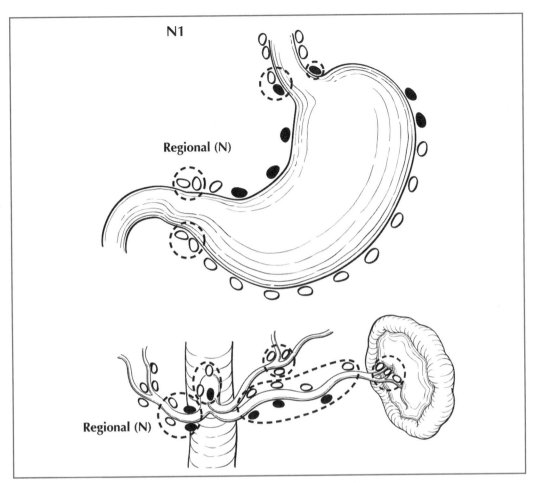

FIGURE 17.10. *For stomach N1 is defined as regional lymph node metastasis.*

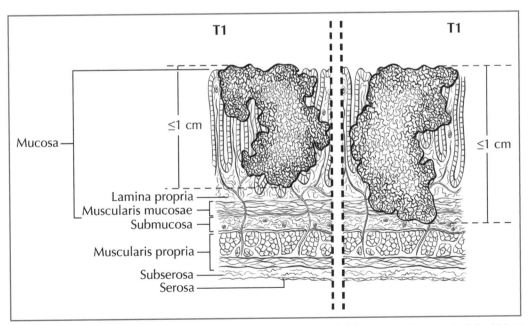

FIGURE 17.11. *For duodenum/jejunum/ileum T1 is defined as tumor that invades lamina propria (left side) or submucosa (right side) and size 1 cm or less. For ampulla T1 is defined as tumor 1 cm or less.*

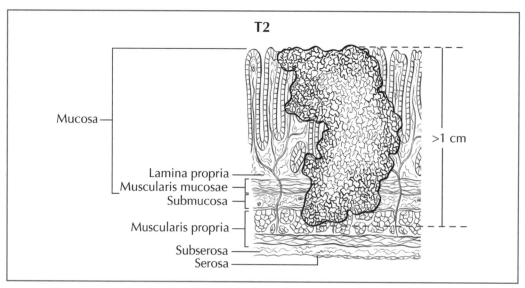

FIGURE 17.12. *For duodenum/jejunum/ileum T2 is defined as tumor that invades muscularis propria or size > 1 cm. For ampulla T2 is defined as tumor > 1 cm (ampullary tumors).*

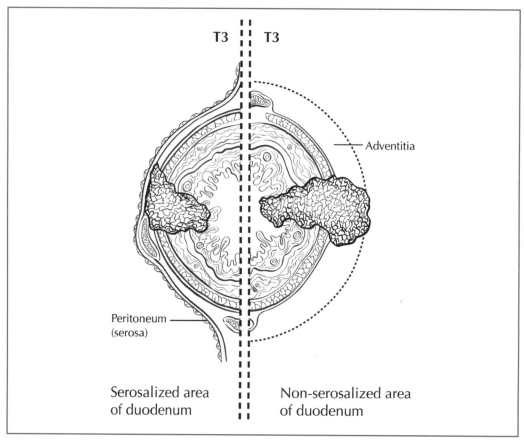

FIGURE 17.13. *For jejunum/ileum T3 is defined as tumor that invades through the muscularis propria into subserosal tissue (left side) without penetration of overlying serosa or for duodenum/ampulla invades pancreas or retroperitoneum or for all small bowel sites and ampulla, into non-peritonealized tissues (right side).*

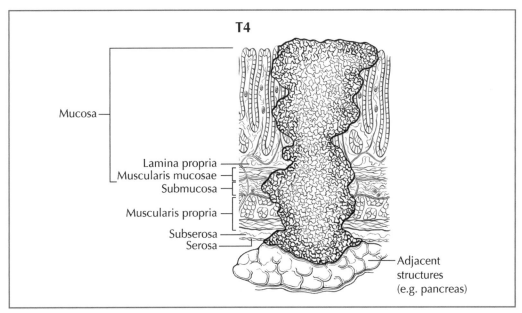

FIGURE 17.14. *For duodenum/ampulla/jejunum/ileum T4 is defined as tumor that invades visceral peritoneum (serosa) or invades other organs.*

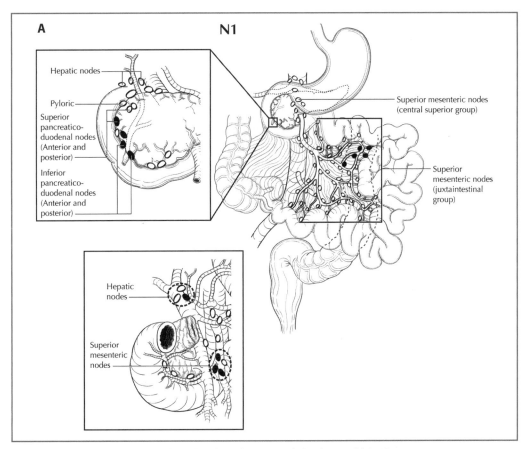

FIGURE 17.15A. *N1 is defined as regional lymph node metastasis for the small intestine.*

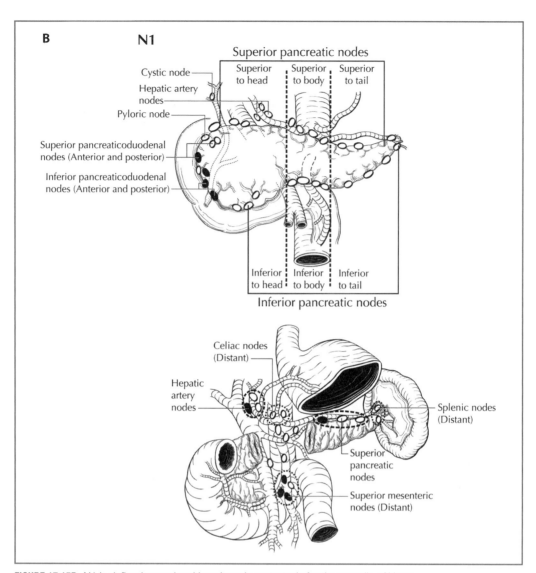

FIGURE 17.15B. *N1 is defined as regional lymph node metastasis for the ampulla of Vater.*

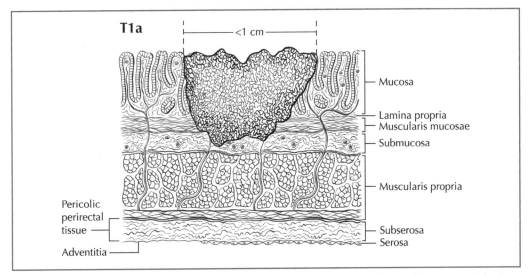

FIGURE 17.16. *For colon or rectum T1 is defined as tumor that invades lamina propria or submucosa and size 2 cm or less. T1a is defined as tumor size less than 1 cm in greatest dimension.*

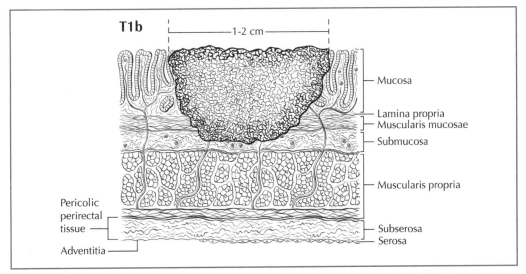

FIGURE 17.17. *For colon or rectum T1b is defined as tumor that is size 1–2 cm in greatest dimension.*

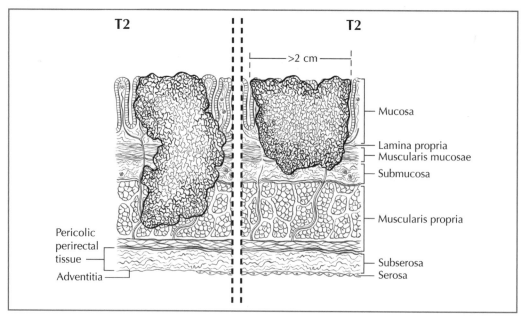

FIGURE 17.18. *For colon or rectum T2 is defined as tumor that invades muscularis propria (left side) or size more than 2 cm with invasion of lamina propria or submucosa (right side).*

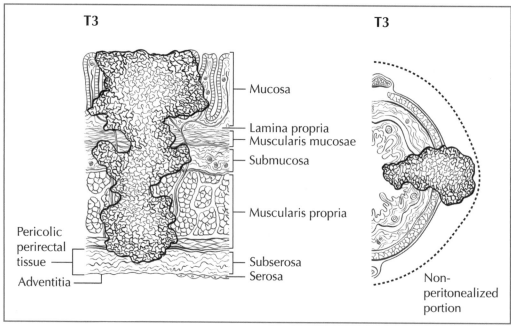

FIGURE 17.19. *For colon or rectum T3 is defined as tumor that invades through the muscularis propria into the subserosa (left side), or into non-peritonealized pericolic or perirectal tissues (right side).*

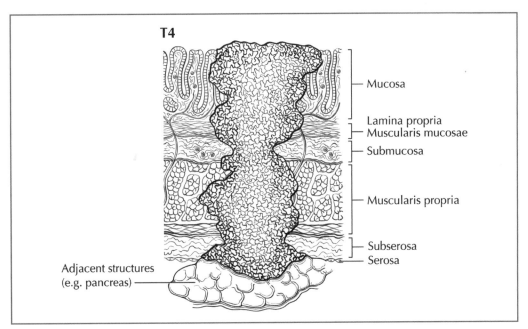

FIGURE 17.20. *For colon or rectum T4 is defined as tumor that invades peritoneum or other organs.*

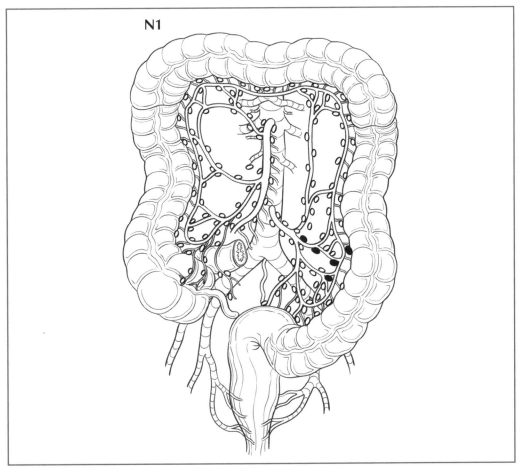

FIGURE 17.21. *For colon or rectum N1 is defined as regional lymph node metastasis.*

PROGNOSTIC FACTORS (SITE-SPECIFIC FACTORS)

(Recommended for Collection)

Required for staging	None
Clinically significant	Preoperative plasma chromogranin A level (CgA) Urinary 5-hydroxyindolacetic acid (5-HIAA) level Mitotic count

Liver

(Excluding intrahepatic bile ducts; sarcomas and tumors metastatic to the liver are not included)

18

SUMMARY OF CHANGES

Intrahepatic bile ducts are no longer included in this staging chapter. The staging of liver cancer now includes only hepatocellular carcinoma

T Category Changes

- In the T3 category, patients with invasion of major vessels are distinguished from patients with multiple tumors, of which any are >5 cm, but lack major vessel invasion because of the markedly different prognosis of these subgroups

  - T3a includes multiple tumors, any >5 cm
  - T3b includes tumors of any size involving a major portal vein or hepatic vein

- T4 category unchanged

N Category Changes

- Inferior phrenic lymph nodes were reclassified to regional lymph nodes from distant lymph nodes

Stage Grouping Changes

- Changes in T3 classification led to changes in Stage III groupings

  - Stage IIIA now includes only T3a; patients with major vessel invasion are removed from the IIIA stage grouping
  - Stage IIIB now includes only T3b (major vessel invasion)
  - T4 is shifted to Stage IIIC

- Stage IV includes all patients with metastasis, whether nodal or distant, separated into IVA and B to permit identification of each subgroup

  - Stage IVA now includes node-positive disease (N1)
  - Stage IVB now includes distant metastasis (M1)

ICD-O-3 TOPOGRAPHY CODE

C22.0   Liver

ICD-O-3 HISTOLOGY CODE RANGES

8170–8175

C.C. Compton et al. (eds.), *AJCC Cancer Staging Atlas: A Companion to the Seventh Editions of the AJCC Cancer Staging Manual and Handbook*, DOI 10.1007/978-1-4614-2080-4_18,
© 2012 American Joint Committee on Cancer

ANATOMY

Primary Site. The liver has a dual blood supply: the hepatic artery, which typically branches from the celiac artery, and the portal vein, which drains the intestine. Blood from the liver passes through the hepatic veins and enters the inferior vena cava. The liver is divided into right and left liver by a plane (Rex-Cantlie line) projecting between the gallbladder fossa and the vena cava and defined by the middle hepatic vein (Figure 18.1). Couinaud refined knowledge about the functional anatomy of the liver and proposed division of the liver into four sectors (formerly called segments) and eight segments. In this nomenclature, the liver is divided by vertical and oblique planes or scissurae defined by the three main hepatic veins and a transverse plane or scissura that follows a line drawn through the right and left portal branches. Thus, the four traditional segments (right anterior, right posterior, left medial, and left lateral) are replaced by sectors (right anterior, right posterior, left medial, and left posterior), and these sectors are divided into segments by the transverse scissura (Figure 18.2). The eight segments are numbered clockwise in a frontal plane. Recent advances in hepatic surgery have made possible anatomic (also called typical) resections along these planes.

Histologically, the liver is divided into lobules with central veins draining each lobule. The portal triads between the lobules contain the intrahepatic bile ducts and the blood supply, which consists of small branches of the hepatic artery and portal vein and intrahepatic lymphatic channels.

Regional Lymph Nodes. The regional lymph nodes are the hilar, hepatoduodenal ligament lymph nodes, inferior phrenic, and caval lymph nodes, among which the most prominent are the hepatic artery and portal vein lymph nodes (Figure 18.3). Nodal involvement should be coded as N1. Nodal involvement is now considered stage IV disease.

Distant Metastatic Sites. The main mode of dissemination of liver carcinomas is via the portal veins (intrahepatic) and hepatic veins. Intrahepatic venous dissemination cannot be differentiated from satellitosis or multifocal tumors and is classified as multiple tumors. The most common sites of extrahepatic dissemination are the lungs and bones. Tumors may extend through the liver capsule to adjacent organs (adrenal, diaphragm, and colon) or may rupture, causing acute hemorrhage and peritoneal metastasis.

PROGNOSTIC FEATURES

Clinical factors predictive of decreased survival duration include an elevated serum alpha-fetoprotein level and Child-Pugh class B and C liver disease. For patients who undergo tumor resection, the main predictor of poor outcome is a positive surgical margin (grossly or microscopically involved tumors indicative of incomplete resection). The effect of the extent of surgical clearance at the closest margin (<10 mm vs. >10 mm) remains controversial. Other prognostic factors associated with decreased survival include major vessel invasion and tumor size >5 cm in patients with multiple tumors.

FIBROSIS SCORE (F)

The fibrosis score as defined by Ishak is recommended because of its prognostic value in overall survival. This scoring system uses a 0–6 scale.

F0   Fibrosis score 0–4 (none to moderate fibrosis)

F1   Fibrosis score 5–6 (severe fibrosis or cirrhosis)

DEFINITIONS OF TNM

Primary Tumor (T)

TX	Primary tumor cannot be assessed
T0	No evidence of primary tumor
T1	Solitary tumor without vascular invasion (Figure 18.4)
T2	Solitary tumor with vascular invasion or multiple tumors none more than 5 cm (Figure 18.5A, B)
T3a	Multiple tumors more than 5 cm (Figure 18.6A)
T3b	Single tumor or multiple tumors of any size involving a major branch of the portal vein or hepatic vein (Figure 18.6B)
T4	Tumor(s) with direct invasion of adjacent organs other than the gallbladder or with perforation of visceral peritoneum (Figure 18.7)

Regional Lymph Nodes (N)

NX	Regional lymph nodes cannot be assessed
N0	No regional lymph node metastasis
N1	Regional lymph node metastasis (Figure 18.8)

Distant Metastasis (M)

M0	No distant metastasis
M1	Distant metastasis

ANATOMIC STAGE/PROGNOSTIC GROUPS

Stage	T	N	M
Stage I	T1	N0	M0
Stage II	T2	N0	M0
Stage IIIA	T3a	N0	M0
Stage IIIB	T3b	N0	M0
Stage IIIC	T4	N0	M0
Stage IVA	Any T	N1	M0
Stage IVB	Any T	Any N	M1

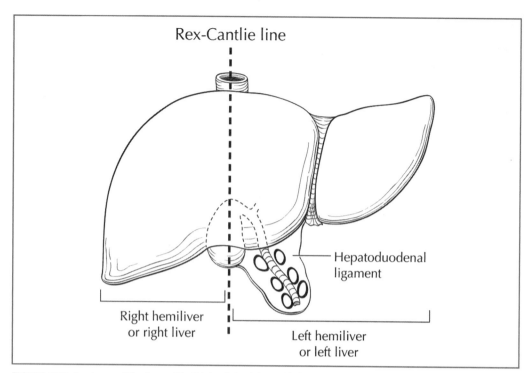

FIGURE 18.1. *Anatomy of the liver with division into right and left lobes by the plane of Rex-Cantlie line.*

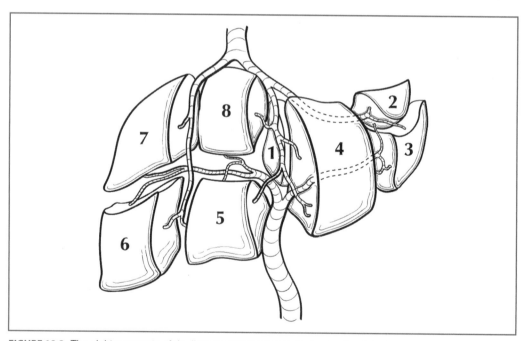

FIGURE 18.2. *The eight segments of the liver are numbered clockwise in a frontal plane.*

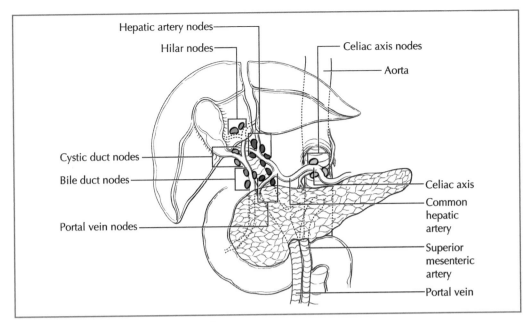

FIGURE 18.3. *Regional lymph nodes of the liver.*

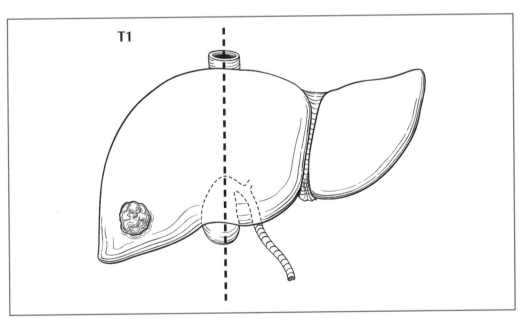

FIGURE 18.4. *T1 is defined as a solitary tumor without vascular invasion, regardless of size.*

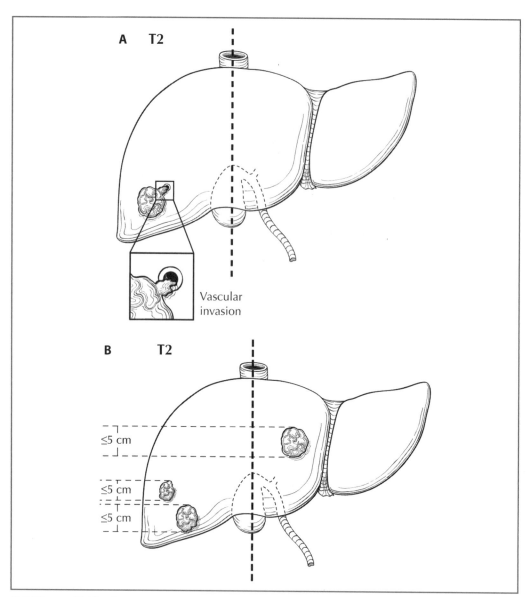

FIGURE 18.5. *(A) All solitary tumors with vascular invasion, regardless of size, are classified T2. (B) Multiple tumors, with none more than 5 cm, are classified T2.*

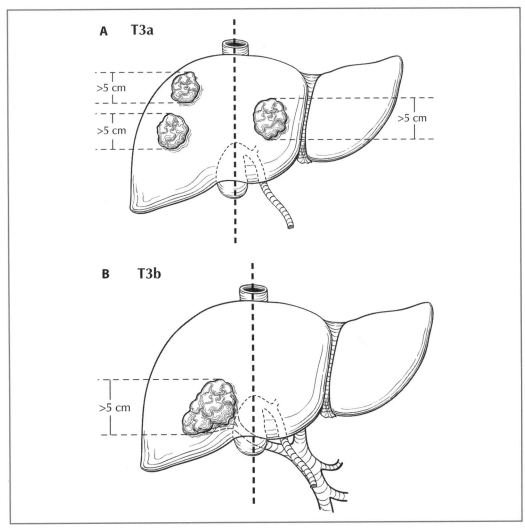

FIGURE 18.6. *(A) Multiple tumors more than 5 cm are classified T3a. (B) A tumor involving a major branch of the portal or hepatic vein(s) is classified T3b.*

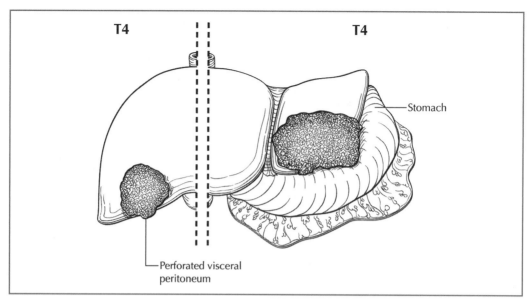

FIGURE 18.7. *Two views of T4: tumor with perforation of the visceral peritoneum (left of dotted line); tumor directly invading adjacent organs other than the gallbladder (right of dotted line, tumor invades stomach).*

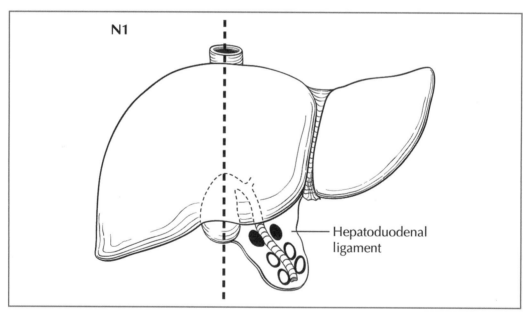

FIGURE 18.8. *N1 is defined as metastasis to regional lymph nodes.*

PROGNOSTIC FACTORS (SITE-SPECIFIC FACTORS)

(Recommended for Collection)

Required for staging	None
Clinically significant	Alpha fetoprotein (AFP)
	Fibrosis score
	Hepatitis serology
	Creatinine (part of the Model for End Stage Liver Disease score)
	Bilirubin (part of the Model for End Stage Liver Disease score)
	Prothrombin time international normalized ratio (INR) (part of the Model for End Stage Liver Disease score)

Intrahepatic Bile Ducts

19

SUMMARY OF CHANGES

- This is a novel staging system that is independent of the staging system for hepatocellular carcinoma and independent of the staging system for extrahepatic bile duct malignancy, including hilar bile duct cancers. The rare combined hepatocellular and cholangiocarcinoma (mixed hepatocholangio carcinomas) are included with the intrahepatic bile duct cancer staging classification
- The tumor category (T) is based on three major prognostic factors including tumor number, vascular invasion, and direct extrahepatic tumoral extension
- The nodal category (N) is a binary classification based on the presence or absence of regional lymph node metastasis
- The metastasis category (M) is a binary classification based on the presence or absence of distant disease
- Recommend collection of preoperative or pretreatment serum CA19–9

ICD-O-3 TOPOGRAPHY CODES

C22.0   Liver
C22.1   Intrahepatic bile duct

ICD-O-3 HISTOLOGY CODE RANGES

8160, 8161, 8180

ANATOMY

Primary Site. At the hilar plate, the right and left hepatic bile ducts enter the liver parenchyma (Figure 19.1). Histologically these bile ducts are lined by a single layer of tall uniform columnar cells. The mucosa usually forms irregular pleats or small longitudinal folds. The walls of the bile ducts have a layer of subepithelial connective tissue and muscle fiber. However, these muscle fibers are typically sparse or absent within the hepatic parenchyma. There is a periductal neural component, which is frequently involved by cholangiocarcinomas.

The tumor growth patterns of intrahepatic cholangiocarcinoma include the mass forming type, the periductal infiltrating type, and a mixed type. Mass forming intrahepatic cholangiocarcinoma shows a radial growth pattern invading into the adjacent liver parenchyma with well-demarcated gross margins. On histopathologic examination, these are nodular sclerotic masses with distinct borders. In contrast, the periductal infiltrating type of cholangiocarcinoma demonstrates a diffuse longitudinal growth pattern along the bile duct.

The percentage of patients with the purely mass forming type is estimated to be 60% of all patients with intrahepatic cholangiocarcinoma, while the purely periductal infiltrating type represents 20% of all cases and a mixed pattern of mass forming and periductal infiltrating type represents the remaining 20% of cases of intrahepatic cholangiocarcinoma. Limited analyses suggest that the diffuse periductal infiltrating type is associated with a poor prognosis. However, comparison of the prognostic significance of this variable to other prognostic factors is lacking. Either histologic type may invade vascular structures, although this is less commonly observed for mass forming intrahepatic cholangiocarcinoma. Anatomically, the intrahepatic bile ducts extend from the periphery of the liver to the second order bile duct ducts (see perihilar bile duct definition, Chap. 21).

Regional Lymph Nodes. Compared with primary hepatocellular carcinoma, regional lymph node metastases are more commonly associated with intrahepatic cholangiocarcinoma. The lymph node drainage patterns from the intrahepatic bile ducts demonstrate laterality. Tumors in the left lateral bi-segment (segment 2–3) of the liver may preferentially drain to lymph nodes along the lesser curvature of the stomach and subsequently to the celiac nodal basin. In contrast, intrahepatic cholangiocarcinomas of the right liver (segment 5–8) may primarily drain to hilar lymph nodes and subsequently to caval and periaortic lymph nodes (Figures 19.2 and 19.3).

For right liver (segment 5–8) intrahepatic cholangiocarcinomas, the regional lymph nodes include the hilar (common bile duct, hepatic artery, portal vein, and cystic duct) periduodenal and peripancreatic lymph nodes. For left liver (segment 2–4) intrahepatic cholangiocarcinomas, regional lymph nodes include hilar, and gastrohepatic lymph nodes. For intrahepatic cholangiocarcinomas, disease spread to the celiac and/or periaortic and caval lymph nodes are considered distant metastases (M1). Inferior phrenic nodes are considered regional, not distant nodes.

Metastatic Sites. Intrahepatic cholangiocarcinomas usually metastasize to other intrahepatic locations (classified in the T category as multiple tumors) and to the peritoneum, and subsequently, to the lungs and pleura (classified in the M category as distant metastasis).

PROGNOSTIC FEATURES

Clinical factors predictive of decreased survival include serum CA 19-9 level, the presence of underlying liver disease, and multiple tumors. For patients treated with surgical resection, the main predictors of poor outcome include regional lymph node involvement and incomplete resection. Other important prognostic factors include the finding of satellitosis or multiple intrahepatic tumors, vascular invasion, and periductal infiltrating tumor growth pattern.

DEFINITIONS OF TNM

Primary Tumor (T)	
TX	Primary tumor cannot be assessed
T0	No evidence of primary tumor
Tis	Carcinoma in situ (intraductal tumor)
T1	Solitary tumor without vascular invasion (Figure 19.4)
T2a	Solitary tumor with vascular invasion (Figure 19.5A)
T2b	Multiple tumors, with or without vascular invasion (Figure 19.5B)
T3	Tumor perforating the visceral peritoneum or involving the local extra hepatic structures by direct invasion (Figures 19.6)
T4	Tumor with periductal invasion (Figure 19.7)

Regional Lymph Nodes (N)

NX	Regional lymph nodes cannot be assessed
N0	No regional lymph node metastasis
N1	Regional lymph node metastasis present (Figure 19.8)

Distant Metastasis (M)

M0	No distant metastasis
M1	Distant metastasis present

ANATOMIC STAGE/PROGNOSTIC GROUPS

Stage 0	Tis	N0	M0
Stage I	T1	N0	M0
Stage II	T2	N0	M0
Stage III	T3	N0	M0
Stage IVA	T4	N0	M0
Stage IVB	Any T	N1	M0
	Any T	Any N	M1

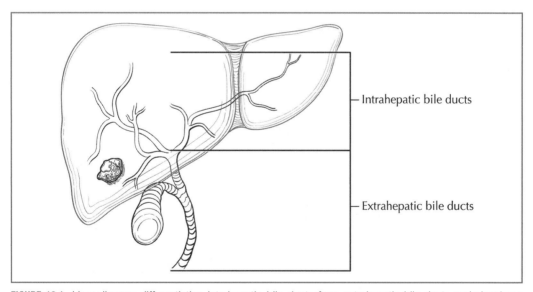

FIGURE 19.1. *Liver diagram differentiating intrahepatic bile ducts from extrahepatic bile ducts and showing a mass-forming type of intrahepatic cholangiocarcinoma. The intrahepatic bile ducts extend from the periphery of the liver and include the right and left hepatic ducts.*

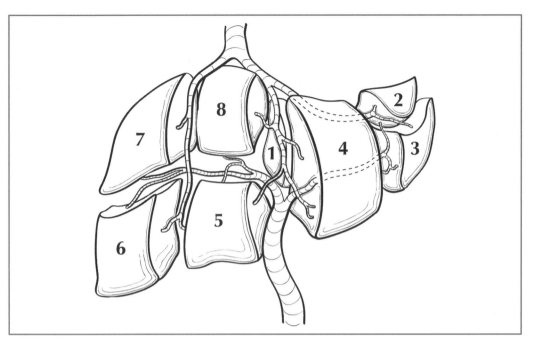

FIGURE 19.2. Segmental anatomy of the liver. The eight segments of the liver are numbered clockwise in a frontal plane.

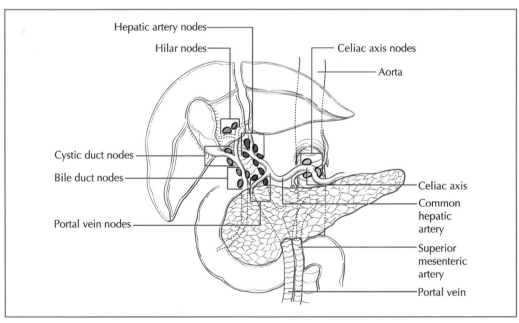

FIGURE 19.3. Lymph node drainage patterns for intrahepatic carcinomas vary with tumor location within the liver. Segments 2 and 3 drain to lymph nodes along the lesser curvature of the stomach and subsequently to the celiac nodal basin. Intrahepatic cholangiocarcinomas of the right liver (segments 5-8) may preferentially drain to hilar lymph nodes and subsequently to caval and periaortic lymph nodes.

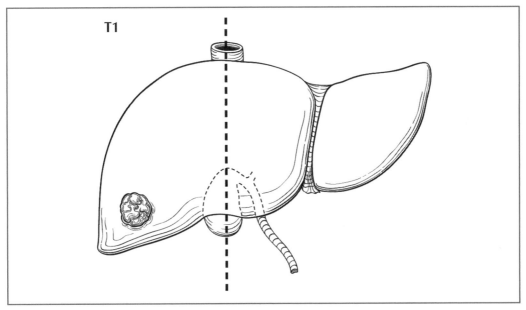

FIGURE 19.4. *T1 is defined as a solitary tumor without vascular invasion, regardless of size.*

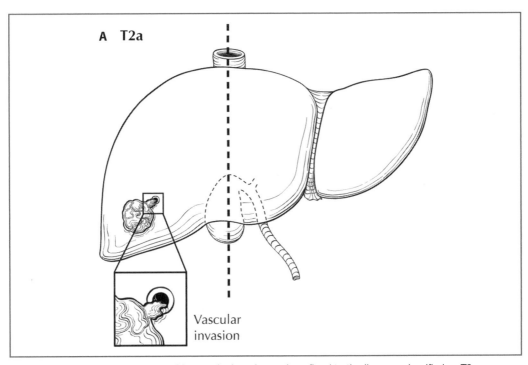

FIGURE 19.5. *(A) All solitary tumors with vascular invasion and confined to the liver are classified as T2a.*

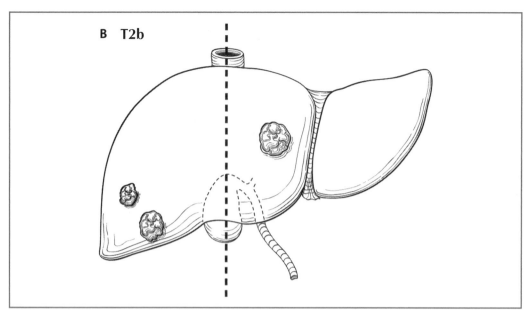

FIGURE 19.5. *(continued) (B) Multiple tumors confined to the liver, with or without vascular invasion, are classified as T2b.*

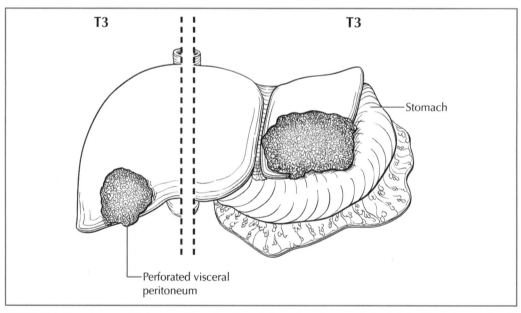

FIGURE 19.6. *Two views of T3: tumor with perforation of visceral peritoneum (left of dotted line); tumor directly invading adjacent organs (right of dotted line, tumor invades stomach).*

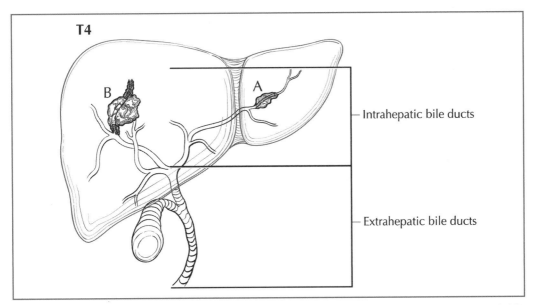

FIGURE 19.7. *Periductal infiltrating tumors exhibit diffuse longitudinal growth pattern along the intrahepatic bile ducts on both gross and microscopic examination. T4 includes diffuse periductal infiltrating tumors (A) and mixed mass-forming and periductal infiltrating tumors (B).*

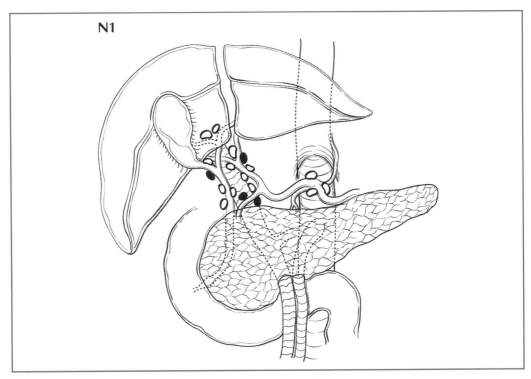

FIGURE 19.8. *N1 is defined as metastasis to regional lymph nodes.*

PROGNOSTIC FACTORS (SITE-SPECIFIC FACTORS)
(Recommended for Collection)

Required for staging	None
Clinically significant	Tumor growth pattern
	Primary sclerosing cholangitis
	CA 19-9

Gallbladder

(Carcinoid tumors and sarcomas are not included)

20

SUMMARY OF CHANGES

- The cystic duct is now included in this classification scheme
- The N classification now distinguishes hilar nodes (N1: lymph nodes adjacent to the cystic duct, bile duct, hepatic artery, and portal vein) from other regional nodes (N2: celiac, peridu- odenal, and peripancreatic lymph nodes, and those along the superior mesenteric artery)
- Stage groupings have been changed to better correlate with surgical resectability and patient outcome; locally unresectable T4 tumors have been reclassified as Stage IV
- Lymph node metastasis is now classified as Stage IIIB (N1) or Stage IVB (N2)

ICD-O-3 TOPOGRAPHY CODES
C23.9   Gallbladder
C24.0   Cystic duct only

ICD-O-3 HISTOLOGY CODE RANGES
8000–8152, 8154–8231, 8243–8245, 8250–8576, 8940–8950, 8980–8981

ANATOMY

Primary Site. The gallbladder is a pear-shaped saccular organ located under the liver situated in line with the physiologic division of the right and left lobes of the liver (Cantlie's line). It straddles Couinaud segments IVb and V. The organ can be divided into three parts: a fundus, a body, and a neck, which tapers into the cystic duct (Figure 20.1). The wall is considerably thinner than that of other hollow organs and lacks a submucosal layer. Its make up consists of a mucosa, a muscular layer, perimuscular connective tissue, and a serosa on one side (serosa is lacking on the side embed- ded in the liver). An important anatomic consideration is that the serosa along the liver edge is more densely adherent to the liver (cystic plate) and much of this is often left behind at the time of chole- cystectomy. For this reason, partial hepatic resection incorporating portions of segments IVb and V is undertaken for some cases. Primary carcinomas of the cystic duct are included in this staging classification schema.

Regional Lymph Nodes. For accurate staging, all nodes removed at operation should be assessed for metastasis. Regional lymph nodes are limited to the hepatic hilus (including nodes along the common bile duct, hepatic artery, portal vein, and cystic duct) (Figure 20.2). Celiac and superior mesenteric artery node involvement is now considered distant metastatic disease.

Metastatic Sites. Cancers of the gallbladder usually metastasize to the peritoneum and liver and occasionally to the lungs and pleura.

C.C. Compton et al. (eds.), *AJCC Cancer Staging Atlas: A Companion to the Seventh Editions of the AJCC Cancer Staging Manual and Handbook*, DOI 10.1007/978-1-4614-2080-4_20,
© 2012 American Joint Committee on Cancer

PROGNOSTIC FEATURES

In as many as 50% of cases, gallbladder cancers are discovered at pathologic analysis after simple cholecystectomy for presumed gallstone disease. Five-year survival is 50% for patients with T1 tumors. Patients with T2 tumors have a 5-year survival rate of 29%, which appears to be improved with more radical resection. Patients with lymph node metastases (Stage IIIB or higher) or locally advanced tumors (Stage IVA or higher) rarely experience long-term survival. The site-specific prognostic factors include histologic type, histologic grade, and vascular invasion. Papillary carcinomas have the most favorable prognosis. Unfavorable histologic types include small cell carcinomas and undifferentiated carcinomas. Lymphatic and/or blood vessel invasion indicate a less favorable outcome. Histologic grade also correlates with outcome.

Patients with T2–T3 cancers discovered at pathologic analysis are usually offered a second operation for radical resection of residual tumor. This may include nonanatomic resection of the gallbladder bed (segments IVB and V of the liver) or more formal anatomic resection such as a right hepatectomy. Resection of the biliary tree is dependent on surgical decision making at the time of the definitive procedure and may be based on cystic duct margin status. Staging classification should be reported for tumors removed by either a single operation or a staged surgical procedure (cholecystectomy followed by definitive resection). In cases where the surgical procedure was staged, it should be noted whether the cholecystectomy was performed laparoscopically or via an open approach. Finally, comment should be made as to whether the primary tumor was located on the free peritoneal or the hepatic side of the gallbladder.

DEFINITIONS OF TNM

Primary Tumor (T)

TX	Primary tumor cannot be assessed
T0	No evidence of primary tumor
Tis	Carcinoma in situ
T1	Tumor invades lamina propria or muscular layer (Figure 20.3)
T1a	Tumor invades lamina propria (Figure 20.3)
T1b	Tumor invades muscular layer (Figure 20.3)
T2	Tumor invades perimuscular connective tissue; no extension beyond serosa or into liver (Figure 20.4)
T3	Tumor perforates the serosa (visceral peritoneum) and/or directly invades the liver and/or one other adjacent organ or structure, such as the stomach, duodenum, colon, pancreas, omentum, or extrahepatic bile ducts (Figure 20.5A, B)
T4	Tumor invades main portal vein or hepatic artery or invades two or more extrahepatic organs or structures (Figure 20.6)

Regional Lymph Nodes (N)

NX	Regional lymph nodes cannot be assessed
N0	No regional lymph node metastasis
N1	Metastases to nodes along the cystic duct, common bile duct, hepatic artery, and/or portal vein (Figure 20.7A)
N2	Metastases to periaortic, pericaval, superior mesenteric artery, and/or celiac artery lymph nodes (Figure 20.7B)

Distant Metastasis (M)

M0	No distant metastasis
M1	Distant metastasis

ANATOMIC STAGE/PROGNOSTIC GROUPS

Stage 0	Tis	N0	M0
Stage I	T1	N0	M0
Stage II	T2	N0	M0
Stage IIIA	T3	N0	M0
Stage IIIB	T1-3	N1	M0
Stage IVA	T4	N0-1	M0
Stage IVB	Any T	N2	M0
	Any T	Any N	M1

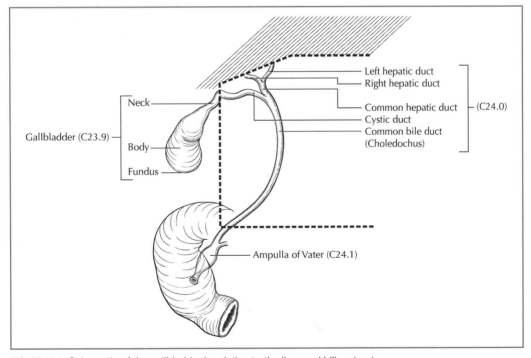

FIGURE 20.1. *Schematic of the gallbladder in relation to the liver and biliary tract.*

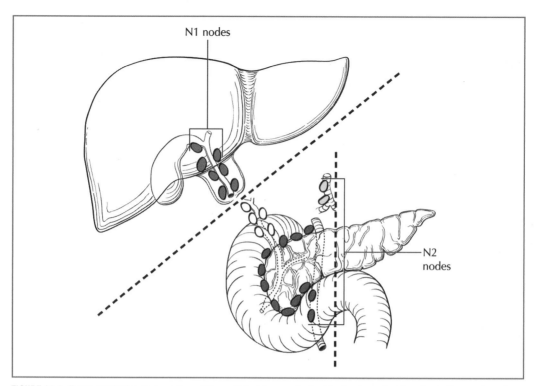

FIGURE 20.2. *Regional (N1) lymph nodes of the gallbladder are limited to the hepatic hilus (including nodes along the common bile duct, hepatic artery, portal vein, and cystic duct). Metastases to celiac, periduodenal, peripancreatic, and superior mesenteric artery lymph nodes are considered N2 disease.*

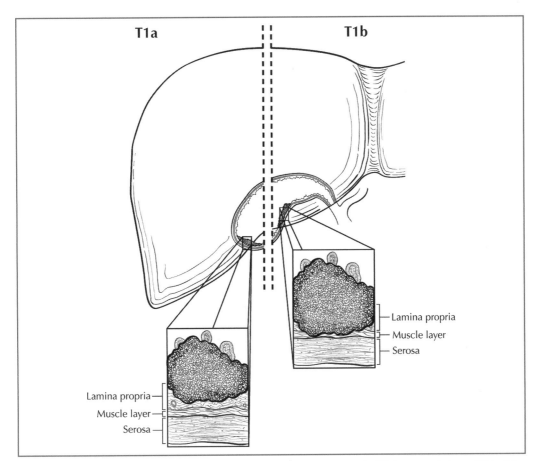

FIGURE 20.3. *Schematic of T1, showing the tumor invading the lamina propria (T1a) or muscle layer (T1b) of the gallbladder.*

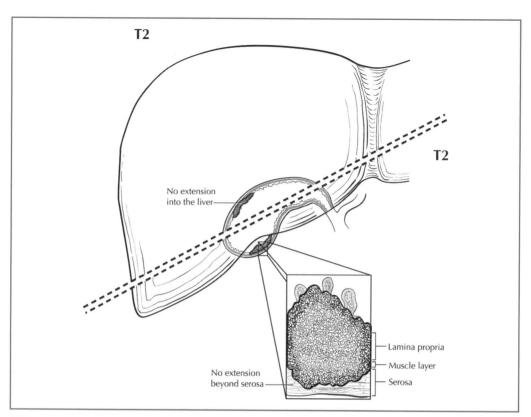

FIGURE 20.4. *Two views of T2: tumor invading perimuscular connective tissue, with no invasion beyond serosa (illustration below dotted line) or into the liver (above dotted line).*

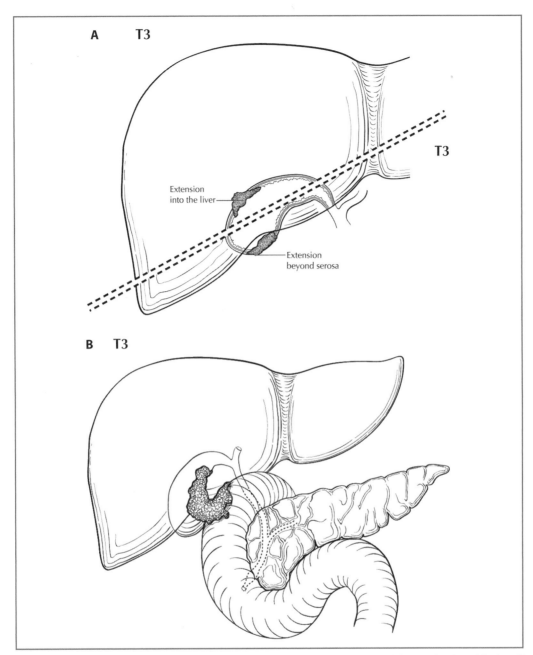

FIGURE 20.5. *(A) Two views of T3: tumor perforating the serosa (visceral peritoneum) (below the dotted line) and/ or directly invading the liver (above the dotted line). (B) T3 may also be defined as tumor invading one other adjacent organ or structure, such as the duodenum (as illustrated), or the stomach, colon, pancreas, omentum, or extrahepatic bile ducts.*

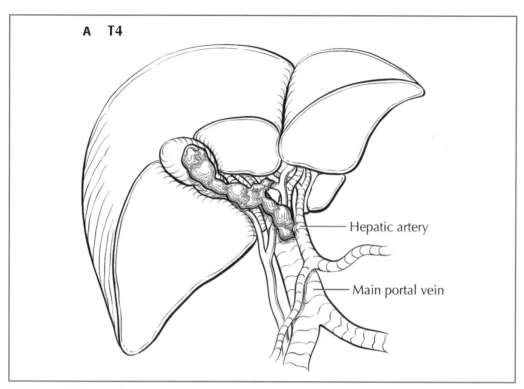

FIGURE 20.6. (A) T4 is defined as tumor invading main portal vein or hepatic artery.

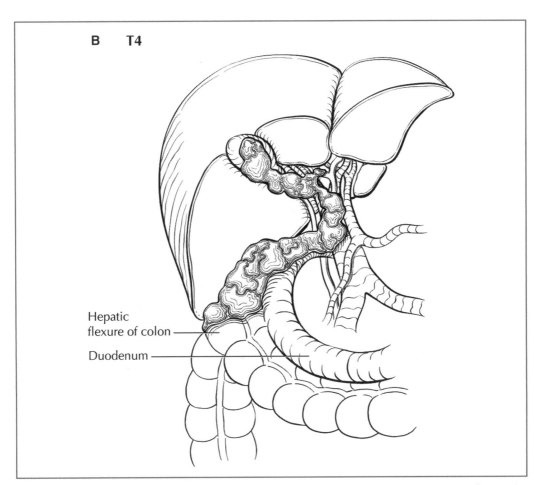

B   T4

Hepatic
flexure of colon

Duodenum

FIGURE 20.6. *(continued) (B) T4 is defined as invading two or more extrahepatic organs or structures (here, colon and duodenum).*

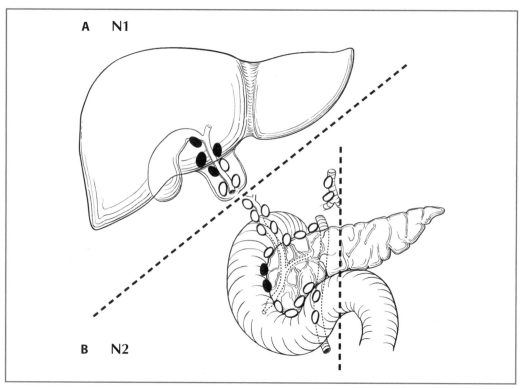

FIGURE 20.7. *(A) N1 is defined as metastasis to hepatic hilar (regional) lymph nodes. (B) N2 is defined as metastasis to periaortic, pericaval, superior mesenteric artery and/or celiac artery lymph nodes.*

PROGNOSTIC FACTORS (SITE-SPECIFIC FACTORS)
(Recommended for Collection)

Required for staging	None
Clinically significant	Tumor location
	Specimen type
	Extent of liver resection
	Free peritoneal side vs. hepatic side for T2

Perihilar Bile Ducts

(Sarcoma and carcinoid tumors are not included)

21

SUMMARY OF CHANGES

- Extrahepatic bile duct tumors have been separated into perihilar (proximal) and distal groups and separate staging classifications defined for each
- T1 (confined to bile duct) and T2 (beyond the wall of the bile duct) have been specified histologically
- T2 includes invasion of adjacent hepatic parenchyma
- T3 is defined as unilateral vascular invasion
- T4 is defined on the basis of bilateral biliary and/or vascular invasion
- Lymph node metastasis has been reclassified as stage III (upstaged from stage II)
- The stage IV grouping defines unresectability based on local invasion (IVA) or distant disease (IVB)

ICD-O-3 TOPOGRAPHY CODES

C24.0   Extrahepatic bile duct (proximal or perihilar only)

ICD-O-3 HISTOLOGY CODE RANGES

8000–8152, 8154–8231, 8243–8245, 8250–8576, 8940–8950, 8980–8981

ANATOMY

Primary Site. Cholangiocarcinoma can develop anywhere along the biliary tree, from proximal peripheral intrahepatic ducts to the distal intraduodenal bile duct. Extrahepatic bile duct tumors have traditionally been separated into perihilar (or proximal), middle, and distal subgroups. However, middle lesions are rare and managed either as a proximal tumor with combined hepatic and hilar resection or as a distal tumor with pancreaticoduodenectomy. In this edition of the *AJCC Cancer Staging Manual*, extrahepatic cholangiocarcinoma is divided into perihilar and distal subgroups, with middle lesions classified according to their treatment. Perihilar cholangiocarcinomas are defined anatomically as tumors located in the extrahepatic biliary tree proximal to the origin of the cystic duct (Figure 21.1). They may extend proximally into either the right hepatic duct, the left hepatic duct, or both. Laterally refers to tumor extension related to either right or left periductal regions.

The sixth edition of the *AJCC Cancer Staging Manual* classified invasion of adjacent hepatic parenchyma and unilateral vascular involvement as T3. However, patients with invasion of adjacent hepatic parenchyma have been found to have a better prognosis than patients with vascular invasion (Figure 21.2). Thus, adjacent hepatic invasion is now classified T2, whereas unilateral vascular involvement is classified as T3.

T4 tumors are defined as those with bilateral hepatic involvement of vascular structures, bilateral tumor expansion into secondary biliary radicals, or extension to secondary biliary radicals with contralateral vascular invasion. The median survival of patients with T4 tumors is 8–13 months, and in this edition of the *AJCC Cancer Staging Manual*, T4 tumors are classified as stage IVA. However, highly

C.C. Compton et al. (eds.), *AJCC Cancer Staging Atlas: A Companion to the Seventh Editions of the AJCC Cancer Staging Manual and Handbook*, DOI 10.1007/978-1-4614-2080-4_21,
© 2012 American Joint Committee on Cancer

selected patients with T4 tumors may be candidates for protocol-based chemoradiation followed by liver transplantation.

Regional Lymph Nodes. In perihilar cholangiocarcinoma, the prevalence of lymphatic metastasis increases directly with T category and ranges from 30% to 53% overall. Hilar and pericholedochal nodes in the hepatoduodenal ligament are most often involved (Figure 21.2).

Metastatic Sites. Perihilar cholangiocarcinoma is characterized by intrahepatic ductal extension, as well as spread along perineural and periductal lymphatic channels. While the liver is a common site of metastases, spread to other organs, especially extra-abdominal sites, is uncommon. Extrahepatic metastases have been reported in the peritoneal cavity, lung, brain, and bone.

PROGNOSTIC FEATURES

Patients who undergo surgical resection for localized perihilar cholangiocarcinoma have a median survival of approximately 3 years and a 5-year survival rate of 20% to 40%. In carefully selected patients with primary sclerosing cholangitis and early-stage perihilar cholangiocarcinoma, preliminary data report excellent results with neoadjuvant chemoradiation and liver transplantation. Complete resection with negative histologic margins is the major predictor of outcome, and liver resection is essential to achieve negative margins. Factors adversely associated with survival include high tumor grade, vascular invasion, lobar atrophy, and lymph node metastasis. Papillary morphology carries a more favorable prognosis than nodular or sclerosing tumors.

DEFINITIONS OF TNM

Primary Tumor (T)

TX	Primary tumor cannot be assessed
T0	No evidence of primary tumor
Tis	Carcinoma in situ
T1	Tumor confined to the bile duct, with extension up to the muscle layer or fibrous tissue (Figure 21.3)
T2a	Tumor invades beyond the wall of the bile duct to surrounding adipose tissue (Figure 21.4)
T2b	Tumor invades adjacent hepatic parenchyma (Figure 21.4)
T3	Tumor invades unilateral branches of the portal vein or hepatic artery (Figure 21.5)
T4	Tumor invades main portal vein or its branches bilaterally; or the common hepatic artery; or the second-order biliary radicals bilaterally; or unilateral second-order biliary radicals with contralateral portal vein or hepatic artery involvement (Figure 21.6)

Regional Lymph Nodes (N)

NX	Regional lymph nodes cannot be assessed
N0	No regional lymph node metastasis
N1	Regional lymph node metastasis (including nodes along the cystic duct, common bile duct, hepatic artery, and portal vein) (Figure 21.7A)
N2	Metastasis to periaortic, pericaval, superior mesenteric artery, and/or celiac artery lymph nodes (Figure 21.7B)

Distant Metastasis (M)

M0   No distant metastasis

M1   Distant metastasis

ANATOMIC STAGE/PROGNOSTIC GROUPS

Stage 0	Tis	N0	M0
Stage I	T1	N0	M0
Stage II	T2a-b	N0	M0
Stage IIIA	T3	N0	M0
Stage IIIB	T1-3	N1	M0
Stage IVA	T4	N0-1	M0
Stage IVB	Any T	N2	M0
	Any T	Any N	M1

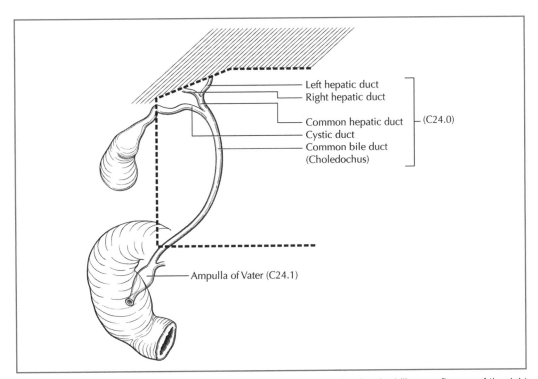

FIGURE 21.1. *Anatomy of bile duct cancers. Perihilar bile duct cancers involve the biliary confluence of the right and left hepatic ducts.*

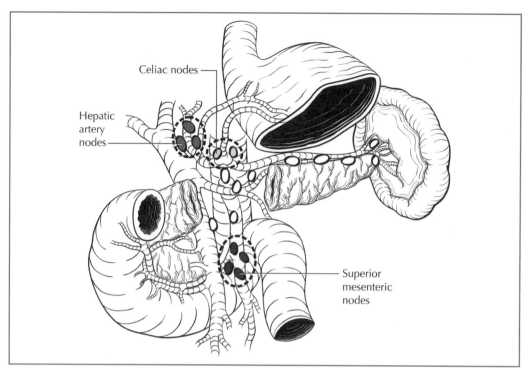

FIGURE 21.2. *Regional lymph nodes of the perihilar bile duct.*

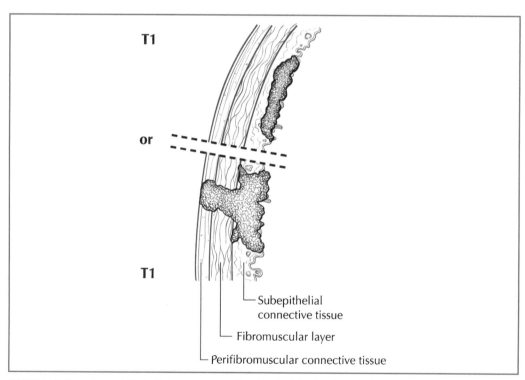

FIGURE 21.3. *Two views of T1: both tumors are confined to the bile duct histologically.*

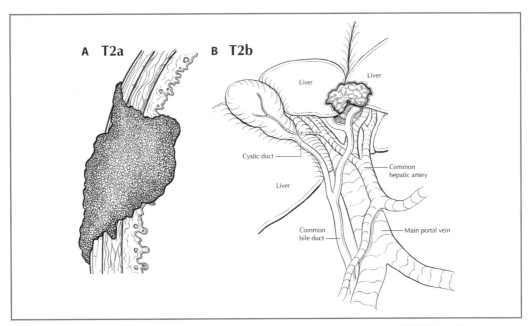

FIGURE 21.4. *(A) T2a is defined as tumor that invades beyond the wall of the bile duct. (B) T2b is defined as tumor that invades the adjacent hepatic parenchyma.*

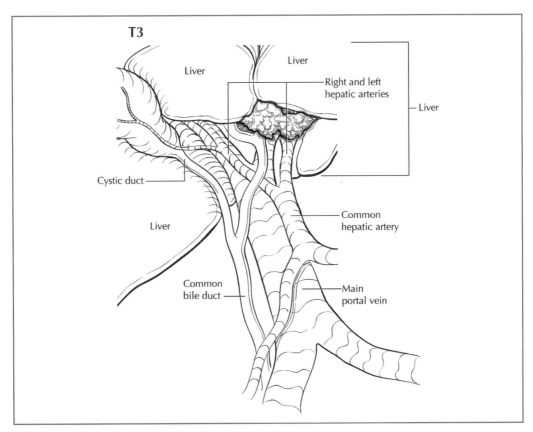

FIGURE 21.5. *T3 tumor invading unilateral branch of hepatic artery.*

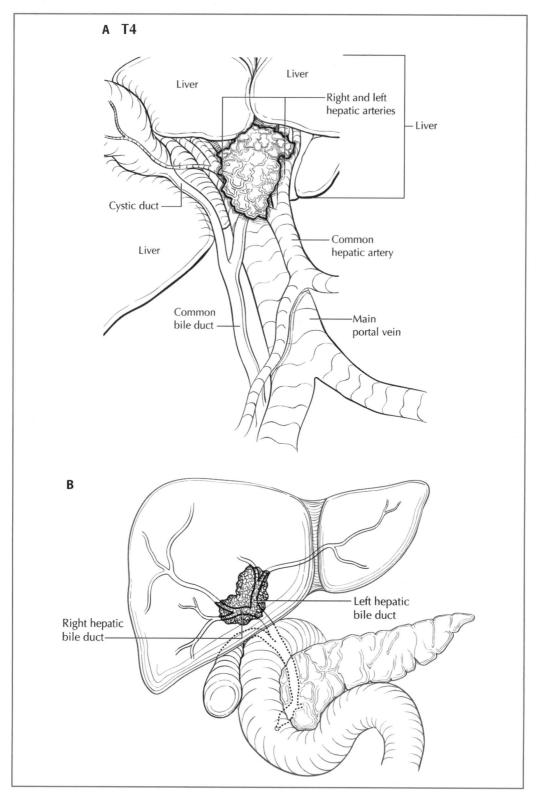

FIGURE 21.6. *T4 is defined as tumor invading main portal vein or its branches bilaterally; or the common hepatic artery or its branches bilaterally; or the second-order biliary radicals bilaterally; or unilateral second-order biliary radicals with contralateral portal vein or hepatic artery involvement. (A) T4 tumor invading bilateral branches of portal vein and hepatic artery. (B) T4 tumor invades the second-order biliary radicals bilaterally.*

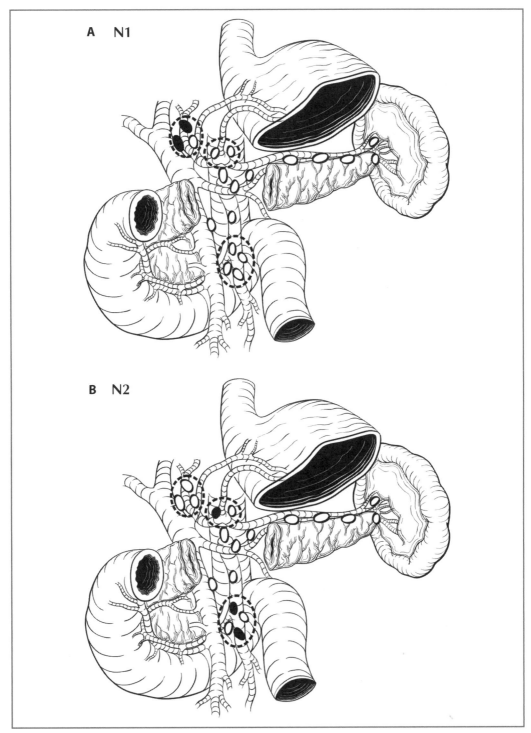

FIGURE 21.7. (A) N1 is defined as metastases to hepatic hilar nodes, including nodes along the cystic duct, common bile duct, hepatic artery and portal vein. (B) N2 is defined as metastases to periaortic, pericaval, superior mesenteric artery, and/or celiac artery lymph nodes.

PROGNOSTIC FACTORS (SITE-SPECIFIC FACTORS)

(Recommended for Collection)

Required for staging	None
Clinically significant	Tumor location
	Papillary variant
	Tumor growth pattern
	Primary sclerosing cholangitis
	CA 19-9

Distal Bile Duct

(Sarcoma and carcinoid tumors are not included)

22

SUMMARY OF CHANGES

- Extrahepatic bile duct was a single chapter in the sixth edition, this has been divided into two chapters for the seventh edition [Perihilar Bile Ducts (see Chap. 21) and Distal Bile Duct]
- Two site-specific prognostic factors, preoperative or pretreatment serum carcinoembryonic antigen and CA19-9, are recommended for collection

ICD-O-3 TOPOGRAPHY CODE

C24.0   Distal bile duct only

ICD-O-3 HISTOLOGY CODE RANGES

8000–8152, 8154–8231, 8243–8245, 8250–8576, 8940–8950, 8980–8981

ANATOMY

Primary Site. The cystic duct connects to the gallbladder and joins the common hepatic duct to form the common bile duct, which passes posterior to the first part of the duodenum, traverses the head of the pancreas, and then enters the second part of the duodenum through the ampulla of Vater (Figure 22.1). Histologically, the bile ducts are lined by a single layer of tall, uniform columnar cells. The mucosa usually forms irregular pleats or small longitudinal folds. The walls of the bile ducts have a layer of subepithelial connective tissue and muscle fibers. It should be noted that the muscle fibers are most prominent in the distal segment of the common bile duct. The extrahepatic ducts lack a serosa but are surrounded by varying amounts of adventitial adipose tissue. Adipose tissue surrounding the fibromuscular wall is not considered part of the bile duct mural anatomy. Invasion of the perimural adventitial adipose tissue is considered extension beyond the bile duct wall.

Regional Lymph Nodes. Accurate tumor staging requires that all lymph nodes that are removed be analyzed. Optimal histologic examination of a pancreaticoduodenectomy specimen should include analysis of a minimum of 12 lymph nodes. If the resected lymph node is negative but this number examined is not met, pN0 should still be assigned. The regional lymph nodes are the same as those resected for cancers of the head of the pancreas; i.e., nodes along the common bile duct, hepatic artery, and back toward the celiac trunk, the posterior and anterior pancreaticoduodenal nodes, and the nodes along the superior mesenteric vein and the right lateral wall of the superior mesenteric artery (Figure 22.2A, B). Anatomic division of regional lymph nodes is not necessary; however, separately submitted lymph nodes should be reported as submitted.

Metastatic Sites. Carcinomas that arise in the distal segment of the common bile duct can spread to the pancreas, duodenum, stomach, colon, or omentum. Distant metastases usually occur late in the course of the disease and are most often found in the liver, lungs, and peritoneum.

C.C. Compton et al. (eds.), *AJCC Cancer Staging Atlas: A Companion to the Seventh Editions of the AJCC Cancer Staging Manual and Handbook*, DOI 10.1007/978-1-4614-2080-4_22, © 2012 American Joint Committee on Cancer

PROGNOSTIC FEATURES

Patients who undergo surgical resection for localized bile duct adenocarcinoma have a median survival of approximately 2 years and a 5-year survival of 20–40% based on extent of disease at the time of surgery. Several adverse prognostic factors based on the pathologic characteristics of the primary tumor have been reported for carcinomas of the extrahepatic bile ducts. These include histologic type, histologic grade, and vascular, lymphatic, and perineural invasion. Papillary carcinomas have a more favorable outcome than other types of carcinoma. High-grade tumors (grades 3–4) have a less favorable outcome than low-grade tumors (grades 1–2). Positive surgical margins have emerged as a very important prognostic factor. Residual tumor classification (R0, R1, R2) should be reported if the margins are involved.

Patients who undergo pancreaticoduodenectomy for localized periampullary adenocarcinoma of nonpancreatic origin have a superior survival duration compared with similarly treated patients who have adenocarcinoma of pancreatic origin (median survival 3–4 years compared with 18–24 months; 5-year survival 35–45% compared with 10–20%). However, as is true of the natural history of pancreatic adenocarcinoma, extent of disease and the histologic characteristics of the primary tumor predict survival duration. Even in patients who undergo a potentially curative resection, the presence of lymph node metastasis, poorly differentiated histology, positive margins of resection, and tumor invasion into the pancreas are associated with a less favorable outcome. Histologic evidence of tumor extension from the ampulla into the pancreatic parenchyma appears to reflect the extent of both local and regional disease. Perineural invasion, ulceration, and high histopathologic grade are also adverse prognostic factors. Although tumor size is not part of the TNM classification, it has prognostic significance.

Preoperative or pretreatment level of two serum markers, carcinoembryonic antigen and CA19-9, may have prognostic significance and their collection is recommended.

DEFINITIONS OF TNM

Primary Tumor (T)

TX	Primary tumor cannot be assessed
T0	No evidence of primary tumor
Tis	Carcinoma in situ
T1	Tumor confined to the bile duct histologically (Figure 22.3)
T2	Tumor invades beyond the wall of the bile duct (Figure 22.4)
T3	Tumor invades the gallbladder, pancreas, duodenum, or other adjacent organs without involvement of the celiac axis, or the superior mesenteric artery (Figure 22.5)
T4	Tumor involves the celiac axis, or the superior mesenteric artery (Figure 22.6)

Regional Lymph Nodes (N)

NX	Regional lymph nodes cannot be assessed
N0	No regional lymph node metastasis
N1	Regional lymph node metastasis (Figure 22.7A, B)

Distant Metastasis (M)

M0	No distant metastasis
M1	Distant metastasis

ANATOMIC STAGE/PROGNOSTIC GROUPS

Stage 0	Tis	N0	M0
Stage IA	T1	N0	M0
Stage IB	T2	N0	M0
Stage IIA	T3	N0	M0
Stage IIB	T1	N1	M0
	T2	N1	M0
	T3	N1	M0
Stage III	T4	Any N	M0
Stage IV	Any T	Any N	M1

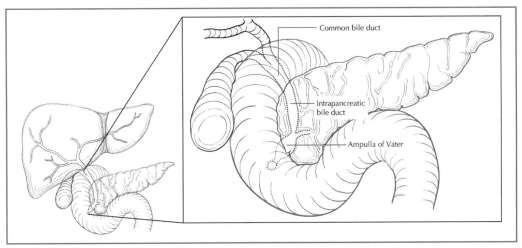

FIGURE 22.1. *Anatomy bile duct cancers. Distal bile duct tumors are defined as those lesions arising between the junction of the cystic duct-common hepatic duct and the ampulla of Vater. Malignant tumors that develop in congenital choledochal cysts and tumor arising in the intrapancreatic portion of the common bile duct are also classified as distal bile duct cancers.*

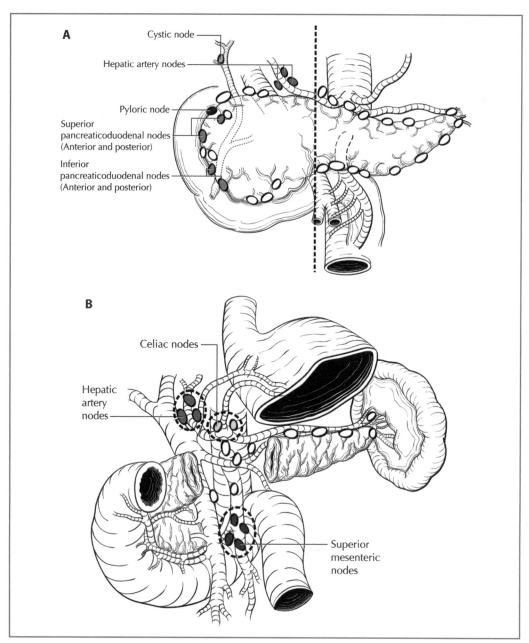

FIGURE 22.2. *(A) Regional lymph nodes for distal bile duct cancers are the same as those for cancers of the head of the pancreas (left of dashed line). (B) Regional lymph nodes of the distal bile duct (anterior view with pancreatic body removed to reveal retroperitoneal vessels and lymph nodes).*

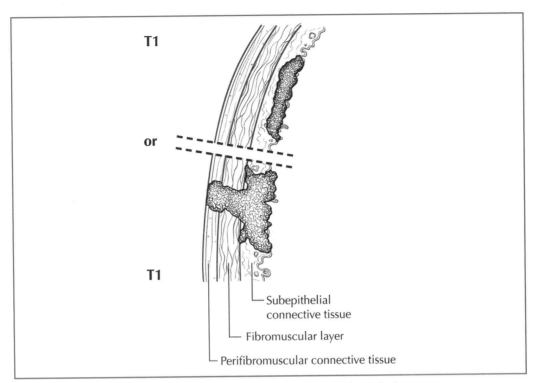

FIGURE 22.3. *Two views of T1: both tumors are confined to the bile duct histologically.*

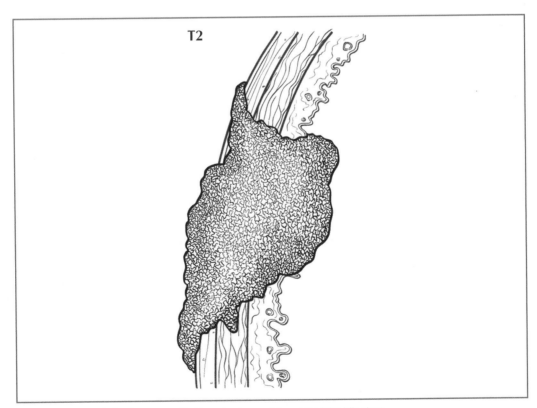

FIGURE 22.4. *T2 is defined as tumor that invades beyond the wall of the bile duct.*

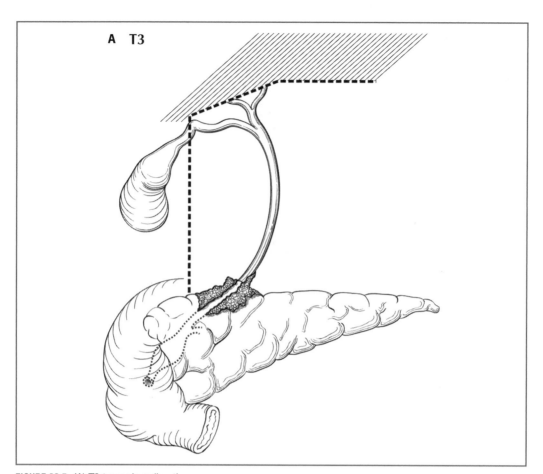

FIGURE 22.5. (A) T3 tumor invading the pancreas.

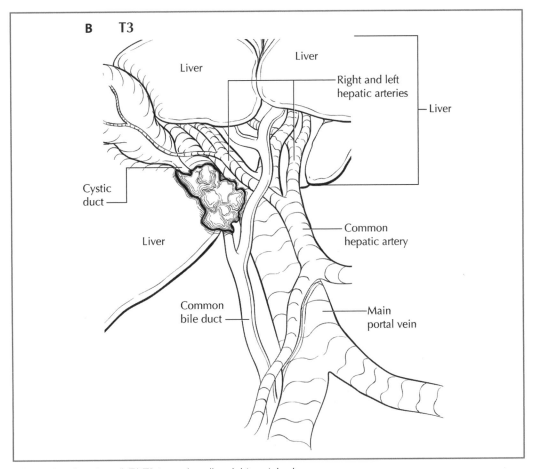

FIGURE 22.5. *(continued) (B) T3 tumor invading right portal vein.*

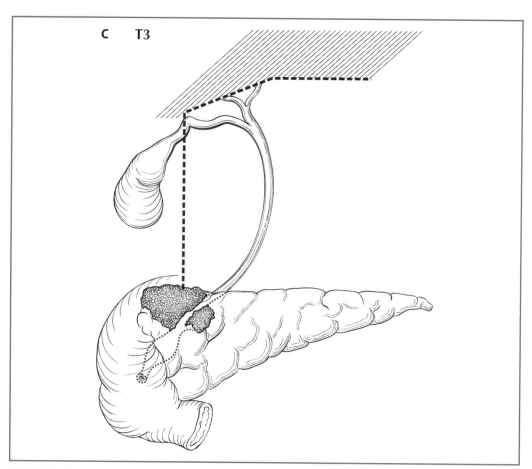

FIGURE 22.5. *(continued) (C) T3 tumor invading duodenum.*

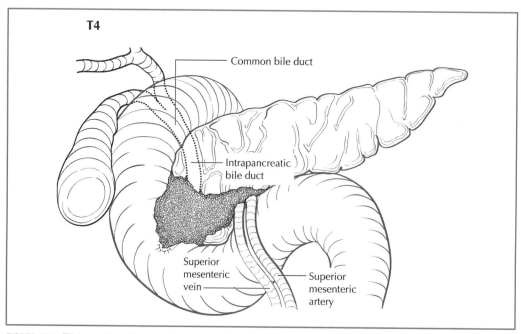

FIGURE 22.6. *T4 tumor invading superior mesenteric artery.*

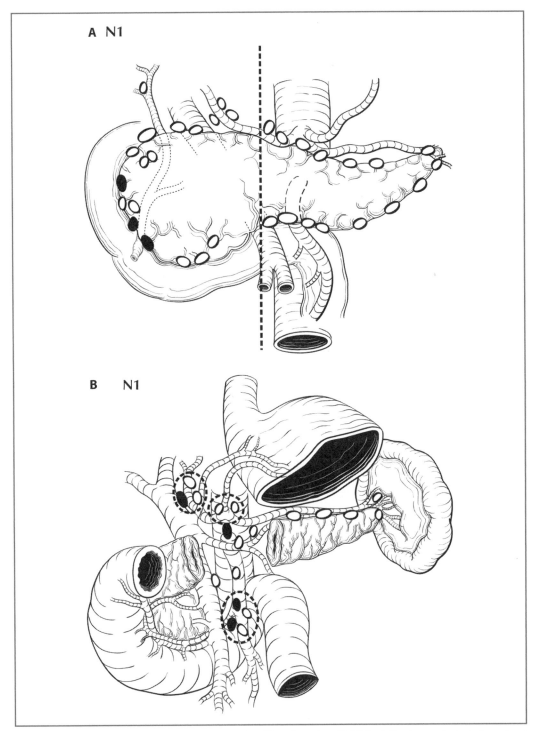

A N1

B N1

FIGURE 22.7. *(A) N1 is defined as metastasis to regional lymph nodes. (B) N1 is defined as metastasis to regional lymph nodes.*

PROGNOSTIC FACTORS (SITE-SPECIFIC FACTORS)

(Recommended for Collection)

Required for staging   None

Clinically significant   Tumor location
                              Carcinoembryonic antigen (CEA)
                              CA 19-9

Ampulla of Vater

23

ICD-O-3 TOPOGRAPHY CODE

C24.1   Ampulla of Vater

ICD-O-3 HISTOLOGY CODE RANGES

8000–8152, 8154–8231, 8243–8245, 8250–8576, 8940–8950, 8980–8981

ANATOMY

Primary Site. The ampulla is a small dilated duct less than 1.5 cm long, formed in most individuals by the union of the terminal segments of the pancreatic and common bile ducts (Figure 23.1). In 42% of individuals, however, the ampulla is the termination of the common duct only, the pancreatic duct having its own entrance into the duodenum adjacent to the ampulla. In these individuals, the ampulla may be difficult to locate or even nonexistent. The ampulla opens into the duodenum, usually on the posterior-medial wall, through a small mucosal elevation, the duodenal papilla, which is also called the papilla of Vater. Although carcinomas can arise either in the ampulla or on the papilla, they most commonly arise near the junction of the mucosa of the ampulla with that of the papilla. It may not be possible to determine the exact site of origin for large tumors. Nearly all cancers that arise in this area are well-differentiated adenocarcinomas.

Regional Lymph Nodes. A rich lymphatic network surrounds the pancreas and periampullary region, and accurate tumor staging requires that all lymph nodes that are removed be analyzed. The regional lymph nodes are the peripancreatic lymph nodes, which also include the lymph nodes along the hepatic artery and portal vein (Figures 23.2, 23.3). Anatomic division of regional lymph nodes is not necessary. However, separately submitted lymph nodes should be reported as submitted. Optimal histologic examination of a pancreaticoduodenectomy specimen should include analysis of a minimum of 12 lymph nodes. If the resected lymph nodes are negative, but this number examined is not met, pN0 should still be assigned. The number of lymph nodes sampled and the number of involved lymph nodes should be recorded.

Metastatic Sites. Tumors of the ampulla may infiltrate adjacent structures, such as the wall of the duodenum, the head of the pancreas, and extrahepatic bile ducts. Metastatic disease is most commonly found in the liver and peritoneum and is less commonly seen in the lungs and pleura.

PROGNOSTIC FEATURES

Patients who undergo pancreaticoduodenectomy for localized periampullary adenocarcinoma of nonpancreatic origin have a superior survival duration compared with similarly treated patients who have adenocarcinoma of pancreatic origin (median survival 3–4 years compared with 18–24 months; 5-year survival 35–45% compared with 10–20%). However, as is true of the natural history of pancreatic adenocarcinoma, extent of disease and the histologic characteristics of the primary tumor predict survival duration. Even in patients who undergo a potentially curative resection, the presence of lymph node metastases, poorly differentiated histology, positive margins of resection, and tumor invasion into the pancreas are associated with a less favorable outcome. Histologic evidence of tumor extension from the ampulla into the pancreatic parenchyma appears to reflect the extent of both local and regional disease. Perineural invasion, ulceration, and high histopathologic grade are also adverse prognostic factors.

Although tumor size is not part of the TNM classification, it has prognostic significance. Tumor involvement (positivity) of resection margins repeatedly has been demonstrated to be an adverse prognostic factor. The residual tumor classification (R1, or R2) should be reported if the margins are involved.

Lymph node metastasis in patients with adenocarcinoma of the ampulla of Vater is consistently reported to be a predictor of poor outcome, although it does not appear to be as powerful a predictor of disease recurrence or short survival duration as for pancreatic carcinoma. The actuarial 5-year survival following potentially curative surgery in node-positive patients with pancreatic adenocarcinoma is 0–5%; in those with ampullary adenocarcinoma it is 15–30%. Extended retroperitoneal lymphadenectomy has not been shown to improve survival. Tumors with papillary histology have a better outcome than non-papillary tumors. Two serum markers may have prognostic significance and should be routinely collected before surgery or treatment begins and may be useful to assess treatment response. These are carcinoembryonic antigen (CEA) and CA19-9.

DEFINITIONS OF TNM

Primary Tumor (T)

TX	Primary tumor cannot be assessed
T0	No evidence of primary tumor
Tis	Carcinoma in situ
T1	Tumor limited to ampulla of Vater or sphincter of Oddi (Figure 23.4)
T2	Tumor invades duodenal wall (Figure 23.5)
T3	Tumor invades pancreas (Figure 23.6)
T4	Tumor invades peripancreatic soft tissues or other adjacent organs or structures other than pancreas (Figure 23.7)

Regional Lymph Nodes (N)

NX	Regional lymph nodes cannot be assessed
N0	No regional lymph node metastasis
N1	Regional lymph node metastasis (Figure 23.8A, B, C)

Distant Metastasis (M)

M0   No distant metastasis

M1   Distant metastasis (Figure 23.9A, B)

ANATOMIC STAGE/PROGNOSTIC GROUPS

Stage 0	Tis	N0	M0
Stage IA	T1	N0	M0
Stage IB	T2	N0	M0
Stage IIA	T3	N0	M0
Stage IIB	T1	N1	M0
	T2	N1	M0
	T3	N1	M0
Stage III	T4	Any N	M0
Stage IV	Any T	Any N	M1

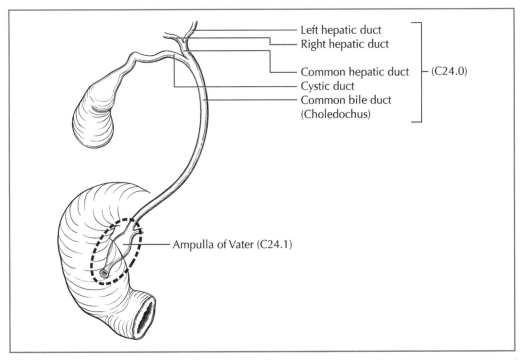

FIGURE 23.1. *Anatomy of the ampulla of Vater, strategically located at the confluence of the pancreatic and common bile ducts.*

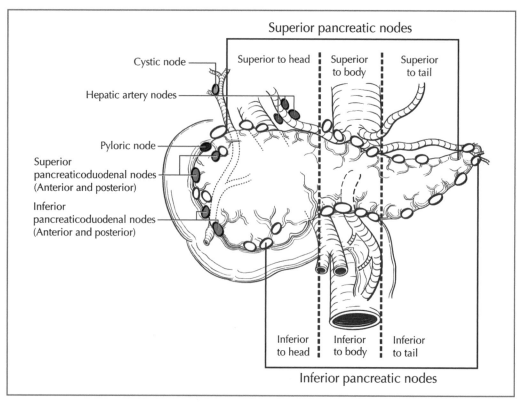

FIGURE 23.2. *Regional lymph nodes of the ampulla of Vater include lymph nodes in the region of the head of the pancreas, and those of the hepatic artery and pyloric regions. Lymph nodes along the distal body and tail of the pancreas are not considered regional lymph nodes for the ampulla of Vater.*

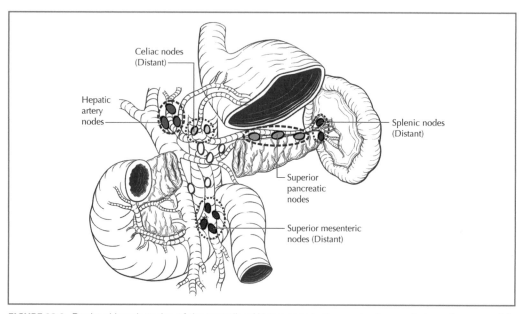

FIGURE 23.3. *Regional lymph nodes of the ampulla of Vater, namely the proximal mesenteric and common bile duct lymph nodes. The celiac axis lymph nodes, the splenic lymph nodes and lymph nodes along the distal body and tail of the pancreas are not considered regional lymph nodes for the ampulla of Vater.*

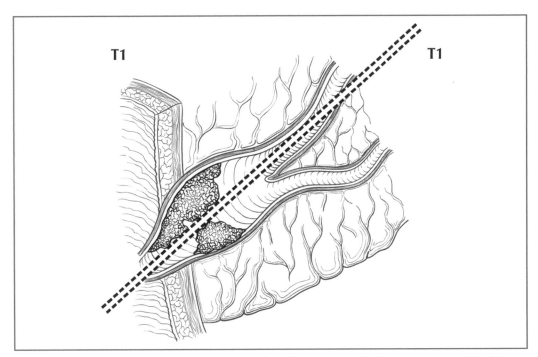

FIGURE 23.4. *Two views of T1: tumor limited to ampulla of Vater (below dotted line) or sphincter of Oddi (tumor shown above dotted line).*

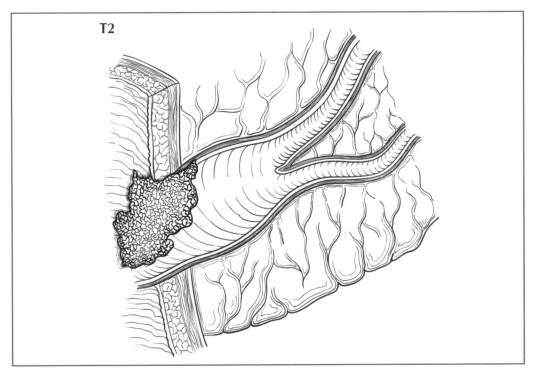

FIGURE 23.5. *T2 is defined as tumor invading duodenal wall.*

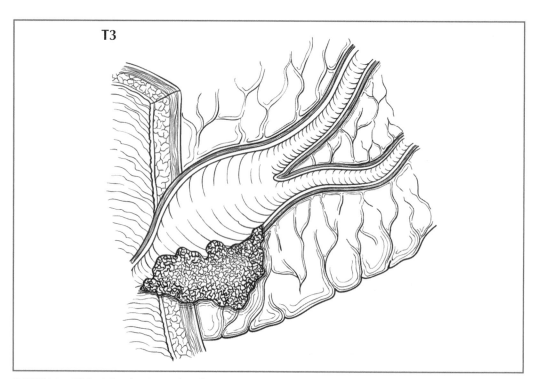

FIGURE 23.6. *T3 is defined as tumor invading pancreas.*

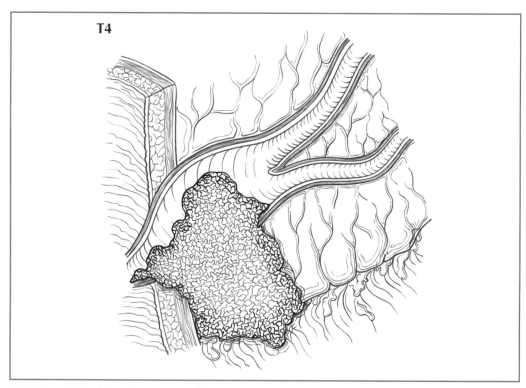

FIGURE 23.7. *T4 is defined as tumor invading peripancreatic soft tissues or other adjacent organs or structures.*

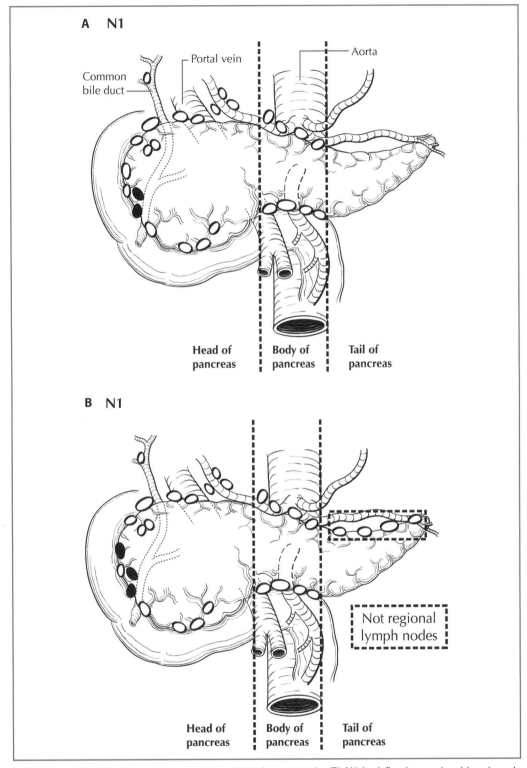

FIGURE 23.8. *(A) N1 is defined as regional lymph node metastasis. (B) N1 is defined as regional lymph node metastasis. This image highlights some nodes that are not considered regional.*

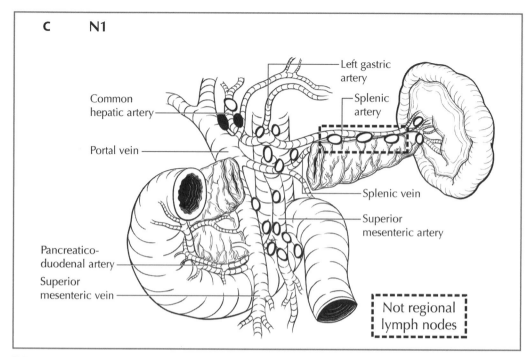

C N1

Left gastric artery

Common hepatic artery

Splenic artery

Portal vein

Splenic vein

Superior mesenteric artery

Pancreatico-duodenal artery

Superior mesenteric vein

Not regional lymph nodes

FIGURE 23.8. *(continued) (C) N1 is defined as regional lymph node metastasis.*

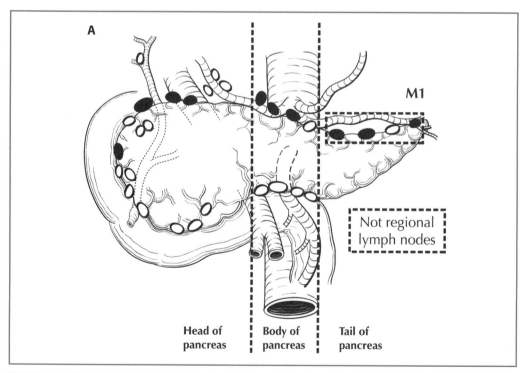

A

M1

Not regional lymph nodes

Head of pancreas **Body of pancreas** **Tail of pancreas**

FIGURE 23.9. *(A) M1 is defined as distant metastasis, here to lymph nodes of the tail of the pancreas.*

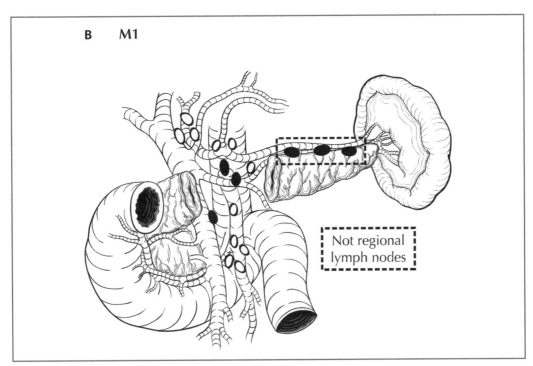

B   M1

Not regional lymph nodes

FIGURE 23.9. *(continued) (B) M1 is defined as distant metastasis, here to lymph nodes of the tail of the pancreas.*

PROGNOSTIC FACTORS (SITE-SPECIFIC FACTORS)	
(Recommended for Collection)	
Required for staging	None
Clinically significant	Preoperative or pretreatment carcinoembryonic antigen (CEA)
	Preoperative or pretreatment CA 19-9

Exocrine and Endocrine Pancreas

24

SUMMARY OF CHANGES

- Pancreatic neuroendocrine tumors (including carcinoid tumors) are now staged by a single pancreatic staging system
- The definition of TNM and the Anatomic Stage/Prognostic Groupings for this chapter have not changed from the sixth edition for exocrine tumors

---

ICD-O-3 TOPOGRAPHY CODES

C25.0   Head of pancreas
C25.1   Body of pancreas
C25.2   Tail of pancreas
C25.3   Pancreatic duct
C25.4   Islets of Langerhans (endocrine pancreas)
C25.7   Other specified parts of pancreas
C25.8   Overlapping lesion of pancreas
C25.9   Pancreas, NOS

ICD-O-3 HISTOLOGY CODE RANGES

8000–8576, 8940–8950, 8971, 8980–8981

ANATOMY

Primary Site. The pancreas is a long, coarsely lobulated gland that lies transversely across the posterior abdomen and extends from the duodenum to the splenic hilum (Figure 24.1). The organ is divided into a head with a small uncinate process, a neck, a body, and a tail. The anterior aspect of the body of the pancreas is in direct contact with the posterior wall of the stomach; posteriorly, the pancreas extends to the inferior vena cava, superior mesenteric vein, splenic vein, and left kidney

Regional Lymph Nodes. A rich lymphatic network surrounds the pancreas, and accurate tumor staging requires that all lymph nodes that are removed be analyzed. Optimal histologic examination of a pancreaticoduodenectomy specimen should include analysis of a minimum of 12 lymph nodes. The standard regional lymph node basins and soft tissues resected for tumors located in the head and neck of the pancreas include lymph nodes along the common bile duct, common hepatic artery, portal vein, posterior and anterior pancreaticoduodenal arcades, and along the superior mesenteric vein and right lateral wall of the superior mesenteric artery (Figures 24.2 and 24.3). For cancers located in body and tail, regional lymph node basins include lymph nodes along the common hepatic artery, celiac axis, splenic artery, and splenic hilum. Anatomic division of regional lymph nodes is not necessary. However, separately submitted lymph nodes should be reported as labeled by the surgeon.

Metastatic Sites. Distant spread is common on presentation and typically involves the liver, peritoneal cavity, and lungs. Metastases to other sites are uncommon.

DEFINITION OF LOCATION

Tumors of the head of the pancreas are those arising to the right of the superior mesenteric–portal vein confluence (Figure 24.1). The uncinate process is part of the pancreatic head. Tumors of the body of the pancreas are defined as those arising between the left edge of the superior mesenteric–portal vein confluence and the left edge of the aorta. Tumors of the tail of the pancreas are those arising to the left of the left edge of the aorta.

Surgical Margins. In pancreaticoduodenectomy specimens, the bile duct, pancreatic duct, and superior mesenteric artery margins should be evaluated grossly and microscopically. The superior mesenteric artery margin has also been termed the retroperitoneal, mesopancreatic, and uncinate margin. In total pancreatectomy specimens, the bile duct and retroperitoneal margins should be assessed. Duodenal (with pylorus-preserving pancreaticoduodenectomy) and gastric (with standard pancreaticoduodenectomy) margins are rarely involved, but their status should be included in the surgical pathology report. Reporting of margins may be facilitated by ensuring documentation of the pertinent margins: (1) Common bile (hepatic) duct, (2) pancreatic neck, (3) superior mesenteric artery margin, (4) other soft tissue margins (i.e., posterior pancreatic), duodenum, and stomach.

Particular attention should be paid to the superior mesenteric artery margin (soft tissue that often contains perineural tissue adjacent to the right lateral wall of the superior mesenteric artery; see Figure 24.4), because most local recurrences arise in the pancreatic bed along this critical margin. The soft tissue between the anterior surface of the inferior vena cava and the posterior aspect of the pancreatic head and duodenum is best referred to as the posterior pancreatic margin (not the retroperitoneal margin). The superior mesenteric artery margin (retroperitoneal or uncinate margin) should be inked as part of the gross evaluation of the specimen; the specimen is then cut perpendicular to the inked margin for histologic analysis. The closest microscopic approach of the tumor to the margin should be recorded in millimeters.

PROGNOSTIC FEATURES

Adenocarcinoma. Patients who undergo surgical resection for localized nonmetastatic adenocarcinoma of the pancreas have a long-term survival rate of approximately 20% and a median survival of 12–20 months. Patients with locally advanced, non-metastatic disease have a median survival of 6–10 months. Patients with metastatic disease have a short survival (3–6 months), the length of which depends on the extent of disease, performance status, and response to systemic therapy.

A number of investigators have examined pathologic factors of the resected tumor (in patients with apparently localized, resectable pancreatic cancer) in an effort to establish reliable prognostic variables associated with decreased survival duration. Metastatic disease in regional lymph nodes, poorly differentiated histology, and increased size of the primary tumor have been associated with decreased survival duration. Perineural invasion, lymphovascular invasion, and elevated CA 19-9 levels are also associated with a poor prognosis. Another prognostic factor of importance in patients who undergo pancreaticoduodenectomy is incomplete resection. Therefore, margin assessment is of major importance in the gross and microscopic evaluation of the pancreaticoduodenectomy specimen. It is important to note that the extent of resection (R0, complete resection with grossly and microscopically negative margins of resection; R1, grossly negative but microscopically positive margins of resection; R2, grossly and microscopically positive margins of resection) is not part of the TNM staging system but is prognostically significant. Retrospective pathologic analysis of archival material does not allow accurate assessment of the margins of resection or of the number of lymph nodes retrieved; this information must be obtained when the specimen is removed and examined in the surgical pathology laboratory. The margin of resection most likely to be positive is the superior mesenteric artery margin along the right lateral border of the superior mesenteric artery. This margin is defined as the soft tissue margin directly adjacent to the proximal 3–4 cm of the superior mesenteric artery and is inked for evaluation of margin status on permanent-section histologic evaluation (see the Pathologic Staging section). Incomplete resection resulting in a grossly positive retroperitoneal margin provides no survival advantage from surgical resection (compared with those who receive chemoradiation and no surgery).

Neuroendocrine Tumors. Patients who undergo surgical resection for localized neuroendocrine carcinoma of the pancreas have a 5-year overall survival rate of approximately 55.4%, significantly better than patients with pancreatic adenocarcinoma. Those who do not undergo resection have 5-year survival of approximately 15.6%. The natural history of these tumors is poorly understood due to their relative rarity, but demonstrated prognostic factors include patient age, distant metastases, tumor functional status, and degree of differentiation. Including these tumors in the pancreatic cancer staging system will allow for improved data collection and subsequent identification of potential prognostic factors. Importantly, the classification of these tumors as "benign" or "malignant" is not consistent, thus all pancreatic neuroendocrine tumors irrespective of being classified as benign or malignant should be staged by this system and reported to cancer registries.

DEFINITIONS OF TNM

Primary Tumor (T)

TX	Primary tumor cannot be assessed
T0	No evidence of primary tumor
Tis	Carcinoma in situ*
T1	Tumor limited to the pancreas, 2 cm or less in greatest dimension (Figure 24.5)
T2	Tumor limited to the pancreas, more than 2 cm in greatest dimension (Figure 24.5)
T3	Tumor extends beyond the pancreas but without involvement of the celiac axis or the superior mesenteric artery (Figure 24.6A, B, C, D)
T4	Tumor involves the celiac axis or the superior mesenteric artery (unresectable primary tumor) (Figure 24.7)

*This also includes the "PanInIII" classification.

Regional Lymph Nodes (N)

NX	Regional lymph nodes cannot be assessed
N0	No regional lymph node metastasis
N1	Regional lymph node metastasis (Figure 24.8A, B, C, D)

Distant Metastasis (M)

M0	No distant metastasis
M1	Distant metastasis

ANATOMIC STAGE/PROGNOSTIC GROUPS

Stage 0	Tis	N0	M0
Stage IA	T1	N0	M0
Stage IB	T2	N0	M0
Stage IIA	T3	N0	M0
Stage IIB	T1	N1	M0
	T2	N1	M0
	T3	N1	M0
Stage III	T4	Any N	M0
Stage IV	Any T	Any N	M1

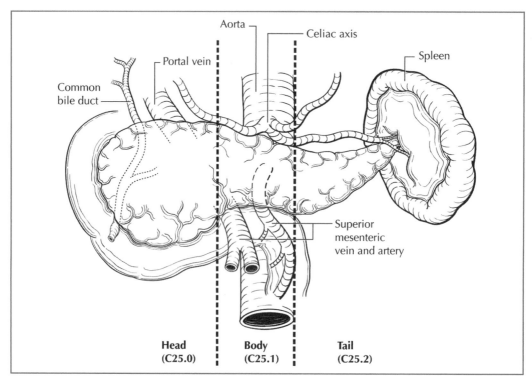

FIGURE 24.1. *Anatomic subsites of the pancreas.*

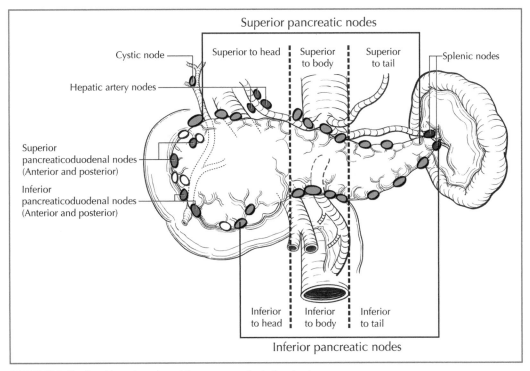

FIGURE 24.2. *Regional lymph nodes of the pancreas (anterior view).*

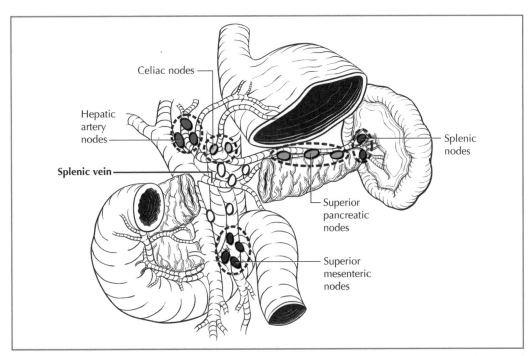

FIGURE 24.3. *Regional lymph nodes of the pancreas (anterior view with pancreatic body removed to reveal retroperitoneal vessels and lymph nodes).*

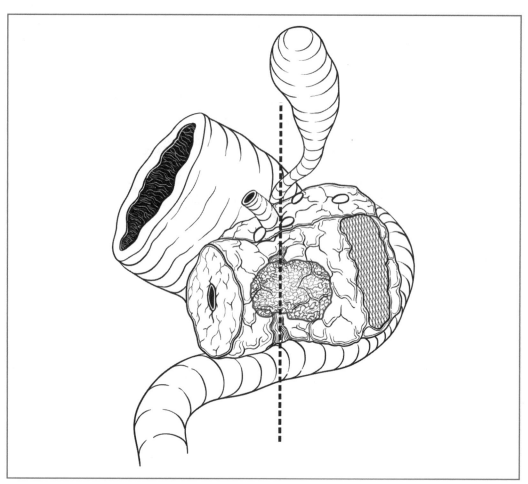

FIGURE 24.4. Posterior view of pancreatic head with dotted line indicating the location of the confluence of the portal and superior mesenteric veins. The hatched area shows the uncinate process margin.

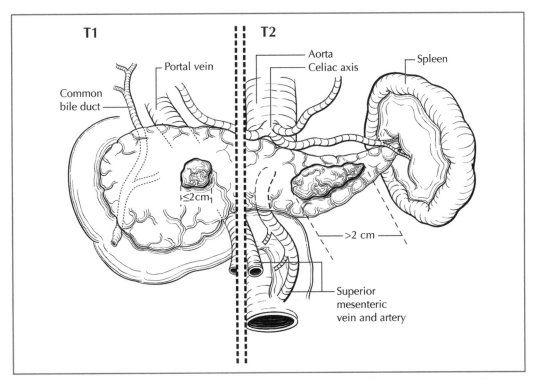

FIGURE 24.5. *T1 (left of dotted line) is defined as tumor limited to the pancreas 2 cm or less in greatest dimension. T2 (right of dotted line) is defined as tumor limited to the pancreas more than 2 cm in greatest dimension.*

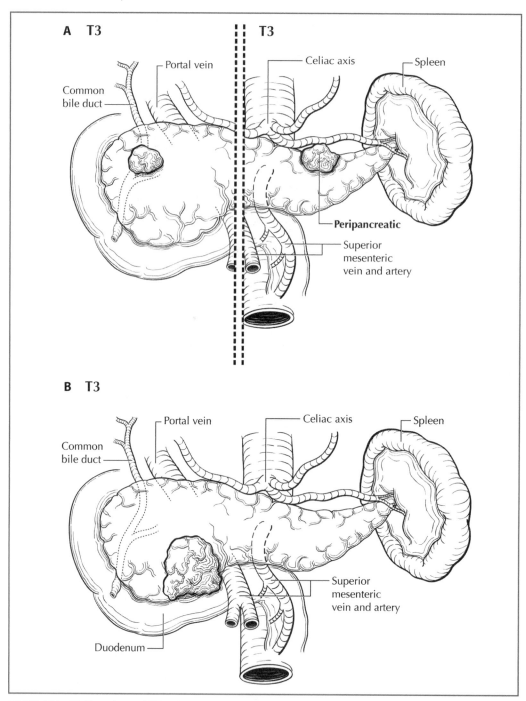

FIGURE 24.6. *(A) Two views of T3, which is defined as tumor that extends beyond the pancreas but without involvement of the celiac axis or the superior mesenteric artery. Left of the dotted line: tumor invades the common bile duct without involving the superior mesenteric artery. Right of the dotted line: tumor invades peripancreatic tissues without involving the celiac axis. (B) T3: tumor invades duodenum without involvement of the superior mesenteric artery.*

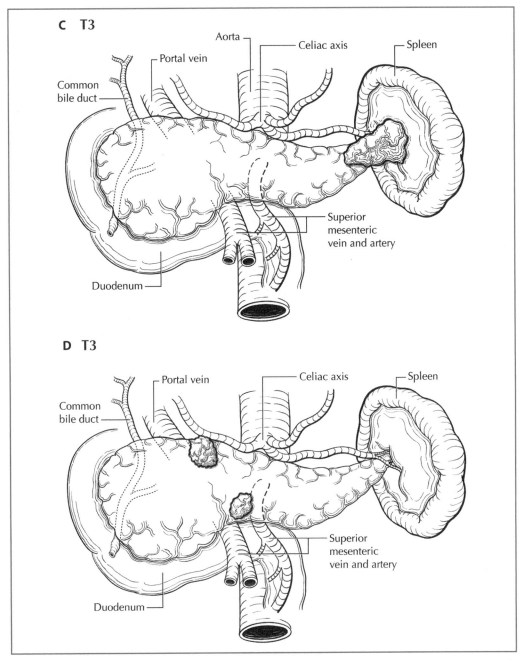

FIGURE 24.6. *(continued) (C) T3: tumor invades spleen without involvement of celiac axis or superior mesenteric artery. (D) Two views of T3 that show tumor abutting but not encasing the superior mesenteric artery and the portal vein.*

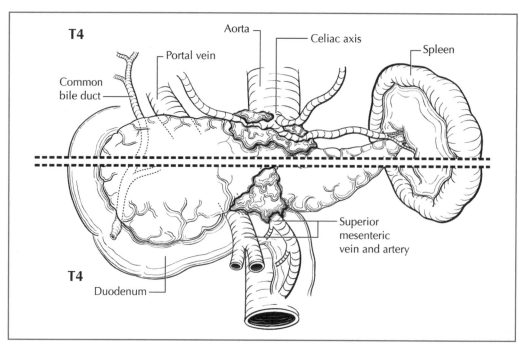

FIGURE 24.7. *Two views of T4, which is defined as tumor encasing the celiac axis (above dotted line) or (below dotted line) the superior mesenteric artery (unresectable primary tumor).*

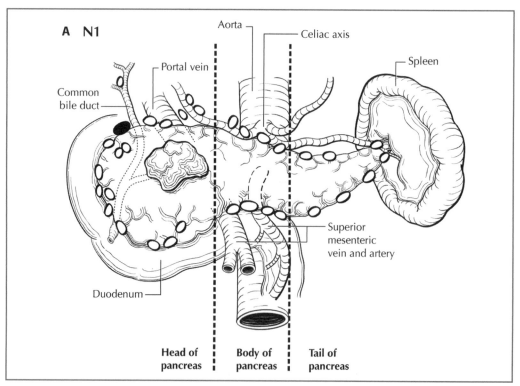

FIGURE 24.8. *N1 is defined as regional lymph node metastasis. (A) Here, the primary tumor and single nodal metastasis are located within the head of pancreas.*

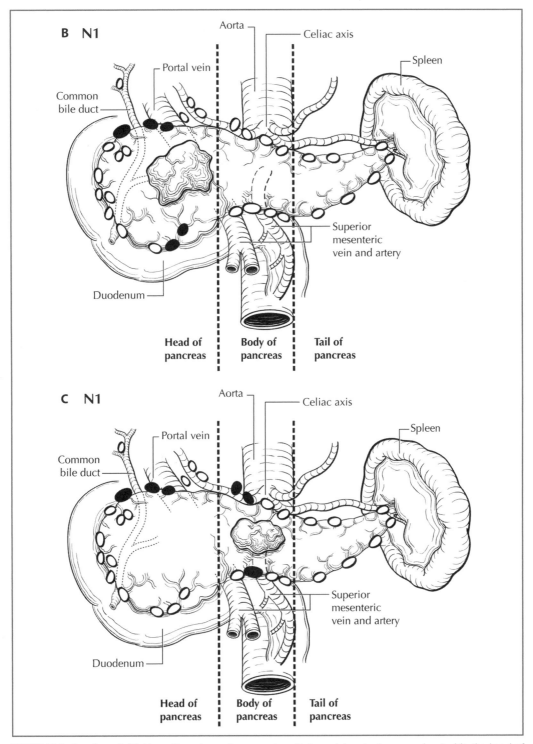

FIGURE 24.8. *(continued) (B) Here, the primary tumor and multiple nodal metastases are located in the head of pancreas. (C) Here, the primary tumor is located in the body of pancreas with multiple nodal metastases in the head and body of pancreas.*

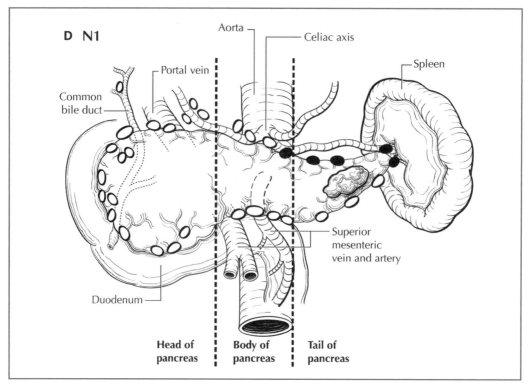

FIGURE 24.8. *(continued) (D) Here, the primary tumor is located in the tail of pancreas with multiple nodal metastases in the tail of pancreas and hilum of spleen.*

PROGNOSTIC FACTORS (SITE-SPECIFIC FACTORS)	
(Recommended for Collection)	
Required for staging	None
Clinically significant	Preoperative CA 19-9
	Preoperative carcinoembryonic antigen (CEA)
	Preoperative plasma chromogranin A level (CgA)
	(endocrine pancreas)
	Mitotic count (endocrine pancreas)

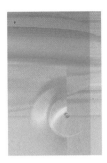

PART IV
Thorax

Lung

(Carcinoid tumors are included. Sarcomas and other rare tumors are not included)

25

SUMMARY OF CHANGES

- This staging system is now recommended for the classification of both non-small cell and small cell lung carcinomas and for carcinoid tumors of the lung
- The T classifications have been redefined:

  - T1 has been subclassified into T1a (≤2 cm in size) and T1b (>2–3 cm in size)
  - T2 has been subclassified into T2a (>3–5 cm in size) and T2b (>5–7 cm in size)
  - T2 (>7 cm in size) has been reclassified as T3
  - Multiple tumor nodules in the same lobe have been reclassified from T4 to T3
  - Multiple tumor nodules in the same lung but a different lobe have been reclassified from M1 to T4

- No changes have been made to the N classification. However, a new international lymph node map defining the anatomical boundaries for lymph node stations has been developed
- The M classifications have been redefined:

  - M1 has been subdivided into M1a and M1b
  - Malignant pleural and pericardial effusions have been reclassified from T4 to M1a
  - Separate tumor nodules in the contralateral lung are considered M1a
  - M1b designates distant metastases

ICD-O-3 TOPOGRAPHY CODES

C34.0 Main bronchus
C34.1 Upper lobe, lung
C34.2 Middle lobe, lung
C34.3 Lower lobe, lung
C34.8 Overlapping lesion of lung
C34.9 Lung, NOS

ICD-O-3 HISTOLOGY CODE RANGES

8000–8576, 8940–8950, 8980–8981

ANATOMY

Primary Site. Carcinomas of the lung arise either from the alveolar lining cells of the pulmonary parenchyma or from the mucosa of the tracheobronchial tree. The trachea, which lies in the middle mediastinum, divides into the right and left main bronchi, which extend into the right and left lungs,

C.C. Compton et al. (eds.), *AJCC Cancer Staging Atlas: A Companion to the Seventh Editions of the AJCC Cancer Staging Manual and Handbook*, DOI 10.1007/978-1-4614-2080-4_25,

respectively. The bronchi then subdivide into the lobar bronchi in the upper, middle, and lower lobes on the right and the upper and lower lobes on the left (Figure 25.1). The lungs are encased in membranes called the visceral pleura. The inside of the chest cavity is lined by a similar membrane called the parietal pleura. The potential space between these two membranes is the pleural space. The mediastinum contains structures in between the lungs, including the heart, thymus, great vessels, lymph nodes, and esophagus.

The great vessels include:

Aorta
Superior vena cava
Inferior vena cava
Main pulmonary artery
Intrapericardial segments of the trunk of the right and left pulmonary artery
Intrapericardial segments of the superior and inferior right and left pulmonary veins

Regional Lymph Nodes. The regional lymph nodes extend from the supraclavicular region to the diaphragm. During the past three decades, two different lymph node maps have been used to describe the regional lymph nodes potentially involved by lung cancers. The first such map, proposed by Naruke and officially endorsed by the Japan Lung Cancer Society, is used primarily in Japan. The second, the Mountain-Dresler modification of the American Thoracic Society (MD-ATS) lymph node map, is used in North America and Europe. The nomenclature for the anatomical locations of lymph nodes differs between these two maps especially with respect to nodes located in the paratracheal, tracheobronchial angle, and subcarinal areas. Recently, the International Association for the Study of Lung Cancer (IASLC) proposed a lymph node map (Figure 25.2) that reconciles the discrepancies between these two previous maps, considers other published proposals, and provides more detailed nomenclature for the anatomical boundaries of lymph nodes stations. Table 25.1 shows the definition for lymph node stations in the IASLC map. The IASLC lymph node map is now the recommended means of describing regional lymph node involvement for lung cancers. Analyses of a large international lung cancer database suggest that for purposes of prognostic classification, it may be appropriate to amalgamate lymph node stations into *zones*. However, the use of lymph node zones for N staging remains investigational and needs to be confirmed by future prospective studies.

There are no evidence-based guidelines regarding the *number* of lymph nodes to be removed at surgery for adequate staging. However, adequate N staging is generally considered to include sampling or dissection of lymph nodes from stations 2R, 4R, 7, 10R, and 11R for right-sided tumors, and stations 5, 6, 7, 10L, and 11L for left-sided tumors. Station 9 lymph nodes should also be evaluated for lower lobe tumors. The more peripheral lymph nodes at stations 12–14 are usually evaluated by the pathologist in lobectomy or pneumonectomy specimens but may be separately removed when sublobar resections (e.g., segmentectomy) are performed. There is evidence to support the recommendation that histological examination of hilar and mediastinal lymphenectomy specimen(s) will ordinarily include 6 or more lymph nodes/stations. Three of these nodes/stations should be mediastinal, including the subcarinal nodes and three from N1 nodes/stations.

Distant Metastatic Sites. The most common metastatic sites are the brain, bones, adrenal glands, contralateral lung, liver, pericardium, kidneys, and subcutaneous tissues. However, virtually any organ can be a site of metastatic disease.

PROGNOSTIC FEATURES

The IASLC lung cancer database, although retrospective, provides the largest published analyses of prognostic factors in both NSCLC and SCLC. Potentially useful prognostic variables for lung cancer survival that were considered included TNM stage; tumor histology; patient age, sex, and performance status; various laboratory values; and molecular markers.

Clinical Factors. Analyses of the IASLC lung cancer database revealed that in addition to clinical stage, performance status and patient age and sex (male gender being associated with a worse survival) were important prognostic factors for both NSCLC and SCLC. In NSCLC, squamous cell carcinoma was associated with a better prognosis for patients with Stage III disease but not in other tumor stages. In advanced NSCLC (Stages IIIB/IV), some laboratory tests (principally white blood cells and hypercalcemia) were also important prognostic variables. In SCLC, albumin was an independent biological factor. Analyses that incorporate these factors along with overall TNM stage stratify both NSCLC and SCLC patients into 4 groups that have distinctly different overall survivals. In addition to these, a recent study of 455 patients with completely resected pathologic Stage I NSCLC suggests that high preoperative serum carcinoembryonic antigen (CEA) levels identify patients who have a poor prognosis, especially if those levels also remain elevated postoperatively. Other retrospective studies report that the intensity of hypermetabolism on FDG-PET scan is correlated with outcome in NSCLC patients managed surgically. Additional prospective studies are needed to validate these findings and to determine whether FDG-PET is prognostic across all lung cancer stages and histologies.

In the lung, arterioles are frequently invaded by cancers. For this reason, the V classification is applicable to indicate vascular invasion, whether venous or arteriolar.

Biological Factors. In recent years, multiple biological and molecular markers have been found to have prognostic value for survival in lung cancer, particularly NSCLC. Although some molecular abnormalities, for example EGFR and K-ras mutations, are now being used to stratify patients for treatment, none is yet routinely used for lung cancer staging.

Primary Tumor (T)

TX	Primary tumor cannot be assessed, or tumor proven by the presence of malignant cells in sputum or bronchial washings but not visualized by imaging or bronchoscopy
T0	No evidence of primary tumor
Tis	Carcinoma in situ
T1	Tumor 3 cm or less in greatest dimension, surrounded by lung or visceral pleura, without bronchoscopic evidence of invasion more proximal than the lobar bronchus (i.e., not in the main bronchus)*
T1a	Tumor 2 cm or less in greatest dimension (Figure 25.3)
T1b	Tumor more than 2 cm but 3 cm or less in greatest dimension (Figure 25.3)
T2	Tumor more than 3 cm but 7 cm or less or tumor with any of the following features (T2 tumors with these features are classified T2a if 5 cm or less); Involves main bronchus, 2 cm or more distal to the carina; Invades visceral pleura (PL1 or PL2); Associated with atelectasis or obstructive pneumonitis that extends to the hilar region but does not involve the entire lung
T2a	Tumor more than 3 cm but 5 cm or less in greatest dimension (Figure 25.4)
T2b	Tumor more than 5 cm but 7 cm or less in greatest dimension (Figure 25.4)
T3	Tumor more than 7 cm or one that directly invades any of the following: parietal pleural (PL3), chest wall (including superior sulcus tumors), diaphragm, phrenic nerve, mediastinal pleura, parietal pericardium; or tumor in the main bronchus (less than 2 cm distal to the carina* but without involvement of the carina; or associated atelectasis or obstructive pneumonitis of the entire lung or separate tumor nodule(s) in the same lobe (Figures 25.5 and 25.6A)
T4	Tumor of any size that invades any of the following: mediastinum, heart, great vessels, trachea, recurrent laryngeal nerve, esophagus, vertebral body, carina, separate tumor nodule(s) in a different ipsilateral lobe (Figure 25.6A, B, C, D)

*The uncommon superficial spreading tumor of any size with its invasive component limited to the bronchial wall, which may extend proximally to the main bronchus, is also classified as T1a.

Regional Lymph Nodes (N)

NX	Regional lymph nodes cannot be assessed
N0	No regional lymph node metastases
N1	Metastasis in ipsilateral peribronchial and/or ipsilateral hilar lymph nodes and intrapulmonary nodes, including involvement by direct extension (Figure 25.7)
N2	Metastasis in ipsilateral mediastinal and/or subcarinal lymph node(s) (Figure 25.8)
N3	Metastasis in contralateral mediastinal, contralateral hilar, ipsilateral or contralateral scalene, or supraclavicular lymph node(s) (Figure 25.9)

Distant Metastasis (M)

M0	No distant metastasis
M1	Distant metastasis
M1a	Separate tumor nodule(s) in a contralateral lobe tumor with pleural nodules or malignant pleural (or pericardial) effusion* (Figures 25.9 and 25.10)
M1b	Distant metastasis (in extrathoracic organs)

From Goldstraw P, Crowley J, Chansky K, et al.: The IASLC Lung Cancer Staging Project: Proposals for the revision of the TNM stage groupings in the forthcoming (seventh) edition of the TNM classification of malignant tumours. *J Thorac Oncol* 2:706–714, 2007, with permission.

*Most pleural (and pericardial) effusions with lung cancer are due to tumor. In a few patients, however, multiple cytopathologic examinations of pleural (pericardial) fluid are negative for tumor, and the fluid is nonbloody and is not an exudate. Where these elements and clinical judgment dictate that the effusion is not related to the tumor, the effusion should be excluded as a staging element and the patient should be classified as M0.

ANATOMIC STAGE/PROGNOSTIC GROUPS

Occult carcinoma	TX	N0	M0
Stage 0	Tis	N0	M0
Stage IA	T1a	N0	M0
	T1b	N0	M0
Stage IB	T2a	N0	M0
Stage IIA	T2b	N0	M0
	T1a	N1	M0
	T1b	N1	M0
	T2a	N1	M0
Stage IIB	T2b	N1	M0
	T3	N0	M0
Stage IIIA	T1a	N2	M0
	T1b	N2	M0
	T2a	N2	M0
	T2b	N2	M0
	T3	N1	M0
	T3	N2	M0
	T4	N0	M0
	T4	N1	M0
Stage IIIB	T1a	N3	M0
	T1b	N3	M0
	T2a	N3	M0
	T2b	N3	M0
	T3	N3	M0
	T4	N2	M0
	T4	N3	M0
Stage IV	Any T	Any N	M1a
	Any T	Any N	M1b

ADDITIONAL NOTES REGARDING TNM DESCRIPTORS

The T category is defined by the size and extent of the primary tumor. Definitions have changed from the prior edition of TNM. For the T2 category, visceral pleural invasion is defined as invasion to the surface of the visceral pleura or invasion beyond the elastic layer. On the basis of a review of published literature, the IASLC Staging Committee recommends that elastic stains can be used in cases where it is difficult to identify invasion of the elastic layer by hematoxylin and eosin (H&E) stains. A tumor that falls short of completely traversing the elastic layer is defined as PL0. A tumor that extends through the elastic layer is defined as PL1 and one that extends to the surface of the visceral pleural as PL2. Either PL1 or PL2 status allows classification of the primary tumor as T2. Extension of the tumor to the parietal pleura is defined as PL3 and categorizes the primary tumor as T3. Direct tumor invasion into an adjacent ipsilateral lobe (i.e., invasion across a fissure) is classified as T2a (Figure 25.11).

Multiple tumors may be considered to be synchronous primaries if they are of different histological cell types. When multiple tumors are of the same cell type, they should only be considered to be synchronous primary tumors if in the opinion of the pathologist, based on features such as associated carcinoma in situ or differences in morphology, immunohistochemistry, and/or molecular studies, they represent differing subtypes of the same histopathological cell type, and also have no evidence of mediastinal nodal metastases or of nodal metastases within a common nodal drainage. Synchronous primary tumors are most commonly encountered when dealing with either bronchioloalveolar carcinomas or adenocarcinomas of mixed subtype with a bronchioloalveolar component. Multiple synchronous primary tumors should be staged separately. The highest T category and stage of disease should be assigned and the multiplicity or the number of tumors should be indicated in parenthesis, e.g., T2(m) or T2(5).

Vocal cord paralysis (resulting from involvement of the recurrent branch of the vagus nerve), superior vena caval obstruction, or compression of the trachea or esophagus may be related to direct extension of the primary tumor or to lymph node involvement. The treatment options and prognosis associated with this direct extension of the primary tumor fall within the T4N0-1 (Stage IIIA) category; therefore, a classification of T4 is recommended. If the primary tumor is peripheral, vocal cord paralysis is usually related to the presence of N2 disease and should be classified as such.

The designation of "Pancoast" tumors relates to the symptom complex or syndrome caused by a tumor arising in the superior sulcus of the lung that involves the inferior branches of the brachial plexus (C8 and/or T1) and, in some cases, the stellate ganglion. Some superior sulcus tumors are more anteriorly located and cause fewer neurological symptoms but encase the subclavian vessels. The extent of disease varies in these tumors, and they should be classified according to the established rules. If there is evidence of invasion of the vertebral body or spinal canal, encasement of the subclavian vessels, or unequivocal involvement of the superior branches of the brachial plexus (C8 or above), the tumor is then classified as T4. If no criteria for T4 disease pertain, the tumor is classified as T3.

Tumors directly invading the diaphragm in the absence of other signs of locally advanced disease are rare, constituting less than 1% of all cases of potentially resectable NSCLC. These tumors are considered to be T3, but appear to have a poor prognosis, even after complete resection and in the absence of N2 disease. The classification of such tumors may need to be reevaluated in the future as more survival data become available.

The term *satellite nodules* was included in the 6th edition of the *AJCC Cancer Staging Manual*. It was defined as additional small nodules in the same lobe as the primary tumor but anatomically distinct from it that could be recognized grossly. Additional small nodules that could be identified only microscopically were not included in this definition. The term *satellite nodules* is being deleted from this edition of the *Staging Manual* because it is confusing, has no scientific basis, and is at variance with the UICC Staging Manual. The term *additional tumor nodules* should be used to describe grossly recognizable multiple carcinomas in the same lobe. Such nodules are classified as T3. This definition does not apply to one grossly detected tumor associated with multiple separate microscopic foci.

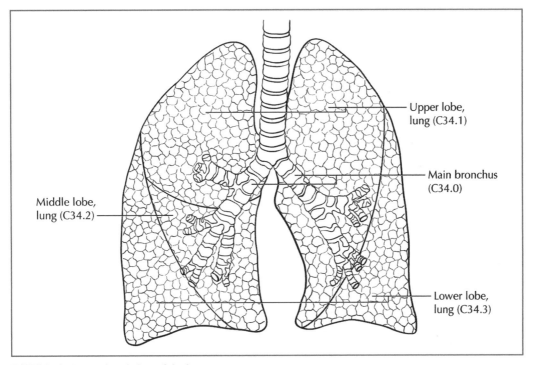

FIGURE 25.1. *Anatomic subsites of the lung.*

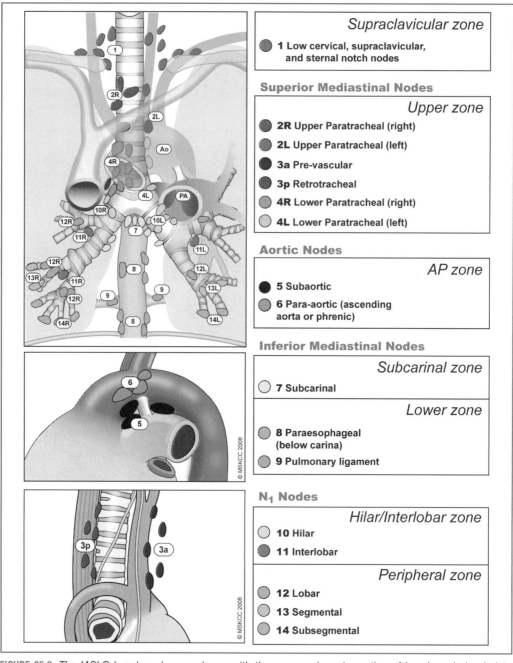

FIGURE 25.2. *The IASLC lymph node map shown with the proposed amalgamation of lymph node levels into zones. (Reprinted with permission courtesy of the International Association for the Study of Lung Cancer. Copyright © 2009 Memorial Sloan-Kettering Cancer Center).*

TABLE 25.1. *Definition for lymph node stations in IASLC Map*

1 Low cervical, supraclavicular and sternal notch nodes

Upper border: lower margin of cricoid cartilage

Lower border: clavicles bilaterally and, in the midline, the upper border of the manubrium, 1R designates right-sided nodes, 1L, left-sided nodes in this region

For lymph node station 1, the midline of the trachea serves as the border between 1R and 1L

2 Upper paratracheal nodes

2R: Upper border: apex of the right lung and pleural space, and in the midline, the upper border of the manubrium

Lower border: intersection of caudal margin of innominate vein with the trachea

As for lymph node station 4R, 2R includes nodes extending to the left lateral border of the trachea

2L: Upper border: apex of the left lung and pleural space, and in the midline, the upper border of the manubrium

Lower border: superior border of the aortic arch

3 Pre-vascular and retrotracheal nodes

3a: Prevascular

On the right:

Upper border: apex of chest

Lower border: level of carina

Anterior border: posterior aspect of sternum

Posterior border: anterior border of superior vena cava

On the left:

Upper border: apex of chest

Lower border: level of carina

Anterior border: posterior aspect of sternum

Posterior border: left carotid artery

3p: Retrotracheal

Upper border: apex of chest

Lower border: carina

4 Lower paratracheal nodes

4R: includes right paratracheal nodes, and pretracheal nodes extending to the left lateral border of trachea

Upper border: intersection of caudal margin of innominate vein with the trachea

Lower border: lower border of azygos vein

4L: includes nodes to the left of the left lateral border of the trachea, medial to the ligamentum arteriosum

Upper border: upper margin of the aortic arch

Lower border: upper rim of the left main pulmonary artery

5 Subaortic (aorto-pulmonary window)

Subaortic lymph nodes lateral to the ligamentum arteriosum

Upper border: the lower border of the aortic arch

Lower border: upper rim of the left main pulmonary artery

(continued)

TABLE 25.1. *(continued)*

6 Para-aortic nodes (ascending aorta or phrenic)

Lymph nodes anterior and lateral to the ascending aorta and aortic arch

Upper border: a line tangential to the upper border of the aortic arch

Lower border: the lower border of the aortic arch

7 Subcarinal nodes

Upper border: the carina of the trachea

Lower border the upper border of the lower lobe bronchus on the left; the lower border of the bronchus intermedius on the right

8 Para-esophageal nodes (below carina)

Nodes lying adjacent to the wall of the esophagus and to the right or left of the midline, excluding subcarinal nodes

Upper border: the upper border of the lower lobe bronchus on the left the lower border of the bronchus intermedius on the right

Lower border the diaphragm

9 Pulmonary ligament nodes

Nodes lying within the pulmonary ligament

Upper border: the inferior pulmonary vein

Lower border: the diaphragm

10 Hilar nodes

Includes nodes immediately adjacent to the mainstem bronchus and hilar vessels including the proximal portions of the pulmonary veins and main pulmonary artery

Upper border: the lower rim of the azygos vein on the right; upper rim of the pulmonary artery on the left

Lower border: interlobar region bilaterally

11 Interlobar nodes

Between the origin of the lobar bronchi

11s: between the upper lobe bronchus and bronchus intermedius on the right

11i: between the middle and lower lobe bronchi on the right

12 Lobar nodes

Adjacent to the lobar bronchi

13 Segmental nodes

Adjacent to the segmental bronchi

14 Subsegmental nodes

Adjacent to the subsegmental bronchi

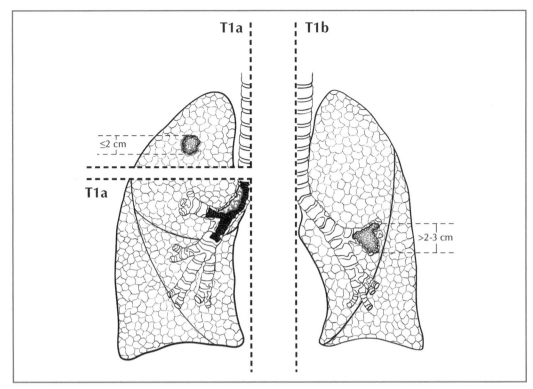

FIGURE 25.3. *T1 is defined as a tumor 3 cm or less in greatest dimension, surrounded by lung or visceral pleura, without bronchoscopic evidence of invasion more proximal than the lobar bronchus (i.e., not in the main bronchus). T1a is defined as a tumor 2 cm or less in greatest dimension (upper left). T1a is also defined as a superficial spreading tumor of any size with its invasive component limited to the bronchial wall, which may extend proximally to the main bronchus (lower left). T1b is defined as a tumor more than 2 cm but 3 cm or less in greatest dimension (right).*

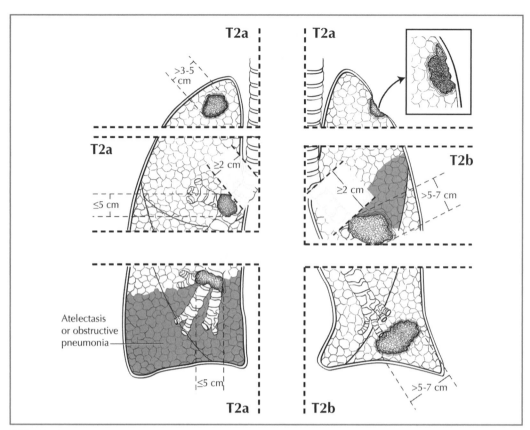

FIGURE 25.4. *T2 is defined as a tumor more than 3 cm but 7 cm or less or tumor with any of the following features (T2 tumors with these features are classified T2a if 5 cm or less); involves main bronchus, 2 cm or more distal to the carina (middle left and middle right); invades visceral pleura (PL1 or PL2) (upper right); associated with atelectasis or obstructive pneumonitis that extends to the hilar region but does not involve the entire lung (bottom left). T2a is defined as tumor more than 3 cm but 5 cm or less in greatest dimension (upper left). T2b is defined as tumor more than 5 cm but 7 cm or less in greatest dimension (bottom right).*

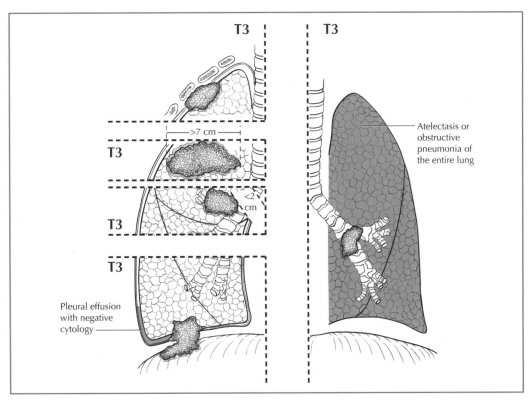

FIGURE 25.5. *T3 is defined as a tumor more than 7 cm (upper middle left) or one that directly invades any of the following: parietal pleural (PL3), chest wall (including superior sulcus tumors) (upper left), diaphragm (lower left), phrenic nerve, mediastinal pleura, parietal pericardium; or tumor in the main bronchus (less than 2 cm distal to the carina but without involvement of the carina) (lower middle left); or associated atelectasis or obstructive pneumonitis of the entire lung (right) or separate tumor nodule(s) in the same lobe.*

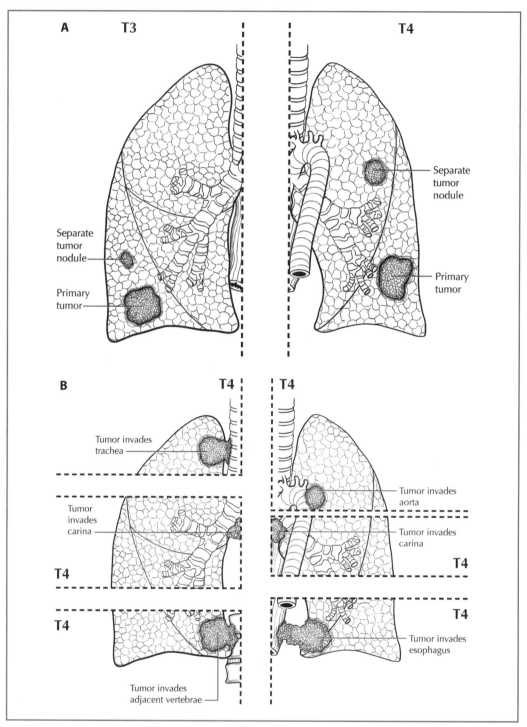

FIGURE 25.6. *(A) T3 includes separate tumor nodule(s) in the same lobe. T4 includes separate tumor nodule(s) in a different ipsilateral lobe. (B) T4 is defined as tumor of any size that invades any of the following: mediastinum, heart, great vessels (upper right), trachea (upper left), recurrent laryngeal nerve, esophagus (lower right), vertebral body (lower left), carina (middle left and right), separate tumor nodule(s) in a different ipsilateral lobe.*

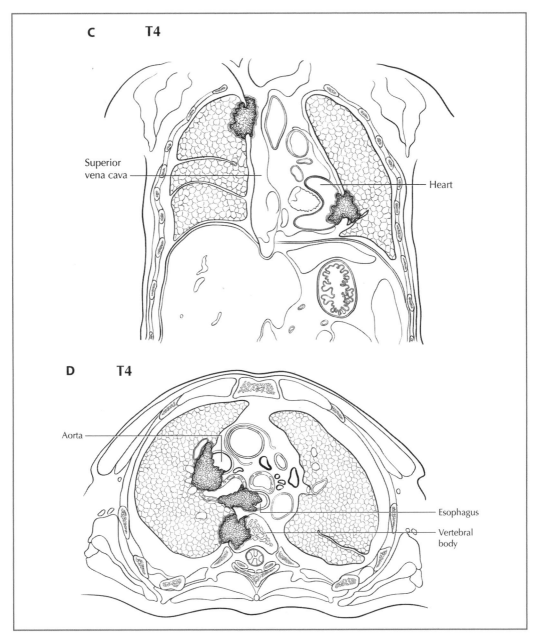

FIGURE 25.6. *(continued) (C) T4 includes tumor invasion of the superior vena cava and heart. (D) T4 includes tumor invasion of the aorta, esophagus, and vertebral body.*

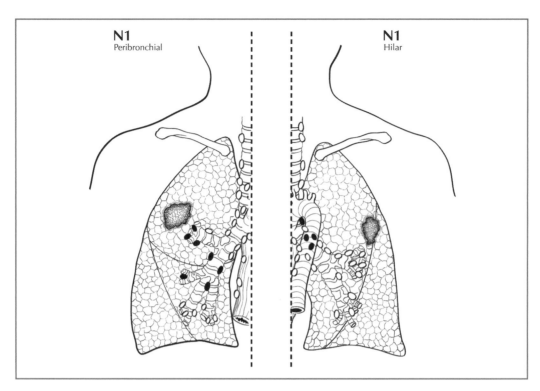

FIGURE 25.7. *N1 is defined as metastasis in ipsilateral peribronchial (left side of diagram) and/or ipsilateral hilar lymph nodes (right side of diagram) and intrapulmonary nodes, including involvement by direct extension of the primary tumor.*

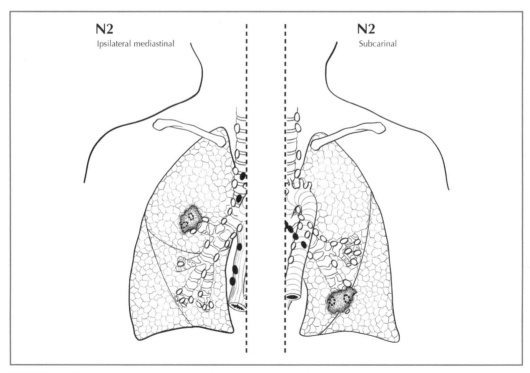

FIGURE 25.8. *N2 is defined as metastasis in ipsilateral mediastinal (left side of diagram) and/or subcarinal lymph node(s) (right side of diagram).*

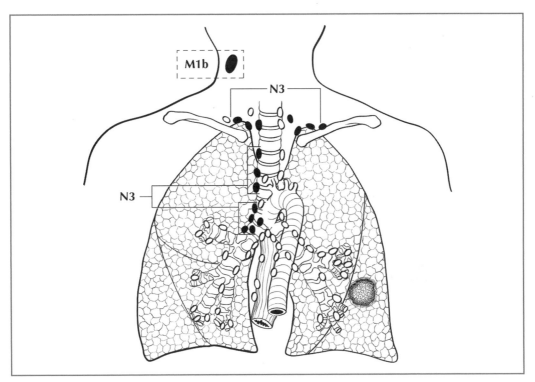

FIGURE 25.9. *N3 is defined as metastasis in contralateral mediastinal, contralateral hilar, ipsilateral or contralateral scalene, or supraclavicular lymph node(s), whereas M1b is defined as distant metastasis (in extrathoracic organs), and this would include distant lymph nodes.*

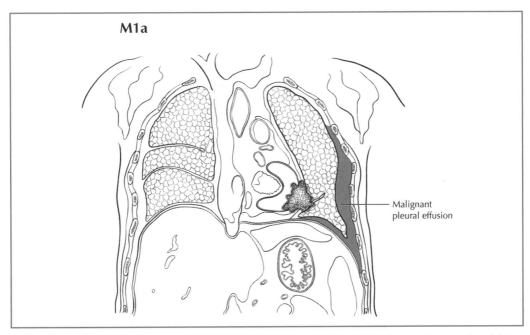

FIGURE 25.10. *M1a is defined as separate tumor nodule(s) in a contralateral lobe; tumor with pleural nodules or malignant pleural (or pericardial) effusion. This is an image of tumor with malignant pleural effusion.*

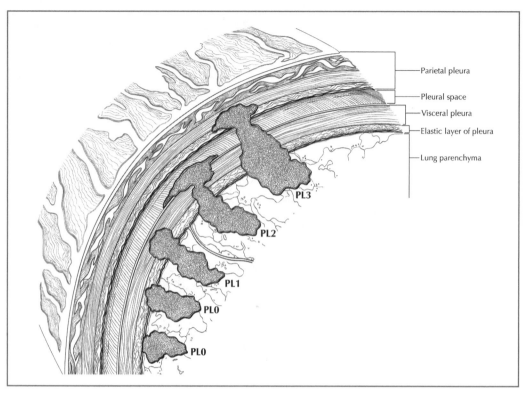

FIGURE 25.11. *A tumor that falls short of completely traversing the elastic layer of the visceral pleura is defined as PL0. A tumor that extends through the elastic layer is defined as PL1 and one that extends to the surface of the visceral pleural as PL2. Extension of the tumor to the parietal pleura is defined as PL3.*

PROGNOSTIC FACTORS (SITE-SPECIFIC FACTORS)	
(Recommended for Collection)	
Required for staging	None
Clinically significant	Pleural/elastic layer invasion (based on H&E and elastic stains)
	Separate tumor nodules
	Vascular invasion – V classification (venous or arteriolar)

Pleural Mesothelioma

26

ICD-O-3 TOPOGRAPHY CODE

C38.4   Pleura, NOS

ICD-O-3 HISTOLOGY CODE RANGES

9050–9053

ANATOMY

Primary Site. The mesothelium covers the external surface of the lungs and the inside of the chest wall (Figure 26.1). It is usually composed of flat tightly connected cells no more than one layer thick.

Regional Lymph Nodes. The regional lymph nodes include (Figure 26.2):

Intrathoracic
Scalene
Supraclavicular
Internal mammary
Peridiaphragmatic

The regional lymph node map and nomenclature adopted for the mesothelioma staging system is identical to that used for lung cancer. See Chap. 25 for a detailed list of intrathoracic lymph nodes. For pN, histologic examinvation of a mediastinal lymphadenectomy or lymph node sampling specimen will ordinarily include regional nodes taken from the ipsilateral N1 and N2 nodal stations. In addition, mesotheliomas often metastasize to lymph nodes not involved by lung cancers, most commonly the internal mammary and peridiaphragmatic nodes. These latter two regions also are classified as N2 nodal stations. Contralateral mediastinal and supraclavicular nodes may be available if a mediastinoscopy or node biopsy is also performed. If involved by metastatic disease these would be staged as N3.

Distant Metastatic Sites. Advanced malignant pleural mesotheliomas often metastasize widely to uncommon sites, including retroperitoneal lymph nodes, the brain, and spine, or even to organs such as the thyroid or prostate. However, the most frequent sites of metastatic disease are the peritoneum, contralateral pleura, and lung.

PROGNOSTIC FEATURES

Several factors are reported to have prognostic significance in patients with malignant pleural mesothelioma. Histological subtype and patient performance status are consistently reported as prognostically significant. Patient age, gender, symptoms (absence or presence of chest pain), and history of asbestos exposure are also cited in various studies as potential prognostic factors. The intensity of primary tumor hypermetabolism on FDG-PET scan as measured by the standardized uptake value (SUV) has also been reported to correlate with overall survival, with tumor SUV greater than 10 being associated with a worse outcome. Further analysis of these various factors in a large multicenter database is needed to determine their true prognostic validity.

DEFINITIONS OF TNM

IMIG Staging System for Diffuse Malignant Pleural Mesothelioma

Primary Tumor (T)

TX   Primary tumor cannot be assessed

T0   No evidence of primary tumor

T1   Tumor limited to the ipsilateral parietal pleura with or without mediastinal pleura and with or without diaphragmatic pleural involvement

T1a   No involvement of the visceral pleura (Figure 26.3)

T1b   Tumor also involving the visceral pleura (Figure 26.3)

T2   Tumor involving each of the ipsilateral pleural surfaces (parietal, mediastinal, diaphragmatic, and visceral pleura) with at least one of the following (Figure 26.4):

      Involvement of diaphragmatic muscle

      Extension of tumor from visceral pleura into the underlying pulmonary parenchyma

T3   Locally advanced but potentially resectable tumor

      Tumor involving all of the ipsilateral pleural surfaces (parietal, mediastinal, diaphragmatic, and visceral pleura) with at least one of the following (Figure 26.5):

      Involvement of the endothoracic fascia

      Extension into the mediastinal fat

      Solitary, completely resectable focus of tumor extending into the soft tissues of the chest wall

      Nontransmural involvement of the pericardium

T4   Locally advanced technically unresectable tumor

      Tumor involving all of the ipsilateral pleural surfaces (parietal, mediastinal, diaphragmatic, and visceral pleura) with at least one of the following (Figure 26.6):

      Diffuse extension or multifocal masses of tumor in the chest wall, with or without associated rib destruction

      Direct transdiaphragmatic extension of tumor to the peritoneum

      Direct extension of tumor to the contralateral pleura

      Direct extension of tumor to mediastinal organs

      Direct extension of tumor into the spine

      Tumor extending through to the internal surface of the pericardium with or without a pericardial effusion or tumor involving the myocardium

Regional Lymph Nodes (N)

NX   Regional lymph nodes cannot be assessed

N0   No regional lymph node metastases

N1   Metastases in the ipsilateral bronchopulmonary or hilar lymph nodes (Figure 26.7)

N2   Metastases in the subcarinal or the ipsilateral mediastinal lymph nodes including the ipsilateral internal mammary and peridiaphragmatic nodes (Figure 26.8)

N3   Metastases in the contralateral mediastinal, contralateral internal mammary, ipsilateral or contralateral supraclavicular lymph nodes (Figure 26.9)

Distant Metastasis (M)

M0   No distant metastasis

M1   Distant metastasis present

ANATOMIC STAGE/PROGNOSTIC GROUPS

Stage	T	N	M
Stage I	T1	N0	M0
Stage IA	T1a	N0	M0
Stage IB	T1b	N0	M0
Stage II	T2	N0	M0
Stage III	T1, T2	N1	M0
	T1, T2	N2	M0
	T3	N0, N1, N2	M0
Stage IV	T4	Any N	M0
	Any T	N3	M0
	Any T	Any N	M1

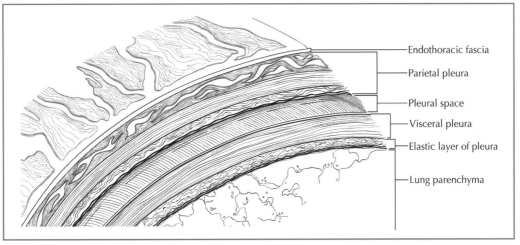

FIGURE 26.1. *Anatomy of the pleura.*

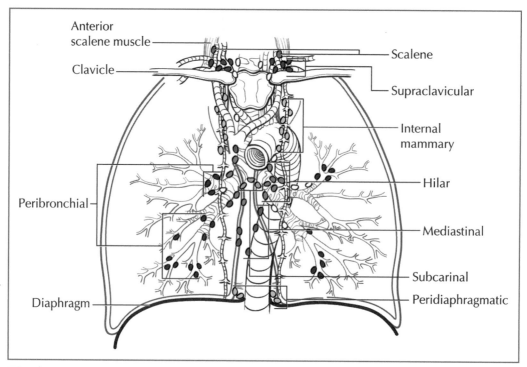

FIGURE 26.2. *Regional lymph nodes of the pleura.*

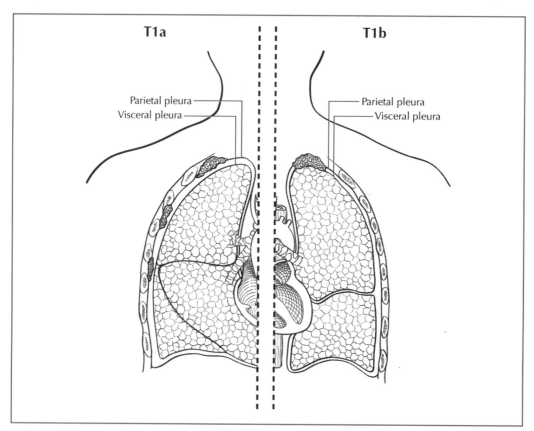

FIGURE 26.3. *T1a (left) shows involvement of the parietal pleura, with no involvement of the visceral pleura. T1b (right) involves ipsilateral visceral pleura with involvement of the parietal pleura.*

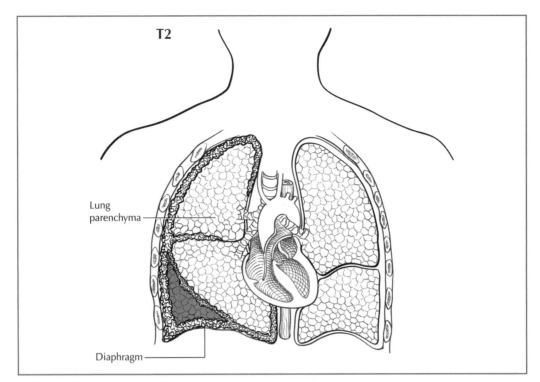

FIGURE 26.4. *T2 is defined as tumor that involves each of the ipsilateral pleural surfaces (parietal, mediastinal, diaphragmatic, and visceral pleura) with at least one of the following: involvement of diaphragmatic muscle (as illustrated); and/or extension of tumor from visceral pleura into the underlying pulmonary parenchyma (as illustrated).*

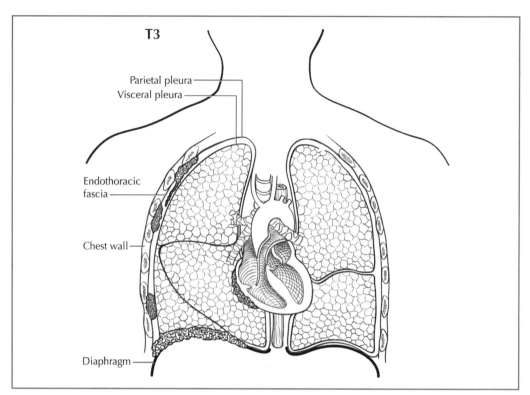

FIGURE 26.5. *T3 is defined as locally advanced but potentially resectable tumor. Tumor involves all of the ipsilateral pleural surfaces (parietal, mediastinal, diaphragmatic, and visceral pleura) with at least one of the following: involvement of the endothoracic fascia (as illustrated); extension into mediastinal fat; solitary, completely resectable focus of tumor extending into the soft tissues of the chest wall (as illustrated); and/or nontransmural involvement of the pericardium (as illustrated).*

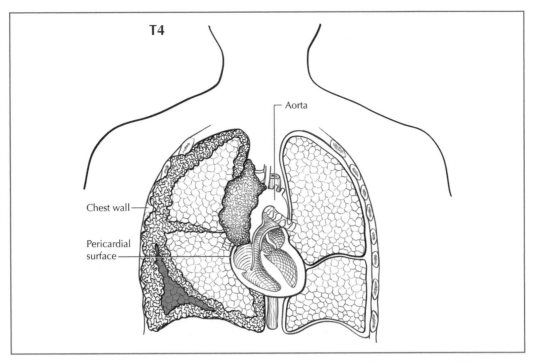

FIGURE 26.6. *T4 is defined as locally advanced technically unresectable tumor. Tumor involves all of the ipsilateral pleural surfaces (parietal, mediastinal, diaphragmatic, and visceral pleura) with at least one additional parameter, such as extension through to the internal surface of the pericardium as illustrated here, and diffuse invasion of chest wall as illustrated here. (The full list of additional parameters is provided under Definition of TNM).*

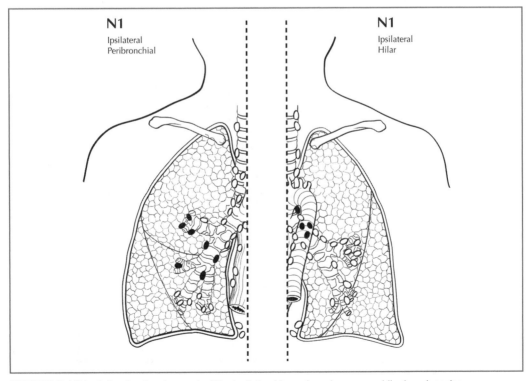

FIGURE 26.7. *N1 is defined as involvement of the ipsilateral bronchopulmonary or hilar lymph nodes.*

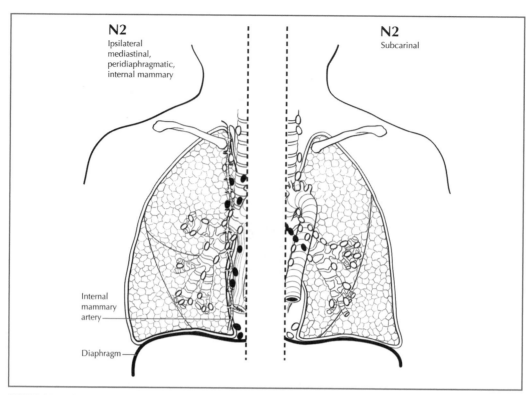

FIGURE 26.8. *N2 is defined as involvement of the subcarinal or the ipsilateral mediastinal lymph nodes including the ipsilateral internal mammary and peridiaphragmatic nodes.*

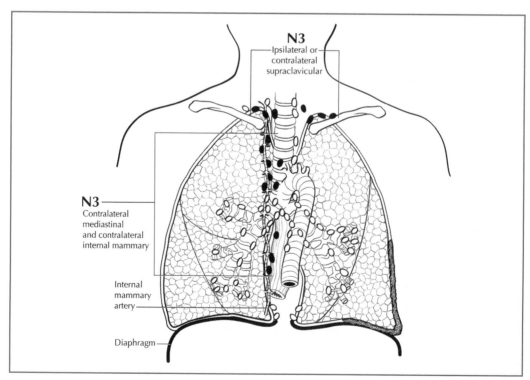

FIGURE 26.9. *N3 is defined as involvement of the contralateral mediastinal, contralateral internal mammary, ipsilateral or contralateral supraclavicular lymph nodes.*

PROGNOSTIC FACTORS (SITE-SPECIFIC FACTORS)
(Recommended for Collection)

Required for staging	None
Clinically significant	Histological subtype (epithelioid, mixed or biphasic, sarcomatoid, desmoplastic) History of asbestos exposure Presence or absence of chest pain FDG-PET SUV

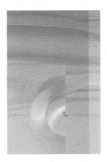

PART V
Musculoskeletal Sites

ICD-O-3 TOPOGRAPHY CODES

C40.0   Long bones of upper limb, scapula, and associated joints
C40.1   Short bones of upper limb and associated joints
C40.2   Long bones of lower limb and associated joints

ICD-O-3 HISTOLOGY CODE RANGES

8800–9136, 9142–9582

ANATOMY

Primary Site. All bones of the skeleton are included in this system (Figure 27.1A). The current staging system does not take into account anatomic site. However, anatomic site is known to influence outcome, and therefore outcome data should be reported specifying site.

Site groups for bone sarcoma (Figure 27.1B):

- Extremity
- Pelvis
- Spine

Regional Lymph Nodes. Regional lymph metastases from bone tumors are extremely rare.

Metastatic Sites. A metastatic site includes any site beyond the regional lymph nodes of the primary site. Pulmonary metastases are the most frequent site for all bone sarcomas. Extra pulmonary metastases occur infrequently, and may include secondary bone metastases, for example.

PROGNOSTIC FEATURES

Known prognostic factors for malignant bone tumors are as follows. (1) T1 tumors have a better prognosis than T2 tumors. (2) Histopathologic low grade (G1, G2) has a better prognosis than high grade (G3, G4). (3) Location of the primary tumor is a prognostic factor. Patients who have an anatomically resectable primary tumor have a better prognosis than those with a non-resectable tumor, and tumors of the spine and pelvis tend to have a poorer prognosis. (4) The size of the primary tumor is a prognostic factor for osteosarcoma and Ewing's sarcoma. Ewing's sarcoma patients with a tumor 8 cm or less in greatest dimension have a better prognosis than those with a tumor greater than 8 cm. Osteosarcoma patients with a tumor 9 cm or less in greatest dimension have a better prognosis than those with a tumor greater than 9 cm. (5) Patients who have a localized primary tumor have a better prognosis than those with metastases. (6) Certain metastatic sites are associated with a poorer prognosis than other sites: bony and hepatic metastases convey a much worse prognosis than do lung metastases, and patients with solitary lung metastases have a better prognosis than those with multiple lung lesions. (7) Histologic response of the primary tumor to chemotherapy is a prognostic factor for osteosarcoma and Ewing's sarcoma. Those patients with a "good" response, >90% tumor necrosis, have a better prognosis than those with less necrosis. (8) Patients with osteosarcoma who experience pathologic fractures may have a poorer prognosis, particularly if their fracture does not heal during chemotherapy. (9) Recent studies have shown that the biologic behavior of osteosarcoma and Ewing's sarcoma is related to specific molecular abnormalities identified in these neoplasms. As with soft tissue sarcomas, investigation has been undertaken to identify molecular markers that are useful both as prognostic tools as well as in directing treatment. The results of this investigation have shown that the biologic behavior of osteosarcoma and Ewing's sarcoma can be related to specific molecular abnormalities. For practical purposes, prognostically relevant molecular aberrations are considered in terms of gene translocations, expression of multidrug resistance genes, expression of growth factor receptors, and mutations in cell cycle regulators.

Investigation as to whether the type of fusion gene detected in Ewing's sarcoma has prognostic significance has been met with mixed results. Initial studies suggested that the EWS-FLI1 type 1 fusion gene was associated with longer relapse-free survival in patients with localized disease and have been confirmed with a subsequent study which found an association between type 1 EWS-FLI1 and overall survival by multivariate analysis. In contrast, a study concluded that no prognostic value was attributed to different fusion genes when evaluated for event-free and overall survival by univariate analysis.

P-glycoprotein, the product of the multidrug resistance 1 gene (MDR1), functions to remove certain chemotherapeutic drugs, such as doxorubicin, from tumor cells. In osteosarcoma, P-glycoprotein status has been noted to be an independent predictor of clinical outcome and to be associated with a ninefold increase in the odds of death and a fivefold increase in the odds of metastases in patients with Stage IIB osteosarcoma. Further investigation showed that P-glycoprotein-positivity at diagnosis emerged as the single factor significantly associated with an unfavorable outcome from survival and multivariate analyses and this association was strong enough to be useful in stratifying patients in whom alternative treatments were being considered.

Also in osteosarcoma, investigation of human epidermal growth factor receptor 2 (HER2)/erbB-2 has led to differing results between investigators as well. Gorlick et al. identified a significant percentage (42.6%) of initial biopsies with high levels of HER2/erbB-2 expression. They noted that there was a correlation with histologic response to neoadjuvant chemotherapy and event-free survival. Zhou et al. noted an association between HER2/erbB-2 expression with an increased risk of metastasis. Scotlandi also confirmed an advantage in event-free survival with HER2 overexpression. Subsequent analysis by Scotlandi has failed to show HER2 amplification/overexpression by immunohistochemistry/CISH and FISH, respectively.

In Ewing's sarcoma, the status of several cell cycle regulators has been shown to correlate with outcome. Aberrant P53, p16INK4A, and p14ARF expression has been shown by several investigators to identify a subset of patients whose tumors will exhibit aggressive behavior and a poor response to chemotherapy. Additional studies revealed that loss of INK4 expression correlated with metastatic disease at presentation and also showed a trend toward shortened survival. Suppression of the cyclin-dependant kinase inhibitor p27(kip1) by EWS-FLI1 has been associated with poor event-free survival in univariate analysis and the expression level of p27 correlates significantly with patient survival. Overall event-free survival has been correlated to P53 alteration in osteosarcoma as well.

A variety of other markers have been described as relevant to the prognosis of osteosarcoma. This includes KI-67, a proliferative marker which has been suggested as a marker for the development of pulmonary metastasis. Heat shock proteins (HSP) have been shown to aid in the growth and development of tumors and overexpression of HSP27 specifically has been shown to carry negative prognostic value. Overexpression of parathyroid hormone Type 1 has been shown to confer an aggressive phenotype in osteosarcoma. Platelet-derived growth factor-AA expression was found to be an independent predictor of tumor progression in osteosarcoma. Nuclear survivin expression/localization has been associated with prolonged survival. Vascular endothelial growth factor expression in untreated osteosarcoma is predictive of pulmonary metastasis and poor prognosis. HLA class I expression has been shown to be associated with significantly better overall and event-free survival than patients lacking HLA class I expression in osteosarcoma. Finally, telomerase expression in osteosarcoma is associated with decreased progression free survival and overall survival.

Investigation to identify molecular markers in chondrosarcoma has progressed at a slower pace. Rozeman et al. investigated a variety of markers, none of which had prognostic importance independent of histologic grade. Decreased Indian Hedgehog signaling and loss of INK4A/p16 has been found to be important in the progression of peripheral chondrosarcoma and enchondroma, respectively.

DEFINITIONS OF TNM

Primary Tumor (T)

TX	Primary tumor cannot be assessed
T0	No evidence of primary tumor
T1	Tumor 8 cm or less in greatest dimension (Figure 27.2)
T2	Tumor more than 8 cm in greatest dimension (Figure 27.3)
T3	Discontinuous tumors in the primary bone site (Figure 27.4)

Regional Lymph Nodes (N)

NX	Regional lymph nodes cannot be assessed
N0	No regional lymph node metastasis
N1	Regional lymph node metastasis

Note: Because of the rarity of lymph node involvement in bone sarcomas, the designation NX may not be appropriate and cases should be considered N0 unless clinical node involvement is clearly evident.

Distant Metastasis (M)

M0	No distant metastasis
M1	Distant metastasis
M1a	Lung (Figure 27.5)
M1b	Other distant sites (Figure 27.6)

ANATOMIC STAGE/PROGNOSTIC GROUPS

Stage IA	T1	N0	M0	G1, 2 Low grade, GX
Stage IB	T2	N0	M0	G1, 2 Low grade, GX
	T3	N0	M0	G1, 2 Low grade, GX
Stage IIA	T1	N0	M0	G3, 4 High grade
Stage IIB	T2	N0	M0	G3, 4 High grade
Stage III	T3	N0	M0	G3, 4 High grade
Stage IVA	Any T	N0	M1a	Any G
Stage IVB	Any T	N1	Any M	Any G
	Any T	Any N	M1b	Any G

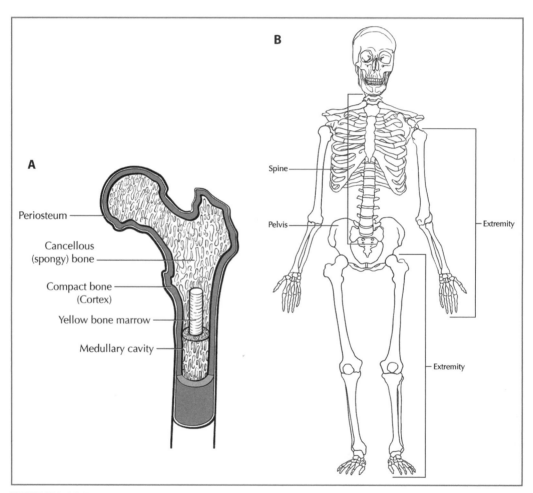

FIGURE 27.1. *(A) The anatomic subsites of the bone. (B) The site groups for bone sarcomas, extremity, pelvis, and spine are illustrated.*

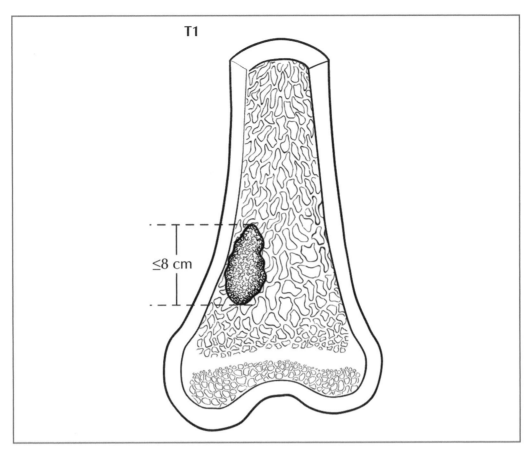

FIGURE 27.2. *T1 is defined as tumor 8 cm or less in greatest dimension.*

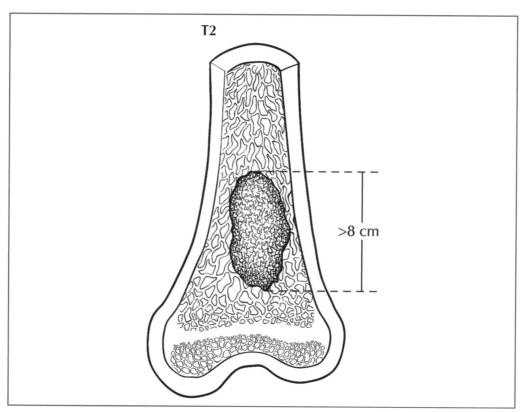

FIGURE 27.3. *T2 is defined as tumor more than 8 cm in greatest dimension.*

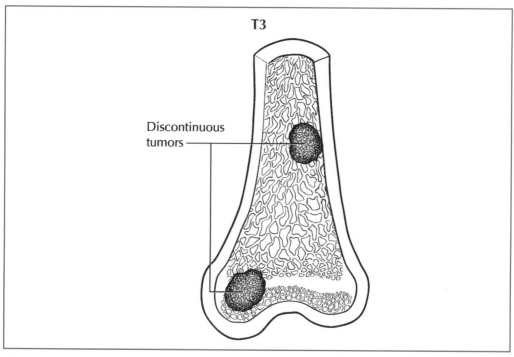

FIGURE 27.4. *T3 is defined as discontinuous tumors in the primary bone site.*

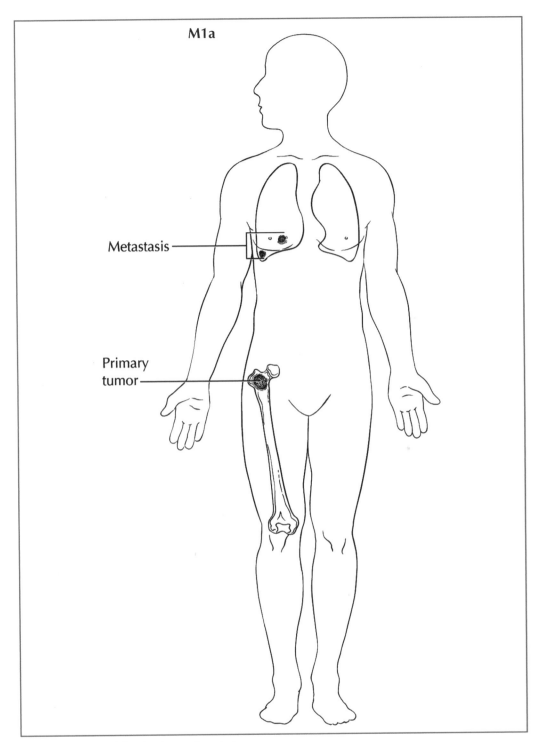

M1a

Metastasis

Primary tumor

FIGURE 27.5. *M1a is defined as lung-only metastases.*

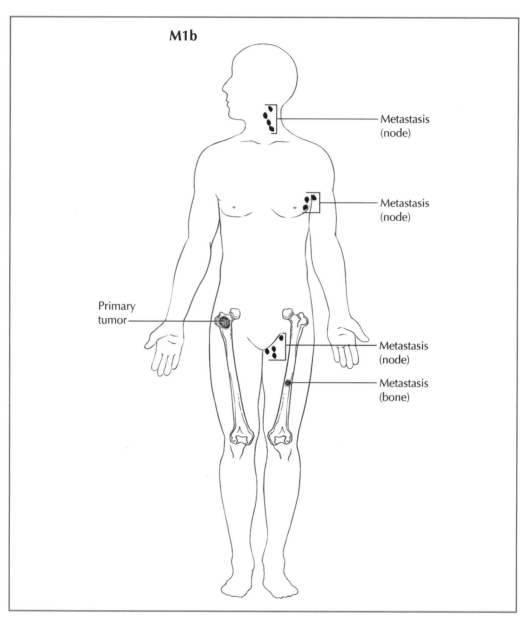

M1b

Metastasis (node)

Metastasis (node)

Primary tumor

Metastasis (node)

Metastasis (bone)

FIGURE 27.6. *M1b is defined as metastases to other distant sites, including lymph nodes.*

PROGNOSTIC FACTORS (SITE-SPECIFIC FACTORS)
(Recommended for Collection)

Required for staging	Grade
Clinically significant	Three dimensions of tumor size
	Percentage necrosis post neoadjuvant systemic therapy from pathology report
	Number of resected pulmonary metastases from pathology report

Soft Tissue Sarcoma

(Kaposi's sarcoma, fibromatosis [desmoid tumor], and sarcoma arising from the dura mater, brain, parenchymatous organs, or hollow viscera are not included)

28

SUMMARY OF CHANGES

- Gastrointestinal stromal tumor (GIST) is now included in Chap. 16; fibromatosis (desmoid tumor), Kaposi's sarcoma, and infantile fibrosarcoma are no longer included in the histological types for this site
- Angiosarcoma, extraskeletal Ewing's sarcoma, and dermatofibrosarcoma protuberans have been added to the list of histologic types for this site
- N1 disease has been reclassified as Stage III rather than Stage IV disease
- Grading has been reformatted from a four grade to a three-grade system as per the criteria recommended by the College of American Pathologists

ICD-O-3 TOPOGRAPHY CODES

C38.0	Heart
C38.1	Anterior mediastinum
C38.2	Posterior mediastinum
C38.3	Mediastinum, NOS
C38.8	Overlapping lesion of heart, mediastinum, and pleura
C47.2	Peripheral nerves and autonomic nervous system of lower limb and hip
C47.3	Peripheral nerves and autonomic nervous system of thorax
C47.4	Peripheral nerves and autonomic nervous system of abdomen
C47.5	Peripheral nerves and autonomic nervous system of pelvis
C47.6	Peripheral nerves and autonomic nervous system of trunk, NOS
C47.8	Overlapping lesion of peripheral nerves and autonomic nervous system
C47.9	Autonomic nervous system, NOS
C48.0	Retro-peritoneum
C48.1	Specified parts of peritoneum
C48.2	Peritoneum, NOS
C48.8	Overlapping lesion of retro-peritoneum and peritoneum
C49.0	Connective, subcutaneous, and other soft tissues of head, face, and neck
C49.1	Connective, subcutaneous, and other soft tissues of upper limb and shoulder
C49.2	Connective, subcutaneous, and other soft tissues of lower limb and hip
C49.3	Connective, subcutaneous, and other soft tissues of thorax
C49.4	Connective, subcutaneous, and other soft tissues of abdomen
C49.5	Connective, subcutaneous, and other soft tissues of pelvis
C49.6	Connective, subcutaneous, and other soft tissues of trunk, NOS
C49.8	Overlapping lesion of connective, subcutaneous, and other soft tissues
C49.9	Connective, subcutaneous, and other soft tissues, NOS

ICD-O-3 HISTOLOGY CODE RANGES

8800–8820, 8823–8935, 8940–9136, 9142–9582

C.C. Compton et al. (eds.), *AJCC Cancer Staging Atlas: A Companion to the Seventh Editions of the AJCC Cancer Staging Manual and Handbook*, DOI 10.1007/978-1-4614-2080-4_28,
© 2012 American Joint Committee on Cancer

ANATOMY

Staging of Soft Tissue Sarcoma

Inclusions. The present staging system applies to soft tissue sarcomas. Primary sarcomas can arise from a variety of soft tissues. These tissues include fibrous connective tissue, fat, smooth or striated muscle, vascular tissue, peripheral neural tissue, and visceral tissue.

Regional Lymph Nodes. Involvement of regional lymph nodes by soft tissue sarcomas is uncommon in adults.

Metastatic Sites. Metastatic sites for soft tissue sarcoma are often dependent on the original site of the primary lesion. For example, the most common site of metastatic disease for patients with extremity sarcoma is the lung, whereas retroperitoneal and gastrointestinal sarcomas often have liver as the first site of metastasis.

Depth. Depth is evaluated relative to the investing fascia of the extremity and trunk. *Superficial* is defined as lack of any involvement of the superficial investing muscular fascia in extremity or trunk lesions. For staging, nonsuperficial head and neck, intrathoracic, intra-abdominal, retroperitoneal, and visceral lesions are considered to be deep lesions.

Depth is also an independent variable and is defined as follows:

1. Superficial – located entirely in the subcutaneous tissues without any degree of extension through the muscular fascia or into underlying muscle. In these cases, pretreatment imaging studies demonstrate a subcutaneous tumor without involvement of muscle, and excisional pathology reports demonstrate a tumor located within the subcutaneous tissues without extension into underlying muscle (Figure 28.1).
2. Deep – located partly or completely within one or more muscle groups within the extremity. Deep tumors may extend through the muscular fascia into the subcutaneous tissues or even to the skin but the critical criterion is location of any portion of the tumor within the muscular compartments of the extremity. In these cases, pretreatment imaging studies demonstrate a tumor located completely or in part within the muscular compartments of the extremity (Figure 28.2).
3. Depth is evaluated in relation to tumor size (T):

   a. Tumor ≤5 cm: T1a = superficial, T1b = deep
   b. Tumor >5 cm: T2a = superficial, T2b = deep

PROGNOSTIC FEATURES

Neurovascular and Bone Invasion. In earlier staging systems, neurovascular and bone invasion by soft tissue sarcomas had been included as a determinant of stage. It is not included in the current staging system, and no plans are proposed to add it at the present time. Nevertheless, neurovascular and bone invasion should always be reported where possible, and further studies are needed to determine whether or not such invasion is an independent prognostic factor.

Molecular Markers. Molecular markers and genetic abnormalities are being evaluated as determinants of outcome. At the present time, however, insufficient data exist to include specific molecular markers in the staging system.

For the present time, molecular and genetic markers should be considered as important information to aid in histopathologic diagnosis, rather than as determinants of stage.

Validation. The current staging system has the capacity to discriminate the overall survival of patients with soft tissue sarcoma. Patients with Stage I lesions are at low risk for disease-related mortality, whereas Stages II and III entail progressively greater risk.

DEFINITION OF TNM

Primary Tumor (T)

TX	Primary tumor cannot be assessed
T0	No evidence of primary tumor
T1	Tumor 5 cm or less in greatest dimension*
T1a	Superficial tumor (Figure 28.3)
T1b	Deep tumor (Figure 28.4)
T2	Tumor more than 5 cm in greatest dimension*
T2a	Superficial tumor (Figure 28.3)
T2b	Deep tumor (Figure 28.5)

*Note: Superficial tumor is located exclusively above the superficial fascia without invasion of the fascia; deep tumor is located either exclusively beneath the superficial fascia, superficial to the fascia with invasion of or through the fascia, or both superficial yet beneath the fascia.

Regional Lymph Nodes (N)

NX	Regional lymph nodes cannot be assessed
N0	No regional lymph node metastasis
N1*	Regional lymph node metastasis

*Note: Presence of positive nodes (N1) in M0 tumors is considered Stage III.

Distant Metastasis (M)

M0	No distant metastasis
M1	Distant metastasis

ANATOMIC STAGE/PROGNOSTIC GROUPS

Stage IA	T1a	N0	M0	G1, GX
	T1b	N0	M0	G1, GX
Stage IB	T2a	N0	M0	G1, GX
	T2b	N0	M0	G1, GX
Stage IIA	T1a	N0	M0	G2, G3
	T1b	N0	M0	G2, G3
Stage IIB	T2a	N0	M0	G2
	T2b	N0	M0	G2
Stage III	T2a, T2b	N0	M0	G3
	Any T	N1	M0	Any G
Stage IV	Any T	Any N	M1	Any G

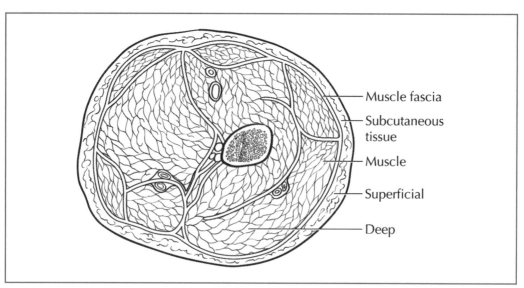

FIGURE 28.1. *Depth is evaluated relative to the investing fascia of the extremity or trunk. Illustrated is superficial depth, which is located entirely in the subcutaneous tissues without any degree of extension through the muscular fascia or into underlying muscle. Illustrated is deep depth, which is located partly or completely within one or more muscle groups within the extremity.*

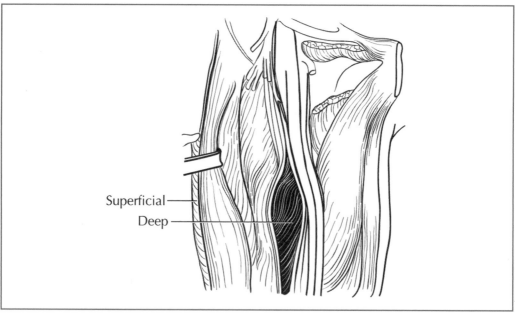

FIGURE 28.2. *Depth is evaluated relative to the investing fascia of the extremity or trunk. Illustrated is superficial depth, which is located entirely in the subcutaneous tissues without any degree of extension through the muscular fascia or into underlying muscle. Illustrated is deep depth, which is located partly or completely within one or more muscle groups within the extremity.*

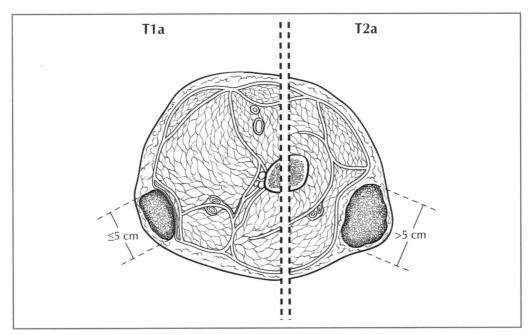

FIGURE 28.3. *T1a is defined as a superficial tumor 5 cm or less in greatest dimension, and T2a is defined as a superficial tumor more than 5 cm in greatest dimension.*

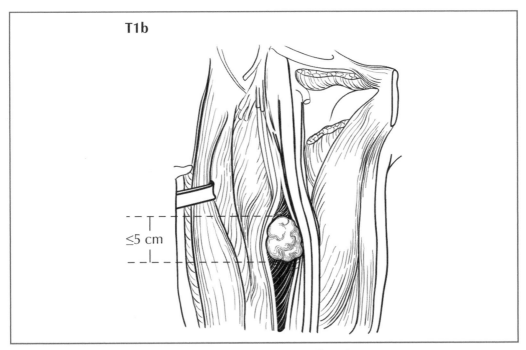

FIGURE 28.4. *T1b is defined as deep tumor 5 cm or less in greatest dimension.*

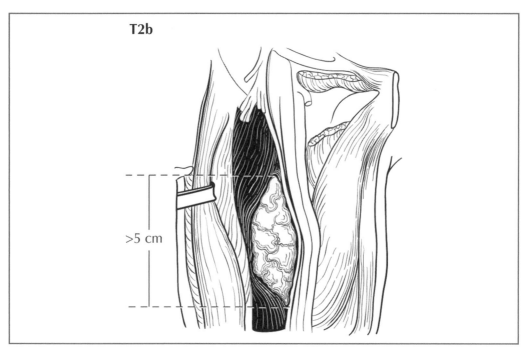

FIGURE 28.5. *T2b is defined as deep tumor more than 5 cm in greatest dimension.*

PROGNOSTIC FACTORS (SITE-SPECIFIC FACTORS)	
(Recommended for Collection)	
Required for staging	Grade
Clinically significant	Neurovascular invasion as determined by pathology
	Bone invasion as determined by imaging
	If pM1, source of pathologic metastatic specimen

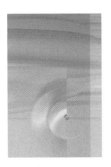

PART VI
Skin

Cutaneous Squamous Cell Carcinoma and Other Cutaneous Carcinomas

29

SUMMARY OF CHANGES

- The previous edition chapter, entitled "Carcinoma of the Skin," has been eliminated and two chapters have been created in its place:

  - Merkel Cell Carcinoma: An entirely new chapter specifically for Merkel cell carcinoma (MCC) has been designed (see Chap. 30)
  - This chapter has been renamed "Cutaneous Squamous Cell Carcinoma and Other Cutaneous Carcinomas" and is an entirely new staging system that, for the first time, reflects a multidisciplinary effort to provide a mechanism for staging nonmelanoma skin cancers according to evidence-based medicine. In total, seven board-certified disciplines collaborated to develop this chapter: Dermatology, Otolaryngology-Head and Neck Surgery, Surgical Oncology, Dermatopathology, Oncology, Plastic Surgery, and Oral and Maxillofacial Surgery. The title of this chapter reflects the basis of the data, which is focused on cutaneous squamous cell carcinoma (cSCC). All other nonmelanoma skin carcinomas (except Merkel cell carcinoma) will be staged according to the cSCC staging system

- Anatomic site of the eyelid is not included – staged by Ophthalmic Carcinoma of the Eyelid (see Chap. 48 in the *AJCC Cancer Staging Manual*)
- The T staging has eliminated the 5-cm-size breakpoint and invasion of extradermal structures for T4. Two cm continues to differentiate T1 and 2, however, a list of clinical and histologic "high-risk features" has been created that can increase the T staging, independent of tumor size
- Grade has been included as one of the "high-risk features" within the T category and now contributes toward the final stage grouping. Other "high-risk features" include primary anatomic site ear or hair-bearing lip, >2 mm depth, Clark level $\geq$ IV, or perineural invasion
- Advanced T stage is reserved for bony extension or involvement (e.g., maxilla, mandible, orbit, temporal bone, or perineural invasion of skull base or axial skeleton for T3 and T4, respectively)
- Nodal (N) staging has been completely revised to reflect published evidence-based data demonstrating that survival decreases with increasing nodal size and number of nodes involved
- Because the majority of cSCC tumors occur on the head and neck, the seventh edition staging system for cSCC and other cutaneous carcinomas was made congruent with the AJCC Head and Neck staging system

ICD-O-3 TOPOGRAPHY CODES

C44.0   Skin of lip, NOS
C44.2   External ear
C44.3   Skin of other and unspecified parts of the face
C44.4   Skin of scalp and neck
C44.5   Skin of trunk
C44.6   Skin of upper limb and shoulder
C44.7   Skin of lower limb and hip
C44.8   Overlapping lesion of skin
C44.9   Skin, NOS
C63.2   Scrotum, NOS

ICD-O-3 HISTOLOGY CODE RANGES

8000–8246, 8248–8576, 8940–8950, 8980–8981

ANATOMY

Primary Site. Cutaneous squamous cell and other carcinomas can occur anywhere on the skin. Cutaneous SCC and BCC most commonly arise on anatomic sites that have been exposed to sunlight. Cutaneous SCC can also arise in skin that was previously scarred or ulcerated – that is, at sites of burns and chronic ulcers (chronic inflammation). All of the components of the skin (epidermis, dermis, and adnexal structures) can give rise to malignant neoplasms.

Nonaggressive NMSC, such as BCC, usually grow solely by local extension, both horizontally and vertically. Continued local extension may result in growth into deep structures, including adipose tissue, cartilage, muscle, and bone. Perineural extension is a particularly insidious form of local extension, as this is often clinically occult. If neglected for an extended length of time, nodal metastasis can occur with nonaggressive NMSC.

Aggressive NMSC, including cSCC and some types of sebaceous and eccrine neoplasms, also grow by local lateral and vertical extension early in their natural history. Once deeper extension occurs, growth may become discontinuous, resulting in deeper local extension, in transit metastasis, and nodal metastasis. In more advanced cases, cSCC and other tumors can extend along cranial foramina through the skull base into the cranial vault. Uncommon types of NMSC vary considerably in their propensity for metastasis.

Regional Lymph Nodes. When deep invasion and eventual metastasis occurs, local and regional lymph nodes are the most common sites of metastasis. Nodal metastasis usually occurs in an orderly manner, initially in a single node, which expands in size. Eventually, multiple nodes become involved with metastasis. Metastatic disease may spread to secondary nodal basins, including contralateral nodes when advanced. Uncommonly, nodal metastases may bypass a primary nodal basin. (Figures 29.1 and 29.2 and Table 29.1).

Metastatic Sites. Nonaggressive NMSC more often involves deep tissue by direct extension than by metastasis. After metastasizing to nodes, cSCC may spread to visceral sites, including lung.

PROGNOSTIC FEATURES

Most studies that analyze early stage cSCC are retrospective in nature and do not rely on multivariate analysis. The revision of the staging system for Stage I and II cSCC was primarily based on consensus opinion of the NMSC Task Force. Poor prognosis for recurrence and metastasis has been correlated with multiple factors such as anatomic site, tumor diameter, poor differentiation, perineural invasion, as well extension >2 mm depth (see High-Risk Features after T classification). These prognostic factors are discussed in detail below. They apply primarily to cSCC and an aggressive subset of NMSC, but rarely to BCC. The following rationale determined the multiple factors used for the T staging:

Tumor Diameter. Tumor size refers to the maximum clinical diameter of the cSCC lesion. In the sixth edition AJCC staging system, 2- and 5-cm tumor size thresholds were used to define the primary tumor (T) and were the sole criteria for T1, T2, and T3. Multiple studies corroborate a correlation between tumor size and more biologically aggressive disease, including local recurrence and metastasis in univariate analysis. Tumor size remains a significant variable on multivariate analysis in some reports. Several published studies point toward 2 cm as a threshold beyond which tumors are more likely to metastasize to lymph nodes. A 3.8-fold risk of recurrence and metastasis for tumors >2 cm was noted by Mullen when reviewing M.D. Anderson Cancer Center's database of 149 cSCC on the trunk and extremities. In a large review of all published literature on the prognosis of SCC occurring on the skin and lip since 1940, Rowe et al. found that among tumors that exceeded 2 cm in diameter, the local recurrence rate was double (15 vs. 7%) and metastatic rates were triple (30 vs. 9%) the rates when the primary was ≤2 cm.

After considering all of this published data, the AJCC cSCC Task Force decided to continue 2 cm as one of the key delineating features between T1 and T2 cSCC staging in the seventh edition AJCC Manual (Table 29.1). This threshold was decided based on the existing published data that ≥2 cm clinical diameter is associated with a poor prognosis. In addition, this breakpoint allowed congruence between cSCC and Head and Neck Staging. Prognostically relevant breakpoints beyond 2 cm are difficult to establish. A limited number of studies suggest 4 cm as significant thresholds, while others show other factors to be important. Therefore, there is a lack of sufficient evidence to support the 5-cm break point featured in the previous NMSC staging system. Thus, a 5-cm breakpoint has been removed from the seventh edition AJCC T staging definitions for cSCC.

High-Risk Tumor Features. Although 2 cm is recognized by many to be an important size cutoff, the metastatic potential of tumors smaller than 2 cm cannot be ignored, as they too can metastasize. In a prospective study of 266 patients with head and neck cSCC metastatic to lymph nodes, the majority of patients had tumors <2 cm in size, leading the investigators to conclude that size alone is a poor predictor of outcome. A review of 915 cSCC in Netherlands' national registry over a 10-year period (comparing nonmetastatic and metastatic lesions matched for gender, location, and other clinicopathologic variables) suggested that the risk of metastasis significantly increased with tumors >1.5 cm. In conceptualizing how to integrate the multiple other clinicopathologic tumor characteristics into the overall staging system, the NMSC Task Force felt that the independent prognostic validity of the multiple other features was insufficient to accurately place them into stage-specific locations. Instead, the Task Force approved a group of "high-risk" features which are combined with diameter to classify tumors as T1 or T2.

Additionally, because of data suggesting that immunosuppression correlates with worse prognosis as described in Lee et al. (in preparation), strong consideration was given toward including immunosuppression as a risk factor. However, because strict TNM criteria preclude inclusion of clinical risk factors in the staging system, this factor should be collected by tumor registries as a site-specific factor rather than incorporated in the final staging system. For centers collecting such data and performing studies, immunosuppressed status may be designated with an "I" after the staging designation.

Depth of Tumor. Recent studies show that both tumor thickness and the depth of invasion are important variables for the prognosis of cSCC. Prospective studies showed that increasing tumor thickness as well as anatomic depth of invasion correlate with an increased risk of metastases. In an initial study, no metastases were associated with primary tumors less than 2 mm in depth (tumor thickness), but a metastatic rate of 15% was noted with tumors greater than 6 mm in depth. This study also reported increasing metastatic rates as tumor invasion progressed from dermis to subcutaneous adipose tissue, to muscle, or bone. Based on the prospective and multivariate data, the seventh edition AJCC cSCC staging system incorporates >2 mm Breslow depth as one of the high-risk features in the T classification. Clark's level IV is included as an additional high-risk feature. Differentiation between the prognostic contributions of Breslow thickness vs. Clark level will depend on future studies.

Anatomic Site. Specific anatomic locations on the hair-bearing lip and ear appear to have an increased local recurrence and metastatic potential and thus have been categorized as high risk in the seventh edition system.

Perineural Invasion. Goepfert et al., in their review of 520 patients with 967 cSCC of the face, found an increased incidence of cervical lymphadenopathy and distant metastasis, as well as significantly reduced survival in patients with tumors that showed perineural invasion. Several univariate studies, all retrospective, have also confirmed that perineural invasion has a negative prognostic impact in cSCC.

Histopathologic Grade or Differentiation. Early studies recognized that the histological grade or degree of differentiation of a cSCC affects prognosis: the more well-differentiated, the less aggressive the clinical course. In 1978, Mohs, in his review of "microscopically controlled surgery," reported significant differences in cure rates for well-differentiated tumors (99.4%) compared with poorly differentiated tumors (42.1%). A multivariate analysis has also confirmed that histopathologic grade correlates with recurrence. The sixth edition staging system used a separate G classification system to denote histopathologic grade, however, grade did not contribute toward overall stage grouping. For the seventh edition AJCC cSCC staging, histopathologic grade includes poorly differentiated tumors as one of the several high-risk features.

Extension to Bony Structures. In the sixth edition T staging system, the T4 designation was used for tumors that "invaded extradermal structures." The most common and important instances of deep anatomic extension for cSCC involve extension to bone of the head and neck and perineural extension to bony structures vs. the skull base. Based on these considerations, in the seventh edition cSCC staging system, T3 designation denotes direct invasion of cSCC into cranial bone structures. The T4 designation is reserved for direct or perineural invasion of the skull base independent of tumor thickness or depth consistent with data from several head and neck studies suggesting that cSCC extending to skull base is associated to poor prognosis similar to advanced lymph node disease. While published studies include facial nerve involvement in nodal staging, the NMSC Task Force decided to separate this factor from nodal status and include it in the T staging in order to understand its unique contribution to prognosis. The NMSC Task Force reached consensus that, similarly, extension of cSCC to axial skeleton should also merit a T4 designation.

Evidence-Based Medicine and Nodal Disease. Since the sixth edition AJCC manual, four studies have examined the outcomes in patients with cSCC and regional lymph node metastasis. Approximately 761 patients from ten centers and three countries have been studied suggesting the number nodes involved and size of lymph node metastasis correlates with poor prognosis.

In 2002, O'Brien et al. conducted a prospective study with multivariate analysis and therein proposed a new clinical staging system for cSCC. He used a new staging system in which he separated the parotid gland involvement from the cervical node metastasis and applied this new P (parotid) N (neck) system to 87 patients with parotid and cervical cSCC metastasis to analyze the influence of clinical stage, extent of surgery, and pathologic findings on outcome by applying this new staging system The multivariate analysis showed that increasing P stage, positive margins, and a failure to have postoperative radiotherapy independently predicted decrease in local control. It also demonstrated that positive surgical margins and the advanced (N2) clinical and pathologic neck disease were independent risk factors for survival. The results from this study concluded that patients with metastatic cSCC in both the parotid gland and neck have significantly worse prognosis than those in the parotid gland only. O'Brien et al. recommended that a new clinical staging system for cSCC of the head and neck should separate parotid (P) and neck disease (N) nodal involvement.

In 2003, Palme et al. in a retrospective, multicenter study, independently tested this new PN staging system on 126 patients with metastatic cSCCs involving the parotid and/or neck. The multivariate analysis showed that advanced P staging (P2 and P3) were independent risk factors for a decrease in local control rate, and the pathologic involvement of neck nodes did not worsen survival of patients with parotid disease. Overall, this analysis concluded that single-modality therapy, P3 stage, and presence of immunosuppression independently predicted a decrease in survival. This study confirmed that the extent of metastatic disease in the parotid gland significantly influences outcome and that separating the parotid from the neck metastasis may be useful.

In 2004, Audet et al., in their retrospective study on 56 patients with previously untreated metastatic head and neck cSCC involving the parotid gland, confirmed that metastatic cSCC to the parotid gland is an aggressive neoplasm that requires combination therapy. They also reported that the presence of a lesion in excess of 6 cm or with facial nerve involvement is associated with a poor prognosis.

In 2006, a larger cohort, multicenter, retrospective study was conducted by Andruchow et al. on 322 patients from six independent institutions to further clarify the clinical behavior of metastatic cSCC and to determine whether or not the proposed changes to the clinical staging system could be validated. In this study, 322 patients with parotid and/or neck metastatic cSCC were restaged with the O'Brien P and N staging system and were followed up for at least 2 years. Both univariate and multivariate analysis confirmed that survival was significantly worse for patients with advanced P stage, suggesting a revised classification of nodal status. This concept of increasing nodal disease correlating with decreased survival was confirmed in a separate prospective analysis of 67 patients with metastatic disease.

Based on patient survival from published studies, the NMSC Task Force decided that there is sufficient evidence to stage patients according to increasing nodal disease. While preliminary data exists to suggest that cervical disease may portend a worse prognosis than similar disease in the parotid, there is insufficient data to support this separation at this time. Separating out facial nerve involvement or involvement of the skull base (now T4) from extensive parotid disease will further clarify the prognosis of these patients.

Immunosuppression and Advanced Disease. It is well known that immunosuppressed patients are at risk for developing malignancies, especially cSCCs. Organ transplant recipients develop squamous cell carcinoma 65 times more frequently than in age-matched controls. The cSCCs in immunocompromised patients are more aggressive: they are numerous, tend to recur, and metastasize at a higher rate. It has been reported that immunocompromised patients have a 7.2 times increased risk of local recurrence and a 5.3 times increased risk of any recurrence of disease. Mortality is also increased with skin cancer, the fourth most common cause of death in a renal transplant cohort. In transplant recipients, cSCC develops 10–30 years earlier than in immunocompetent hosts.

Histopathology of cSCC in an immunocompromised host show more acantholytic changes, early dermal invasion, infiltrative growth pattern, Bowen's disease with carcinoma, and increased depth of the primary. Tumors in immunocompromised patients can range widely in size from 6 to 75 mm; however, Lindelof and colleagues report that most lethal cSCCs in their study were 5–19 mm in diameter. They also point out that focusing on tumor size may be misleading in immunocompromised populations because small tumors can behave very aggressively. For centers prospectively studying cSCC, recording of presence and type of immunosuppression is recommended.

CONCLUSIONS

The seventh edition of the AJCC Staging Manual features MCC as a separate chapter and cSCC is staged in this chapter entitled "Cutaneous Squamous cell and Other Carcinomas." The remainder of NMSC tumors (such as appendageal tumors and BCC) will also be included within the cSCC chapter since those tumors can rarely be advanced and are occasionally described to undergo metastasis. As the first published staging system devoted specifically to cSCC prognosis, this represents an important step for better understanding and studying the prognosis of this potentially metastatic tumor. Additionally, since many cSCC tumors occur on the head and neck, the seventh edition cSCC staging system is congruent with Head and Neck Cancer staging system. Furthermore, the new T staging definitions for the seventh edition for cSCC now capture additional features believed to correlate with high-risk cSCC in order to more meaningfully stratify patients based on prospective systematic data. Certainly there is still a need for multivariate data analysis, particularly to determine the relative contributions of the various described T factors influencing cSCC prognosis. Finally, the new N staging definitions are congruent with Head and Neck staging and reflect recent data that suggests that prognosis is inversely correlated with increasing nodal disease.

DEFINITIONS OF TNM

Definitions for clinical (cTNM) and pathologic (pTNM) classifications are the same. Patients with cSCC in situ are categorized as Tis. Carcinomas that are indeterminate or cannot be staged should be category TX. Carcinomas 2 cm or less in diameter are T1, if they have fewer than two high-risk features. Clinical high-risk features include primary site on ear or hair-bearing lip. Histologic high-risk features include depth >2 mm, Clark level ≥ IV/V, poor differentiation, and the presence of perineural invasion. Tumors greater than 2 cm in diameter are classified as T2. Tumors 2 cm or less in diameter are classified as T2 if the tumor has two or more high-risk features. Invasion into facial bones is classified as T3, while invasion to base of skull or axial skeleton is classified as T4.

Local and regional metastases most commonly present in the regional lymph nodes. The actual status of nodal metastases identified by clinical inspection or imaging and the status and number of positive and total nodes by pathologic analysis must be reported for staging purposes. In instances where lymph node status is not recorded, a designation of NX is used. A solitary parotid or regional lymph node metastasis measuring 3 cm or less in size is given a N1 designation. Several different lymph node states are classified as N2: N2a represents a single ipsilateral lymph node, more than 3 cm but not more than 6 cm in greatest dimension; N2b is defined by multiple ipsilateral lymph nodes, none more than 6 cm in greatest dimension; N2c includes bilateral or contralateral lymph nodes, none more than 6 cm in greatest dimension. Nodal metastases more than 6 cm in greatest dimension are classified as N3.

Distant metastases are staged primarily by the presence (M1) or absence (M0) of metastases in distant organs or sites outside of the regional lymph nodes.

Primary Tumor (T)*

TX	Primary tumor cannot be assessed
T0	No evidence of primary tumor
Tis	Carcinoma in situ (Figure 29.3)
T1	Tumor 2 cm or less in greatest dimension with less than two high-risk features** (Figure 29.4)
T2	Tumor greater than 2 cm in greatest dimension (Figure 29.5) *or*
	Tumor any size with two or more high-risk features**
T3	Tumor with invasion of maxilla, mandible, orbit, or temporal bone (Figure 29.6)
T4	Tumor with invasion of skeleton (axial or appendicular) or perineural invasion of skull base (Figure 29.7)

*Excludes cSCC of the eyelid.
**High-risk features for the primary tumor (T) staging

Depth/invasion	>2 mm thickness
	Clark level $\geq$ IV
	Perineural invasion
Anatomic location	Primary site ear
	Primary site hair-bearing lip
Differentiation	Poorly differentiated or undifferentiated

Regional Lymph Nodes (N)

NX	Regional lymph nodes cannot be assessed
N0	No regional lymph node metastases (Figure 29.8)
N1	Metastasis in a single ipsilateral lymph node, 3 cm or less in greatest dimension (Figure 29.8)
N2	Metastasis in a single ipsilateral lymph node, more than 3 cm but not more than 6 cm in greatest dimension; or in multiple ipsilateral lymph nodes, none more than 6 cm in greatest dimension; or in bilateral or contralateral lymph nodes, none more than 6 cm in greatest dimension (Figure 29.8)
N2a	Metastasis in a single ipsilateral lymph node, more than 3 cm but not more than 6 cm in greatest dimension (Figure 29.8)
N2b	Metastasis in multiple ipsilateral lymph nodes, none more than 6 cm in greatest dimension (Figure 29.8)
N2c	Metastasis in bilateral or contralateral lymph nodes, none more than 6 cm in greatest dimension (Figure 29.8)
N3	Metastasis in a lymph node, more than 6 cm in greatest dimension (Figure 29.8)

Distant Metastasis (M)

M0	No distant metastases
M1	Distant metastases

ANATOMIC STAGE/PROGNOSTIC GROUPS

Patients with primary cSCC or other cutaneous carcinomas with no evidence (clinical, radiologic, or pathologic) of regional or distant metastases are divided into two stages: Stage I for tumors measuring ≤2 cm in size and Stage II for those that are greater than 2 cm in size. In instances where there is clinical concern for extension of tumor into bone and radiologic evaluation has been performed (and is negative), these data may be included to support the Stage I vs. II designation. Tumors that are ≤2 cm in size can be upstaged to Stage II if they contain two or more high-risk features. Stage III patients are those with (1) clinical, histologic, or radiologic evidence of one solitary node measuring ≤3 cm in size or (2) Tumor extension into bone: maxilla, mandible, orbit, or temporal bone. Stage IV patients are those with (1) tumor with direct or perineural invasion of skull base or axial skeleton, (2) ≥2 lymph nodes or (3) single or multiple lymph nodes measuring >3 cm in size or (4) distant metastasis.

Stage	T	N	M
Stage 0	Tis	N0	M0
Stage I	T1	N0	M0
Stage II	T2	N0	M0
Stage III	T3	N0	M0
	T1	N1	M0
	T2	N1	M0
	T3	N1	M0
Stage IV	T1	N2	M0
	T2	N2	M0
	T3	N2	M0
	T Any	N3	M0
	T4	N Any	M0
	T Any	N Any	M1

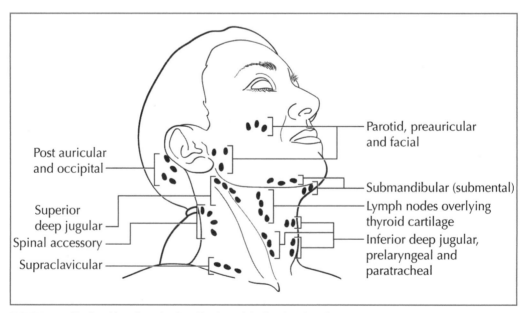

FIGURE 29.1. *Regional lymph nodes for skin sites of the head and neck.*

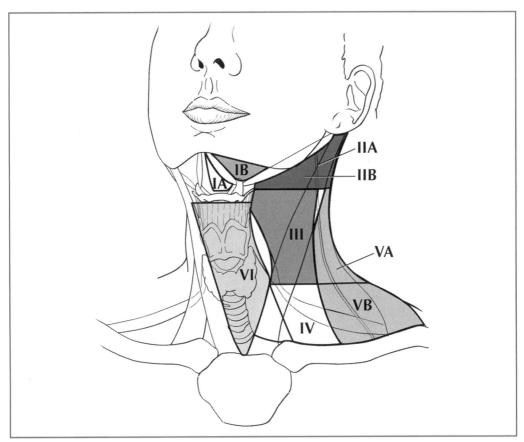

FIGURE 29.2. *Schematic indicating the location of the lymph node levels in the neck as described in Table 29.1.*

TABLE 29.1. *Anatomical Structures Defining the Boundaries of the Neck Levels and Sublevels*

Level	Superior	Inferior	Anterior (Medial)	Posterior (Lateral)
IA	Symphysis of mandible	Body of hyoid	Anterior belly of contralateral digastric muscle	Anterior belly of ipsilateral digastric muscle
IB	Body of mandible	Posterior belly of muscle	Anterior belly of digastric muscle	Stylomyoid muscle
IIA	Skull base	Horizontal plane defined by the inferior body of the hyoid bone	Vertical plane defined by the spinal accessory nerve	Lateral border of the sternocleidomastoid muscle
III	Horizontal planes defined by the inferior body of hyoid	Horizontal plane defined by the inferior border of the cricoid cartilage	Lateral border of the sternohuoid muscle	Lateral border of the sternocleidomastoid or sensory branches of cervical plexus
IV	Horizontal plane defined by the inferior border of the cricoid cartilage	Clavicle	Lateral border of the sternohyoid muscle	Lateral border of the sternocleidomastoid or sensory branches of cervical plexus
VA	Apex of the convergence of the sternocleidomastoid and trapezius muscles	Horizontal plane defined by the lower border of the cricoid cartilage	Posterior border of the sternocleidomastoid muscle or sensory branches of cervical plexus	Anterior border of the the trapezius muscle
VI	Hyoid bone	Suprasternal notch	Common carotid artery	Common carotid artery
VII	Suprasternal notch	Innominate artery	Sternum	Trachea, esophagus, and prevertebral fascia

Modified from Robbins KT, Clayman G, Levine PA, et al.; American Head and Neck Society; American Academy of Otolaryngology--Head and Neck Surgery. Neck dissection classification update: revisions proposed by the American Head and Neck Society and the American Academy of Otolaryngology-Head and Neck Surgery. Arch Otolaryngol Head Neck Surg. 2002 Jul;128(7):751-8, with permission of the American Medical Association.

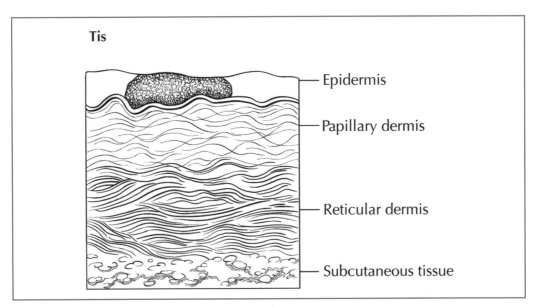

FIGURE 29.3. Carcinoma *in situ*.

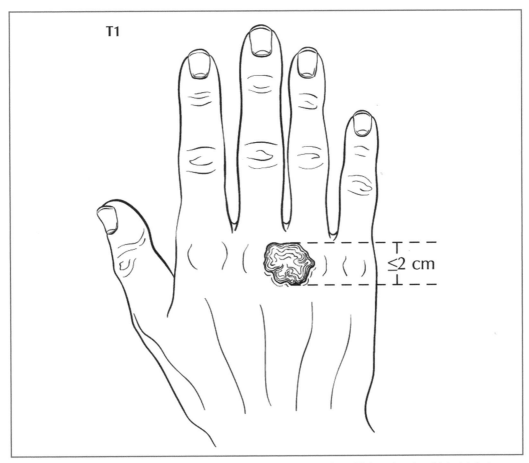

FIGURE 29.4. *T1 is defined as a tumor 2 cm or less in greatest dimension with less than two high-risk features as described in Table 29.2.*

TABLE 29.2. *High-risk features for the primary tumor (T) staging*

Depth/invasion	>2 mm thickness
	Clark level ≥ IV
	Perineural invasion
Anatomic location	Primary site ear
	Primary site hair-bearing lip
Differentiation	Poorly differentiated or undifferentiated

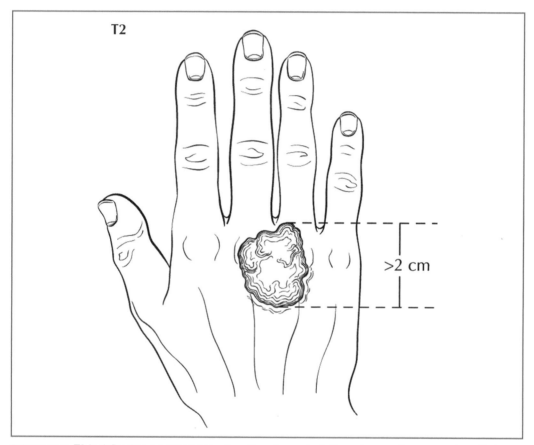

FIGURE 29.5. *T2 is defined as a tumor greater than 2 cm in greatest dimension or a tumor any size with two or more high-risk features as described in Table 29.2.*

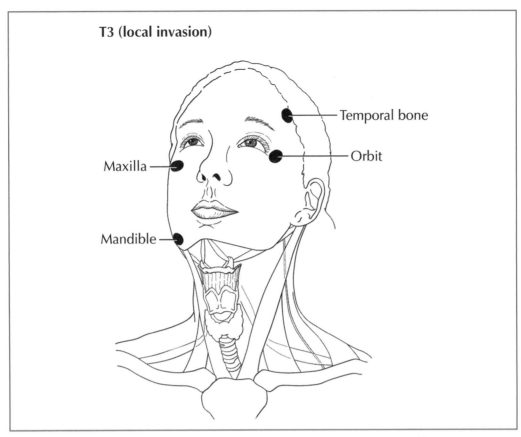

FIGURE 29.6. *T3 is defined as a tumor with invasion of maxilla, mandible, orbit, or temporal bone.*

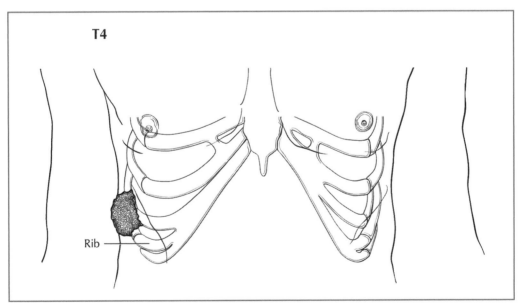

FIGURE 29.7. *T4 is defined as a tumor with invasion of skeleton (axial or appendicular) or perineural invasion of skull base.*

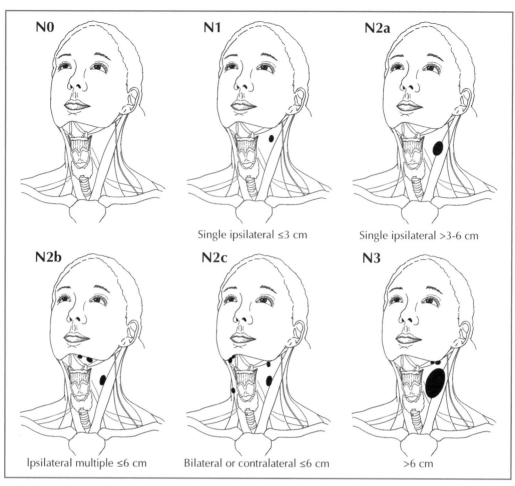

FIGURE 29.8. *Regional lymph node (N) classification for all skin sites, illustrated here for the head and neck skin primary sites.*

PROGNOSTIC FACTORS (SITE-SPECIFIC FACTORS)	
(Recommended for Collection)	
Required for staging	Tumor thickness (in mm)
	Clark's level
	Presence/absence of perineural invasion
	Primary site location on ear or hair-bearing lip
	Histologic grade
	Size of largest lymph node metastasis
Clinically significant	No additional factors

Merkel Cell Carcinoma

(Staging for Merkel Cell of the eyelid [C44.1] is not included in this chapter – see Chap. 48, "Carcinoma of the Eyelid" in the AJCC Cancer Staging Manual)

30

SUMMARY OF CHANGES

- This is the first staging chapter specific for Merkel cell carcinoma. Merkel cell carcinoma was previously included in the "Carcinoma of the Skin" chapter

---

ICD-O-3 TOPOGRAPHY CODES

C44.0   Skin of lip, NOS
C44.2   External ear
C44.3   Skin of other and unspecified parts of face
C44.4   Skin of scalp and neck
C44.5   Skin of trunk
C44.6   Skin of upper limb and shoulder
C44.7   Skin of lower limb and hip
C44.8   Overlapping lesion of skin
C44.9   Skin, NOS
C51.0   Labium majus
C51.1   Labium minus
C51.2   Clitoris
C51.8   Overlapping lesion of vulva
C51.9   Vulva, NOS
C60.0   Prepuce
C60.1   Glans penis
C60.2   Body of penis
C60.8   Overlapping lesion of penis
C60.9   Penis, NOS
C63.2   Scrotum, NOS

ICD-O-3 HISTOLOGY CODE RANGE

8247

ANATOMY

Primary Sites. Merkel cell carcinoma is postulated to arise from the Merkel cell, a neuroendocrine cell of the skin. MCC can occur anywhere on the skin but arises most often in sun-exposed areas. It occurs most commonly on the head and neck, followed by the extremities. In 14% of cases, the primary site remains unknown with MCC presentation in nodal or visceral sites.[4]

Regional Lymph Nodes. The draining regional lymph nodes are the most common site of metastasis (Figures 30.1 and 30.2 and Table 30.1). Regional lymph node metastasis occurs relatively frequently and early, even in the absence of deep local extension or large primary tumor size. Thirty-two percent of clinically negative draining lymph node basins were in fact positive for microscopic

---

C.C. Compton et al. (eds.), *AJCC Cancer Staging Atlas: A Companion to the Seventh Editions of the AJCC Cancer Staging Manual and Handbook*, DOI 10.1007/978-1-4614-2080-4_30,
© 2012 American Joint Committee on Cancer

metastases as revealed by sentinel or elective lymphadenectomy. Intralymphatic "in transit" regional metastases also occur but are uncommon. For MCC, an in transit metastasis is defined as a tumor distinct from the primary lesion and located either (1) between the primary lesion and the draining regional lymph nodes or (2) distal to the primary lesion. In contrast to melanoma, for MCC there is no separate subclassification of in transit metastases based on distance from the primary (i.e., no *satellite* metastasis classification). By convention, the term "regional nodal metastases" refers to disease confined to one nodal basin or two contiguous nodal basins, as in patients with nodal disease in combinations of femoral/iliac, axillary/supraclavicular, or cervical/supraclavicular metastases or in primary truncal disease with axillary/femoral, bilateral axillary, or bilateral femoral metastases.

Metastatic Sites. Merkel cell carcinoma can metastasize to virtually any organ site. Metastases occur most commonly to distant lymph nodes, followed by the liver, lung, bone, and brain.

PROGNOSTIC FEATURES AND SURVIVAL RESULTS

Survival in Merkel cell carcinoma is based on stage at presentation. Overall survival relative to an age- and sex-matched population was determined using 4,700 Merkel cell carcinoma patients in the National Cancer Database registry. Tumor size is a continuous variable with increasing tumor size correlating with modestly poorer prognosis. True lymph node negativity by pathologic evaluation portends a better prognosis compared with patients whose lymph nodes are only evaluated by clinical or radiographic examination. This is in large part likely due to the high rate (33%) of false negative nodal determination by clinical exam alone. Thus, patients should have pathologic evaluation of the draining nodal basin to most accurately predict survival and guide optimal therapy.

Profound immune suppression, such as in HIV/AIDS, chronic lymphocytic leukemia, or solid organ transplantation have all been associated with worse survival in MCC. Further, immunosuppressed patients frequently present with more advanced disease.

DEFINITIONS OF TNM

Those patients with MCC presentations where the primary tumor cannot be assessed should be categorized as TX. Patients with Merkel cell carcinoma in situ are categorized as Tis. The T category of MCC is classified primarily by measuring the maximum dimension of the tumor: 2 cm or less (T1), greater than 2 cm but not more than 5 cm (T2), and greater than 5 cm (T3). Extracutaneous invasion by the primary tumor into bone, muscle, fascia, or cartilage is classified as T4. Inclusion of 2 cm MCC tumors as T1 is consistent with the prior AJCC staging system but differs from other frequently used MCC staging systems that categorize 2 cm tumors as T2. The breakdown of T category is conserved from the prior version of AJCC staging for "Carcinoma of the Skin."

Regional metastases most commonly present in the regional lymph nodes. A second staging definition is related to nodal tumor burden: microscopic vs. macroscopic. Therefore, patients without clinical or radiologic evidence of lymph node metastases but who have pathologically documented nodal metastases are defined by convention as exhibiting "microscopic" or "clinically occult" nodal metastases. In contrast, MCC patients with both clinical evidence of nodal metastases *and* pathologic examination confirming nodal metastases are defined by convention as having "macroscopic" or "clinically apparent" nodal metastases. Nodes clinically positive by exam and negative by pathology would be classified as pN0. Clinically positive nodes in the draining nodal basin that are assumed to be involved with Merkel cell carcinoma but are without pathologic confirmation (no pathology performed) should be classified as N1b and the pathologic classification would be NX. Then in determining the stage grouping, it would be Stage IIIB defaulting to the higher N category.

Distant metastases are defined as metastases that have spread beyond the draining lymph node basin, including cutaneous, nodal, and visceral sites.

Primary Tumor (T)

TX   Primary tumor cannot be assessed

T0   No evidence of primary tumor (e.g., nodal/metastatic presentation without associated primary)

Tis   In situ primary tumor (Figure 30.3)

T1   Less than or equal to 2 cm maximum tumor dimension (Figure 30.4)

T2   Greater than 2 cm but not more than 5 cm maximum tumor dimension (Figure 30.5)

T3   Over 5 cm maximum tumor dimension (Figure 30.6)

T4   Primary tumor invades bone, muscle, fascia, or cartilage (Figure 30.7)

Regional Lymph Nodes (N)

NX   Regional lymph nodes cannot be assessed

N0   No regional lymph node metastasis

cN0   Nodes negative by clinical exam* (no pathologic node exam performed)

pN0   Nodes negative by pathologic exam

N1   Metastasis in regional lymph node(s)

N1a   Micrometastasis** (Figure 30.8)

N1b   Macrometastasis*** (Figure 30.9)

N2   In transit metastasis**** (Figure 30.10)

*Clinical detection of nodal disease may be via inspection, palpation, and/or imaging.

**Isolated tumor cells in a lymph node are classified as micrometastases (N1a) and the presence of isolated tumor cells recorded using the prognostic factor. Micrometastases are diagnosed after sentinel or elective lymphadenectomy.

***Macrometastases are defined as clinically detectable nodal metastases confirmed by therapeutic lymphadenectomy or needle biopsy.

****In transit metastasis: a tumor distinct from the primary lesion and located either (1) between the primary lesion and the draining regional lymph nodes or (2) distal to the primary lesion.

Distant Metastasis (M)

M0   No distant metastasis

M1   Metastasis beyond regional lymph nodes

M1a   Metastasis to skin, subcutaneous tissues or distant lymph nodes

M1b   Metastasis to lung

M1c   Metastasis to all other visceral sites

ANATOMIC STAGE/PROGNOSTIC GROUPS

Patients with primary Merkel cell carcinoma with no evidence of regional or distant metastases (either clinically or pathologically) are divided into two stages: Stage I for primary tumors ≤2 cm in size and Stage II for primary tumors >2 cm in size. Stages I and II are further divided into A and B substages based on method of nodal evaluation. Patients who have pathologically proven node negative disease (by microscopic evaluation of their draining lymph nodes) have improved survival (substaged as A) compared to those who are only evaluated clinically (substaged as B). Stage II has an additional substage (IIC) for tumors with extracutaneous invasion (T4) and negative node status regardless of whether the negative node status was established microscopically or clinically. Stage III is also divided into A and B categories for patients with microscopically positive and clinically occult nodes (IIIA) and macroscopic nodes (IIIB). There are no subgroups of Stage IV Merkel cell carcinoma.

Stage 0	Tis	N0	M0
Stage IA	T1	pN0	M0
Stage IB	T1	cN0	M0
Stage IIA	T2/T3	pN0	M0
Stage IIB	T2/T3	cN0	M0
Stage IIC	T4	N0	M0
Stage IIIA	Any T	N1a	M0
Stage IIIB	Any T	cN1/N1b/N2	M0
Stage IV	Any T	Any N	M1

Note: Isolated tumor cells should be considered positive nodes, similar to melanoma (see Chapter 31).

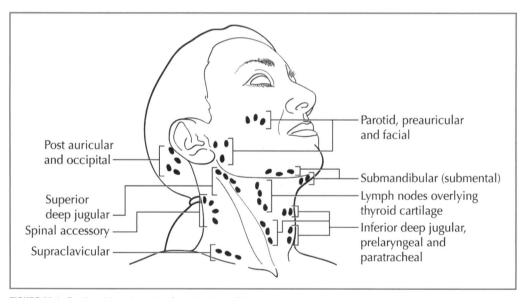

FIGURE 30.1. *Regional lymph nodes for skin sites of the head and neck.*

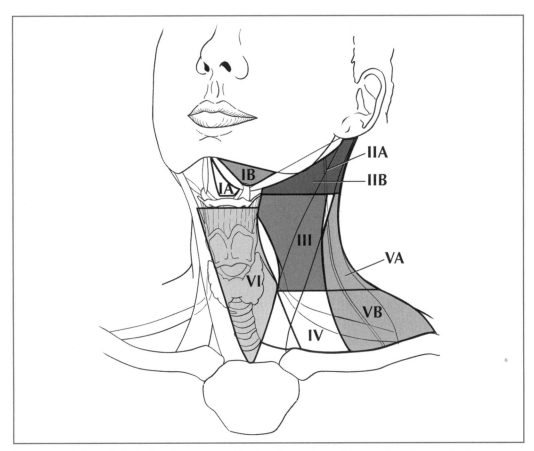

FIGURE 30.2. *Schematic indicating the location of the lymph node levels in the neck as described in Table 30.1.*

TABLE 30.1. *Anatomical Structures Defining the Boundaries of the Neck Levels and Sublevels*

Level	Superior	Inferior	Anterior (Medial)	Posterior (Lateral)
IA	Symphysis of mandible	Body of hyoid	Anterior belly of contralateral digastric muscle	Anterior belly of ipsilateral digastric muscle
IB	Body of mandible	Posterior belly of muscle	Anterior belly of digastric muscle	Stylomyoid muscle
IIA	Skull base	Horizontal plane defined by the inferior body of the hyoid bone	Vertical plane defined by the spinal accessory nerve	Lateral border of the sternocleidomastoid muscle
III	Horizontal planes defined by the inferior body of hyoid	Horizontal plane defined by the inferior border of the cricoid cartilage	Lateral border of the sternohyoid muscle	Lateral border of the sternocleidomastoid or sensory branches of cervical plexus
IV	Horizontal plane defined by the inferior border of the cricoid cartilage	Clavicle	Lateral border of the sternohyoid muscle	Lateral border of the sternocleidomastoid or sensory branches of cervical plexus
VA	Apex of the convergence of the sternocleidomastoid and trapezius muscles	Horizontal plane defined by the lower border of the cricoid cartilage	Posterior border of the sternocleidomastoid muscle or sensory branches of cervical plexus	Anterior border of the the trapezius muscle
VI	Hyoid bone	Suprasternal notch	Common carotid artery	Common carotid artery
VII	Suprasternal notch	Innominate artery	Sternum	Trachea, esophagus, and prevertebral fascia

Modified from Robbins KT, Clayman G, Levine PA, et al.; American Head and Neck Society; American Academy of Otolaryngology–Head and Neck Surgery. Neck dissection classification update: revisions proposed by the American Head and Neck Society and the American Academy of Otolaryngology-Head and Neck Surgery. Arch Otolaryngol Head Neck Surg. 2002 Jul;128(7):751-8, with permission of the American Medical Association.

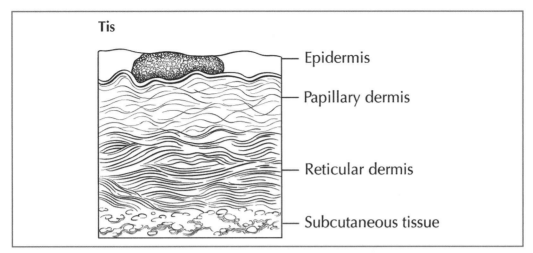

FIGURE 30.3. *Merkel cell carcinoma in situ.*

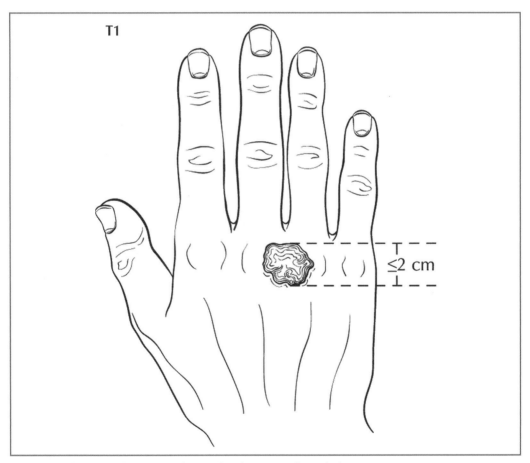

FIGURE 30.4. *T1 is defined as a tumor 2 cm or less in greatest dimension.*

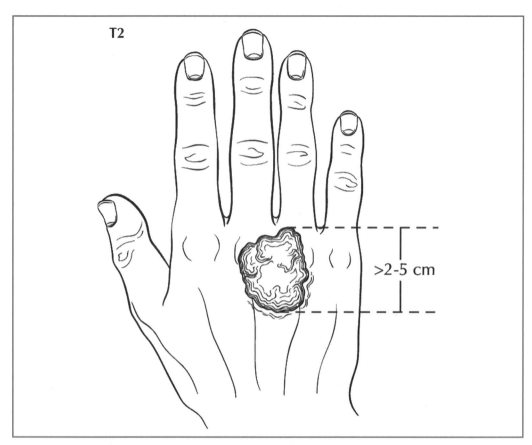

FIGURE 30.5. *T2 is defined as a tumor more than 2 cm, but not more than 5 cm, in greatest dimension.*

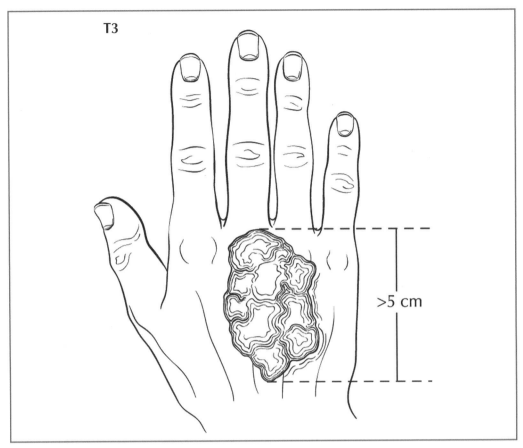

FIGURE 30.6. *T3 is defined as a tumor more than 5 cm in greatest dimension.*

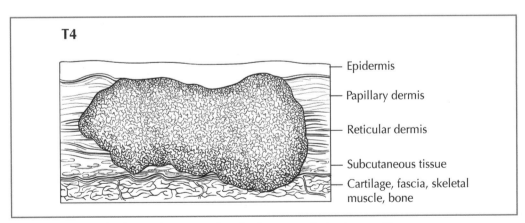

FIGURE 30.7. *T4 is defined as a primary tumor invading bone, muscle, fascia, or cartilage.*

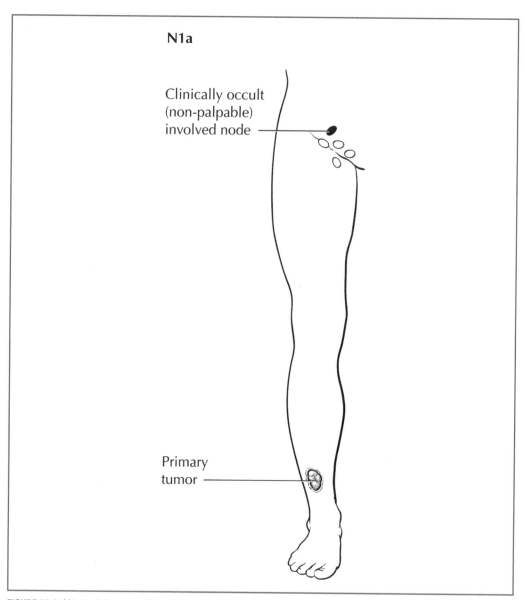

N1a

Clinically occult
(non-palpable)
involved node

Primary
tumor

FIGURE 30.8. *N1a is defined as clinically occult metastasis (micrometastasis): clinically negative node (cN0), pathologic positive node (pN1) in one or more regional nodes.*

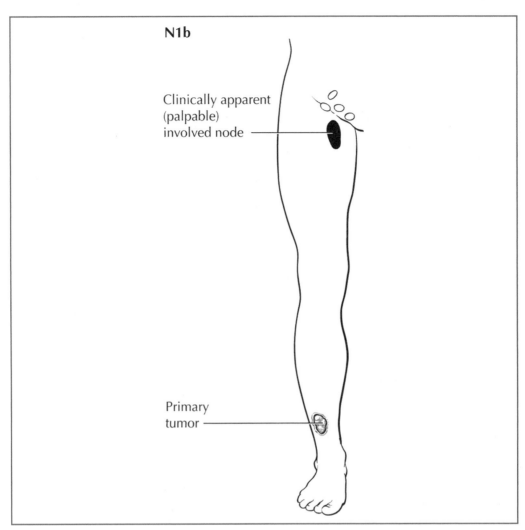

FIGURE 30.9. *N1b is defined as clinically apparent metastasis (macrometastatasis): clinically positive node (cN1), pathologic positive node (pN1) in one or more regional nodes.*

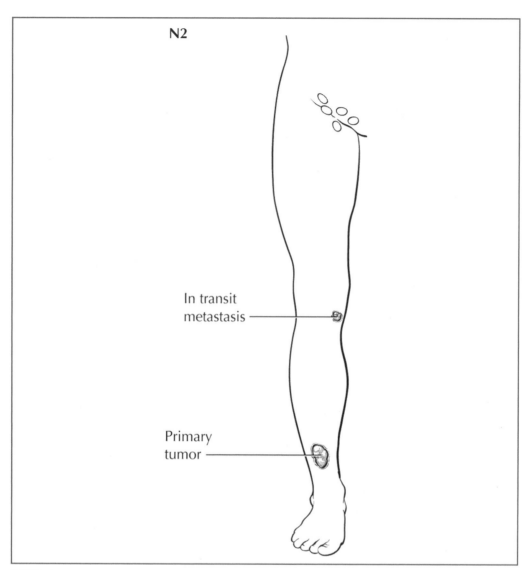

FIGURE 30.10. *N2 is defined as in transit metastasis. This figure illustrates an in transit metastasis which is defined as a tumor distinct from the primary lesion and located either (1) between the primary lesion and the draining regional lymph nodes or (2) distal to the primary lesion.*

PROGNOSTIC FACTORS (SITE-SPECIFIC FACTORS)

(Recommended for Collection)

Required for staging	None
Clinically significant	Measured thickness (depth)
	Tumor base transection status
	Profound immune suppression
	Tumor infiltrating lymphocytes in the primary tumor (TIL)
	Growth pattern of primary tumor
	Size of tumor nests in regional lymph nodes
	Clinical status of regional lymph nodes
	Regional lymph nodes pathological extracapsular extension
	Isolated tumor cells in regional lymph node(s)

Melanoma of the Skin

31

SUMMARY OF CHANGES

- Mitotic rate (histologically defined as mitoses/mm^2, not mitoses/10 HPF) is an important primary tumor prognostic factor. A mitotic rate equal to or greater than 1/mm^2 denotes a melanoma at higher risk for metastasis. It should now be used as one defining criteria of T1b melanomas
- Melanoma thickness and tumor ulceration continue to be used in defining strata in the T category. For T1 melanomas, in addition to tumor ulceration, mitotic rate replaces level of invasion as a primary criterion for defining the subcategory of T1b
- The presence of nodal micrometastases can be defined using either H&E or immunohistochemical staining (previously, only the H&E could be used)
- There is no lower threshold of tumor burden defining the presence of regional nodal metastasis. Specifically, nodal tumor deposits less than 0.2 mm in diameter (previously used as the threshold for defining nodal metastasis) are included in the staging of nodal disease as a result of the consensus that smaller volumes of metastatic tumor are still clinically significant. A lower threshold of clinically insignificant nodal metastases has not been defined based on evidence
- The site of distant metastases [nonvisceral (i.e., skin/soft tissue/distant nodal) vs. lung vs. all other visceral metastatic sites] continues to represent the primary component of categorizing the M category
- An elevated serum lactic dehydrogenase (LDH) level remains a powerful predictor of survival and is also to be used in defining the M category
- Survival estimates for patients with intralymphatic regional metastases (i.e., satellites and in transit metastasis) are somewhat better than for the remaining cohort of Stage IIIB patients. Nevertheless, Stage IIIB still represents the closest statistical fit for this group, so the current staging definition for intralymphatic regional metastasis has been retained
- The prognostic significance of microsatellites has been established less broadly. The Melanoma Task Force recommended that this uncommon feature be retained in the N2c category, largely because the published literature is insufficient to substantiate revision of the definitions used in the Sixth Edition *Staging Manual*
- The staging definition of metastatic melanoma from an unknown primary site was clarified, such that isolated metastases arising in lymph nodes, skin, and subcutaneous tissues are to be categorized as Stage III rather than Stage IV
- The definitions of tumor ulceration, mitotic rate and microsatellites were clarified
- Lymphoscintigraphy followed by lymphatic mapping and sentinel lymph node biopsy (sentinel lymphadenectomy) remain important components of melanoma staging and should be used (or discussed with the patient) in defining occult Stage III disease among patients who present with clinical Stage IB or II melanoma

ICD-O-3 TOPOGRAPHY CODES

C44.0   Skin of lip, NOS
C44.1   Eyelid
C44.2   External ear
C44.3   Skin of other and unspecified parts of face
C44.4   Skin of scalp and neck
C44.5   Skin of trunk
C44.6   Skin of upper limb and shoulder
C44.7   Skin of lower limb and hip
C44.8   Overlapping lesion of skin
C51.0   Labium majus
C51.1   Labium minus
C51.2   Clitoris
C51.8   Overlapping lesion of vulva
C51.9   Vulva, NOS
C60.0   Prepuce
C60.1   Glans penis
C60.2   Body of penis
C60.8   Overlapping lesion of penis
C60.9   Penis, NOS
C63.2   Scrotum, NOS

ICD-O-3 HISTOLOGY CODE RANGES

8720–8790

ANATOMY

Primary Sites. Cutaneous melanoma can occur anywhere on the skin. It occurs most commonly on the extremities in female subjects and on the trunk in male subjects.

Regional Lymph Nodes. The regional lymph nodes are the most common site of metastases (Figures 31.1, 31.2, 31.3, 31.4, and 31.5 and Table 31.1). The widespread use of cutaneous lymphoscintigraphy followed by lymphatic mapping and sentinel lymph node biopsy has greatly enhanced the ability to identify nodal micrometastases and to define the stage of clinically node-negative melanoma patients. Indeed, the distribution of Stage III patients has changed dramatically since the last melanoma staging review; those patients presenting with clinically occult nodal metastases (Stage IIIA) comprise the majority of the Stage III patients, and the number of patients with clinically detectable metastases (Stage IIIB and IIIC) has declined considerably.

Intralymphatic local and regional metastases may also become clinically manifest as (1) *satellite* metastases (defined arbitrarily as grossly visible cutaneous and/or subcutaneous metastases occurring within 2 cm of the primary melanoma); (2) *microsatellites* – microscopic and discontinuous cutaneous and/or subcutaneous metastases found on pathologic examination adjacent to a primary melanoma; or (3) *in transit* metastases (defined arbitrarily as clinically evident cutaneous and/or subcutaneous metastases identified at a distance greater than 2 cm from the primary melanoma in the region between the primary and the first echelon of regional lymph nodes). These manifestations of melanoma constitute a small but clinically significant and distinctive category of patients, with considerable risk of both additional locoregional and distant metastases.

Metastatic Sites. Melanoma can metastasize to virtually any organ site. Distant metastases most commonly occur in the skin or soft tissues, the lung, liver, brain, bone, or gastrointestinal tract.

PROGNOSTIC FEATURES

Melanoma Thickness. The T category of melanoma is classified primarily by measuring the thickness of the melanoma as defined by Dr. Alexander Breslow. In the seventh edition staging version, the T category thresholds of melanoma thickness are still defined in even integers (1.0, 2.0, and 4.0 mm). Although these are arbitrary thresholds for staging purposes, they were previously determined to represent both a statistical "best fit" for the (N0) patient population and the thresholds most compatible with contemporary clinical decision making.

The AJCC Melanoma Staging Database includes prospectively accumulated data on over 27,000 melanoma patients with clinically or pathologically localized melanoma (Stage I and II) for whom tumor thickness and follow-up information is available. As tumor thickness increased, there was a highly significant decline in 5- and 10-year survival ($p < 0.001$). Among the 5,296 patients with 0.01–0.5-mm thick melanomas, the 10-year survival was 96%, while it was 89% in the 6,545 patients with 0.51–1.00 mm thick, 80% in the 8,046 patients with 1.01–2.00 mm thick, 65% in 3,539 patients with 2.01–3.00 mm thick, 57% in the 1,752 patients with 3.01–4.00 mm thick, and 54% in the 1,464 patients with 4.01–6.00-mm thick melanomas. For patients with tumor thickness greater than 6.00 mm, the 10-year survival rate was 42%.

Melanoma Ulceration. The second criterion for determining T category is primary tumor ulceration, i.e., the presence or absence of a completely intact epidermis above the primary melanoma based upon a histopathologic examination. Melanoma ulceration is defined as the combination of the following features: full-thickness epidermal defect (including absence of stratum corneum and basement membrane), evidence of reactive changes (i.e., fibrin deposition and neutrophils), and thinning, effacement, or reactive hyperplasia of the surrounding epidermis in the absence of trauma or a recent surgical procedure.

Survival rates for patients with an ulcerated melanoma are proportionately lower than those of patients with a nonulcerated melanoma of equivalent T category, but are remarkably similar to those of patients with a nonulcerated melanoma of the next highest T category.

Melanoma Mitotic Rate. Primary tumor mitotic rate has been introduced as a required element for the seventh edition melanoma staging system (Figure 31.6). Data from the AJCC Melanoma Staging Database demonstrated a highly significant correlation with increasing mitotic rate and declining survival rates, especially within thin melanoma subgroups. In a multifactorial analysis of 10,233 patients with clinically localized melanoma, mitotic rate was the second most powerful predictor of survival outcome, after tumor thickness. Single institutions have also identified mitotic rate as an adverse prognostic factor.

Mitotic rate should be assessed on all primary melanomas. The recommended approach to enumerating mitoses is to first find the areas in the dermis containing the most mitotic figures, the so-called hot spot. After counting the mitoses in the hot spot, the count is extended to adjacent fields until an area corresponding to 1 mm² is assessed. If no hot spot can be found and mitoses are sparse and randomly scattered throughout the lesion, then a representative mitosis is chosen and beginning with that field the count is then extended to adjacent fields until an area corresponding to 1 mm² is assessed. The count then is expressed as the number of mitoses/mm² (i.e., an area corresponding to approximately four high power fields at 400× in most microscopes). To obtain accurate measurement, calibration of individual microscopes is recommended. For classifying thin ($\leq$1 mm) melanomas, the threshold for a nonulcerated melanoma to be defined as T1b is $\geq$1 mitoses/mm².

When the invasive component of tumor is < 1 mm² (in area), the number of mitoses present in 1 mm² of dermal tissue that includes the tumor should be enumerated and recorded as a number per millimeter squared. Alternatively, in tumors where the invasive component is < 1 mm² in area, the simple presence or absence of a mitosis can be designated as *at least* 1/mm² (i.e., "mitogenic") or

0/mm^2 (i.e., "nonmitogenic"), respectively. At some institutions, when mitotic figures are not found after numerous fields are examined, the mitotic count has been described as "<1/mm^2." For most tumor registries, the designation "<1/mm^2" equals 0 as has been customarily used in the past. This practice may be continued for historical data. For the future, we urge pathologists to list 0 or 1 or more, and this practice should also be demanded by clinicians.

It is common and appropriate practice with small, thin melanomas to have the technician place multiple sections cut from the block on a single slide. As a guide, we suggest that no more than two slides with such multiple sections be evaluated so that exhaustive evaluation of the lesion is not performed. Excellent interobserver reproducibility among specialist, general, and trainee pathologists for their assessment of mitotic rate as defined above has been previously described.

Level of Invasion. The level of invasion, as defined by Dr. Wallace Clark, has been used for over 40 years for various staging systems of melanomas. Although Clark's levels of invasion have prognostic significance in univariate analysis, numerous publications have shown that the level of invasion is less reproducible among pathologists and does not reflect prognosis as accurately as tumor thickness. In the sixth edition of the *Cancer Staging Manual*, level of invasion was used in defining the specific subgroup of thin (T1) melanomas. However, newer information has demonstrated that while level of invasion is an independent prognostic factor, it has the lowest statistical correlation with survival rates compared with the other six independent prognostic variables.

Defining T1 Melanomas. In the T1 cohort of melanomas, the assignment of T1a is restricted to melanomas with three criteria (1) ≤1.0 mm thick, (2) absence of ulceration, and (3) mitotic rate of *less than* 1/mm^2. Thus, T1b melanomas are now defined as those whose tumor thickness is ≤1.0 mm *and* have *at least* 1 mitosis/mm^2 or tumor ulceration. This is a major change from the sixth edition Cancer Staging Manual where the level of invasion was used to define T1b melanomas. In the rare circumstances where the mitotic rate cannot be accurately determined, a level invasion of either IV or V as defined by Clark can be used to categorize patients into the T1b classification.

These recommendations were made after reviewing the statistical information involving 4,861 T1 melanomas from the updated AJCC Melanoma Staging Database demonstrating that mitotic rate was the most powerful predictor of survival outcome for T1 melanoma patients, and conversely, that the level of invasion was no longer statistically significant when mitotic rate and ulceration were included (data not shown). Ten-year survival rates ranged from 97% for T1 melanomas of 0.01–0.50 mm in thickness and <1 mitosis/mm^2 to 87% for 0.51–1.00 mm melanomas with ≥1 mitosis/mm^2. In the latter group, the 10-year survival rates dropped to 85% if the melanoma was also ulcerated.

Sentinel Nodal Staging in T1b Melanoma. In the sixth edition of the AJCC *Staging Manual* it was recommended that sentinel node staging be considered in patients presenting with T1bN0M0 or thicker melanomas, based upon the secondary features of either tumor ulceration or Clark's level IV depth of invasion, which were associated with an approximately 10% yield of occult nodal metastases. The use of mitotic rate for the purpose of classifying thin melanomas as T1b in the seventh edition was based on a survival analysis. The AJCC Melanoma Staging Database did not contain sufficient data for precisely estimating risk for occult nodal micrometastases in this population. However, preliminary evidence from several other large studies would suggest that T1b melanomas (as defined in the new system) of ≥0.76 mm in thickness are associated with an approximately 10% risk of occult nodal metastases. Conversely, T1a melanomas with <1 mitoses/mm^2, or T1b melanomas <0.5 mm in thickness have a very low risk of nodal micrometastases. These data may be helpful when discussing the indications for sentinel lymph node biopsy for staging with individual patients with T1b melanoma.

Melanoma In Situ, Indeterminate Melanomas, Multiple Primary Melanomas. Patients with melanoma in situ are categorized as Tis. Those patients with melanoma presentations that are indeterminate or cannot be microstaged should be categorized as TX. However, when the pathology of the initial biopsy finds that the tumor was transected at the base, the maximal thickness should be recorded without the addition of any residual tumor found in the re-excision. If the total thickness found in the re-excision is greater than the thickness of the original biopsy, then only the maximal thickness in the re-excision should be recorded. When patients present with multiple primary melanomas, the T category staging is based upon the melanoma with the worst prognostic features.

Melanoma Growth Patterns. The data used to derive the TNM categories were largely based on melanomas with superficial spreading and nodular growth patterns. There is some evidence that melanomas of other growth patterns, namely lentigo maligna, acral lentiginous, and desmoplastic melanomas, have a different etiology and natural history. At present, the same staging criteria should be used for melanomas with all growth patterns, even though their prognosis may differ somewhat from the more commonly occurring growth patterns.

Regional Lymph Nodes. The 2008 AJCC Staging Melanoma Database contains over 3,400 Stage III patients, the vast majority of whom presented with micrometastases after a sentinel lymph node biopsy and completion lymphadenectomy. A multivariate Cox regression analysis of the database demonstrated that the number of tumor-bearing nodes, tumor burden at the time of staging (i.e., microscopic vs. macroscopic), and presence or absence of ulceration of the primary melanoma were the most predictive independent factors for survival in these patients. These characteristics were incorporated into the stage grouping criteria. For example, the presence of tumor ulceration was used as a criterion for a higher assigned substage due to lower observed survival rates, such that, there was a uniform 5-year survival probability within each of the Stage III subgroups.

Number of Metastatic Nodes. This factor is the primary criterion for defining the N category, because the number of metastatic nodes correlated best with 10-year survival outcomes in all substages of Stage III in the AJCC analysis. Thus, patients with one node involved by metastasis are categorized as N1, those with 2–3 metastatic nodes as N2 and those with ≥4 metastatic nodes involved (or matted nodes) are defined as N3.

Micrometastases vs. *Macrometastases*. Another significant prognostic feature for patients with nodal metastases is the tumor burden of nodal metastases. This terminology is defined operationally, not by actual measurements. Thus, those patients without clinical or radiographic evidence of lymph node metastases but who have pathologically documented nodal metastases are defined by convention as "microscopic" or "clinically occult" nodal metastases. It is recognized that such nodal metastases may vary in dimensions (especially for deep-seated nodes or in obese patients), but such a delineation can be identified in the medical record, based upon the preoperative clinical exam and the operative notation about the intent of the lymphadenectomy (i.e., whether it is a completion lymphadenectomy after sentinel lymph node biopsy for clinically occult disease or a "therapeutic" lymphadenectomy for clinically detected disease). Survival rates for these two patient groups are significantly different.

Immunohistochemical Detection of Micrometastases. Immunohistology should always be adjunctive to good quality hematoxylin and eosin (H&E) stained sections. That being said, for the purposes of staging for nodal metastases, it is no longer mandatory for histopathologic confirmation using standard H&E staining, although this is highly recommended. With the availability of immunohistochemical (IHC) staining, it is now possible to detect nodal metastases as small as <0.1-mm or even aggregates of a few cells. The availability of immunohistochemical methods to detect melanoma-associated antigens is sufficiently available worldwide, that the AJCC Melanoma Task Force considers it acceptable to classify node-positive metastases based solely on immunohistochemical staining of melanoma-associated markers. In the sixth edition of the *Cancer Staging Manual*, micrometastases were only defined when they were detected by standard H&E staining.

Since some IHC markers are sensitive, but not specific, for staining melanoma cells (e.g., S100, tyrosinase), the definitive diagnosis must include detection with at least one melanoma-associated marker (e.g., HMB-45, Melan-A/MART-1) if cellular morphology is not otherwise diagnostic. These "specific" melanoma markers are of limited sensitivity and may not stain up to 15% of melanomas. In several studies, however, the combination of permanent H&E sections with multiple levels and S-100, Melan-A, and/or HMB-45 IHC increased the overall diagnostic sensitivity of sentinel lymph node biopsy.

The reverse transcriptase polymerase chain reaction (RT-PCR) technique may detect metastases not identifiable by the light microscope. Such sophisticated detection procedures may be incorporated into future staging criteria, but at the present time are associated with conflicting results in the literature and are therefore not sufficiently standardized to warrant their inclusion at this time.

Node Positive Threshold for Defining Nodal Micrometastases. There is no definitive evidence that defines a lower threshold of microscopically identifiable tumor burden that should not be used to define node positive disease for staging purposes. Evidence published in the melanoma literature demonstrates that even small volumes of metastatic tumor (e.g., those of 0.1 mm or less in diameter) are associated with a worse prognosis than pathologically negative nodes over time. The concept that isolated tumor cells in the lymph nodes (especially in subcapsular sinuses) are of no adverse biological significance cannot be substantiated for melanoma at this time, and a lower threshold of clinically insignificant nodal metastases has not been defined based on any evidence known to the AJCC Melanoma Task Force membership. These findings are in contrast to the findings often cited from breast cancer where micrometastases of <0.2 mm are defined as "not clinically relevant" and therefore not used as a criterion for staging node positive breast cancer.

Intralymphatic Metastases. The third criterion for defining the N category is the presence or absence of satellites or in transit metastases, regardless of the number of lesions. The available data show no substantial difference in survival outcome for these two anatomically defined entities. The clinical or microscopic presence of satellites around a primary melanoma or of in transit metastases between the primary melanoma site and the regional lymph node basin represent intralymphatic metastases that portend a relatively poor prognosis.

The sixth edition staging manual classification of Stage III melanoma included those patients with regional lymph node metastases or with metastases within the lymphatics manifesting as either satellite (including microsatellites) or in transit metastases. The latter situation would be designated as "N2c" without nodal metastases or "N3" with synchronous nodal metastasis. The identification of satellite or in transit metastases is associated with a poorer survival rate comparable to that of patients with Stage IIIB melanoma (without concomitant nodal metastases) or IIIC melanoma (with nodal metastases or arising from an ulcerated primary melanoma). The 2008 AJCC Melanoma Staging Database contained new information about patients with intralymphatic metastases (N2c). The 5- and 10-year survival rates were 69% and 52%, respectively. These are somewhat more favorable than that previously reported in the literature and higher than the remaining cohort of Stage IIIB patients. Nonetheless, the AJCC Melanoma Task Force noted that the category of Stage IIIB was presently the closest fit and recommended that the sixth edition staging definition be retained.

The data for microsatellites is less robust, but the more limited evidence shows that the survival outcome is comparable to that of patients with clinically detectable satellite metastases. Microscopic satellites are defined as any discontinuous nest of intralymphatic metastatic cells >0.05 mm in diameter that are clearly separated by normal dermis (not fibrosis or inflammation) from the main invasive component of melanoma by a distance of at least 0.3 mm. The significance of the microscopic satellites relates to their being highly predictive of recurrent locoregional involvement and lower survival rates in patients with otherwise uninvolved lymph nodes.

In the past, the definition of microsatellites has varied and this may account for some of the differences in results regarding their prognostic significance. As a result, the level of evidence regarding the prognostic significance of microsatellites is not as robust, but the available data indicates that this finding is an adverse finding associated with an increased risk of regional recurrences and a decreased disease-free survival rate similar to that of clinically detectable satellites. Whether microsatellites represent an independent predictor of survival outcome is less clear but at present the preponderance of evidence suggests that this feature represents an adverse prognostic factor for survival. Accordingly, the AJCC Melanoma Task Force has recommended that this feature of early lymphatic metastases, as defined above, be retained in the category of N2c melanoma.

Contiguous or Multiple Nodal Basins and Staging. By convention, the term regional nodal metastases refers to disease confined to one nodal basin or two contiguous nodal basins, such as patients with nodal disease involving combinations of femoral/iliac, axillary/supraclavicular, cervical/supraclavicular, axillary/femoral or bilateral axillary/femoral metastases. All such patients would be categorized as having Stage III melanoma.

Distant Metastasis. In patients with distant metastases, the site(s) of metastases and elevated serum levels of lactate dehydrogenase (LDH) are used to delineate the M categories into three groups: M1a, M1b, and M1c, with 1-year survival rates ranging from 40 to 60%.

Site(s) of Distant Metastases. Patients with distant metastasis in the skin, subcutaneous tissue, or distant lymph nodes are categorized as M1a provided the LDH level is normal; they have a relatively better prognosis compared with those patients with metastases located in any other anatomic site. Patients with metastasis to the lung and a normal LDH level are categorized as M1b and have an "intermediate" prognosis when comparing survival rates. Those patients with metastases to any other visceral sites or with an elevated LDH level have a relatively worse prognosis and are designated as M1c.

Elevated Serum Lactate Dehydrogenase. Although it is uncommon in staging classifications to include serum factors, an exception was made for elevated levels of serum LDH. The updated AJCC Melanoma Staging Database clearly demonstrates that this is an independent and highly significant predictor of survival outcome among patients who present with or develop Stage IV disease. The mechanism(s) or source(s) of elevated LDH isoenzymes are unknown, and generally the elevations have a nonspecific pattern of elevation among the various LDH isoenzymes. Nevertheless, the clinical results that have emerged from the assessment of total LDH values in relation to outcome are striking in that survival rates are significantly reduced in those patients with an elevated serum LDH at the time of initial Stage IV diagnosis. Thus 1- and 2-year overall survival rates for those Stage IV patients in the 2008 AJCC Melanoma Staging Database with a normal serum LDH were 65% and 40%, respectively, compared with 32% and 18%, respectively, when the serum LDH was elevated at the time of staging. Furthermore, this factor was among the most predictive independent factors of diminished survival in all published studies when it was analyzed in a multivariate analysis, even after accounting for site and number of metastases. Therefore, when the serum LDH is elevated above the upper limits of normal at the time of staging, such patients with distant metastases are assigned to M1c regardless of the site of their distant metastases. To confirm the elevated serum LDH for staging purposes, it is recommended to obtain two or more determinations obtained more than 24 h apart, since an elevated serum LDH on a single determination can be falsely positive due to hemolysis or other factors unrelated to melanoma metastases.

Number of Metastases. The number of metastases at distant sites has previously been documented as an important prognostic factor. This was also confirmed by preliminary multivariate analyses using the AJCC Melanoma Staging Database. However, this feature was not incorporated into this version of the staging system due to the significant variability in the deployment of diagnostic tests to comprehensively search for distant metastases. These may range from a chest x-ray in some centers to high-resolution double-contrast CT, PET/CT, and MRI in others. Until the indications and types of tests used are better standardized, the number of metastases cannot reliably or reproducibly be used for staging purposes.

Metastatic Melanoma from an Unknown Primary Site. In general, the staging criteria for unknown primary metastatic melanoma should be the same as those for known primary melanomas. Potential sources could be primary cutaneous melanomas that have been previously biopsied or which have regressed, or from mucosal or ocular primary sites. When patients have an initial presentation of metastases in the lymph nodes, these should be presumed to be regional (Stage III instead of Stage IV) if an appropriate staging workup does not reveal any other sites of metastases. These patients have a prognosis and natural history that is similar to, if not more favorable than, patients with the same staging characteristics from a known primary cutaneous melanoma. A careful history should be obtained and a close examination of the skin from which lymphatics drain to that nodal basin should be made for previous biopsy scars or areas of depigmentation. If there have been previous biopsies, the pathology should be reviewed to determine if, in retrospect, any of these may have been a primary melanoma.

When there are localized metastases to the skin or subcutaneous tissues, these should also be presumed to be regional (i.e., Stage III instead of Stage IV) if an appropriate staging workup does not reveal any other sites of metastases. In patients with presumed skin metastases from an unknown primary site, pathology review by an experienced pathologist or dermatopathologist is appropriate to confirm that the lesion is not a variant of a primary melanoma, particularly a melanoma with a regressed junctional component. In some patients, examination of the skin with a Wood's light (Black or UV light) reveals skin changes of a regressed primary melanoma that can be confirmed pathologically.

All other circumstances (i.e., metastases to a visceral site and no known primary melanoma) should be categorized as Stage IV melanoma, using the M1 classification criteria described above reflecting metastatic site and serum LDH status.

STAGE GROUPS

Localized Melanoma (Stages I and II). Patients with primary melanomas with no evidence of regional or distant metastases (either clinically or pathologically) are divided into two stages: Stage I for early-stage patients with relatively "low risk" for metastases and melanoma-specific mortality and Stage II for those with "intermediate risk" for metastases and melanoma-specific mortality. Within each stage, the presence of melanoma ulceration heralds an increased relative risk for metastases compared to patients with melanomas of equivalent thickness without ulceration. Therefore, Stage I patients are subdivided into two subgroups (1) Stage IA are T1 melanomas with mitotic rate of <1/mm^2 and without ulceration (T1aN0M0 melanomas) and (2) Stage IB are either T1 melanomas with mitotic rate of at least 1/mm^2 or histopathologic evidence of ulceration (T1bN0M0) or those T2 melanomas without ulceration regardless of mitotic rate (T2aN0M0). Stage II patients constitute three subgroups (1) Stage IIA are T2 melanomas with ulceration (T2bN0M0) or T3 melanomas without ulceration (T3aN0M0); (2) Stage IIB are either T3 melanomas with ulceration (T3bN0M0) or T4 melanomas without ulceration (T4aN0M0); and (3) Stage IIC are T4 melanomas with ulceration (T4bN0M0).

Regional Metastases (Stage III). There are no substages assigned for clinical Stage III melanoma. The major determinants of outcome for pathologic Stage III melanoma are (1) the number of metastatic lymph nodes, (2) whether the tumor burden is "microscopic" (i.e., clinically occult and detected pathologically by sentinel lymph node biopsy) or "macroscopic" (i.e., clinically apparent physical or radiographic examination and verified pathologically), (3) features of the primary melanoma in the presence of nodal micrometastasis, and (4) the presence or absence of satellite or in transit metastases. Note that primary tumor characteristics, including the presence or absence of ulceration of the primary melanoma, increased mitotic rate, and/or tumor thickness, are significant predictors of an adverse outcome in patients with nodal micrometastases, but does not influence outcome in patients who present with nodal macrometastases.

After accounting for these prognostic features in pathologic Stage III melanoma, there are three definable subgroups with statistically significant differences in survival: Stages IIIA, IIIB, and IIIC. Patients with pathologic Stage IIIA are confined to those who have 1–3 lymph nodes with "microscopic" metastases (detected by sentinel or elective lymphadenectomy), and whose primary melanoma is not ulcerated (T1-4aN1aM0 or T1-4aN2aM0). The 5- and 10-year survival rates for such patients are 78% and 68%, respectively. Patients with pathologic Stage IIIB are those with 1–3 lymph nodes with "macroscopic" metastases and a nonulcerated primary melanoma (i.e., T1-4aN1bM0 or T1-4aN2bM0) or those with 1–3 "microscopic" lymph node metastases and an ulcerated primary melanoma (T1-4bN1aM0 or T1-4bN2aM0) or patients with intralymphatic regional metastases but without nodal metastases (T1-4aN2cM0). The estimated 5- and 10-year survival for Stage IIIB patients is 59% and 43%, respectively. In the sixth edition version of the melanoma staging database, the survival rates for patients with isolated intralymphatic metastases were similar to that of patients in the other two subgroups of Stage IIIB disease described above. In the 2008 Melanoma Staging Database, the results of the N2c melanoma patients were somewhat better, with 5- and 10-year survival rates of 69% and 52%, respectively; a more favorable outcome than those in the other two subgroups comprising Stage IIIB melanoma, but still lower than patients with Stage IIIA melanoma.

Patients grouped as Stage IIIC melanoma are defined as those with a 1–3 "macroscopic" lymph node metastases and an ulcerated primary melanoma (T1-4bN1bM0 or T1-4bN2bM0), patients with satellite(s)/in transit metastases arising from an ulcerated primary melanoma (T1-4bN2cM0), or any patient with N3 disease regardless of T status, including patients with any combination of satellites or in transit metastases and nodal metastases. The estimated 5- and 10-year survival rates for pathologic Stage IIIC patients is significantly lower at 40% and 24%, respectively.

Distant Metastases (Stage IV). Because the survival differences between the M categories are small, there are no stage subgroups of Stage IV melanoma.

DEFINITIONS OF TNM

Primary Tumor (T)

TX	Primary tumor cannot be assessed (e.g., curettaged or severely regressed melanoma)
T0	No evidence of primary tumor
Tis	Melanoma in situ
T1	Melanomas 1.0 mm or less in thickness
T2	Melanomas 1.01–2.0 mm
T3	Melanomas 2.01–4.0 mm
T4	Melanomas more than 4.0 mm

Note: a and b subcategories of T are assigned based on ulceration and number of mitoses per mm² as shown below:

T classification	Thickness (mm)	Ulceration Status/Mitoses
T1	≤1.0	a: w/o ulceration and mitosis < 1/mm^2 (Figure 31.7)
		b: with ulceration or mitoses ≥1/mm^2 (Figure 31.8)
T2	1.01–2.0	a: w/o ulceration (Figure 31.9)
		b: with ulceration (Figure 31.10)
T3	2.01–4.0	a: w/o ulceration (Figure 31.11)
		b: with ulceration (Figure 31.12)
T4	>4.0	a: w/o ulceration (Figure 31.13)
		b: with ulceration (Figure 31.14)

Regional Lymph Nodes (N)

NX	Patients in whom the regional nodes cannot be assessed (e.g., previously removed for another reason)
N0	No regional metastases detected
N1-3	Regional metastases based upon the number of metastatic nodes and presence or absence of intralymphatic metastases (in transit or satellite metastases)

Note: N1-3 and a–c subcategories assigned as shown below:

N Classification	No. of Metastatic Nodes	Nodal Metastatic Mass
N1	1 node	a: micrometastasis* (Figure 31.15)
		b: macrometastasis** (Figure 31.16)
N2	2–3 nodes	a: micrometastasis* (Figure 31.17)
		b: macrometastasis** (Figure 31.18)
		c: in transit met(s)/
		satellite(s) *without*
		metastatic nodes (Figure 31.19)
N3	4 or more metastatic nodes, or matted nodes, or in transit met(s)/satellite(s) *with* metastatic node(s) (Figure 31.20)	

*Micrometastases are diagnosed after sentinel lymph node biopsy and completion lymphadenectomy (if performed).
**Macrometastases are defined as clinically detectable nodal metastases confirmed by therapeutic lymphadenectomy or when nodal metastasis exhibits gross extracapsular extension.

Distant Metastatis (M)

M0	No detectable evidence of distant metastases
M1a	Metastases to skin, subcutaneous, or distant lymph nodes
M1b	Metastases to lung
M1c	Metastases to all other visceral sites or distant metastases to any site combined with an elevated serum LDH

Note: Serum LDH is incorporated into the M category as shown below:

M Classification	Site	Serum LDH
M1a	Distant skin, subcutaneous, or nodal mets	Normal
M1b	Lung metastases	Normal
M1c	All other visceral metastases Any distant metastasis	Normal Elevated

ANATOMIC STAGE/PROGNOSTIC GROUPS

Clinical Staging*				Pathologic Staging**			
Stage 0	Tis	N0	M0	0	Tis	N0	M0
Stage IA	T1a	N0	M0	IA	T1a	N0	M0
Stage IB	T1b	N0	M0	IB	T1b	N0	M0
	T2a	N0	M0		T2a	N0	M0
Stage IIA	T2b	N0	M0	IIA	T2b	N0	M0
	T3a	N0	M0		T3a	N0	M0
Stage IIB	T3b	N0	M0	IIB	T3b	N0	M0
	T4a	N0	M0		T4a	N0	M0
Stage IIC	T4b	N0	M0	IIC	T4b	N0	M0
Stage III	Any T	≥N1	M0	IIIA	T1–4a	N1a	M0
					T1–4a	N2a	M0
				IIIB	T1–4b	N1a	M0
					T1–4b	N2a	M0
					T1–4a	N1b	M0
					T1–4a	N2b	M0
					T1–4a	N2c	M0
				IIIC	T1–4b	N1b	M0
					T1–4b	N2b	M0
					T1–4b	N2c	M0
					Any T	N3	M0
Stage IV	Any T	Any N	M1	IV	Any T	Any N	M1

*Clinical staging includes microstaging of the primary melanoma and clinical/radiologic evaluation for metastases. By convention, it should be used after complete excision of the primary melanoma with clinical assessment for regional and distant metastases.

**Pathologic staging includes microstaging of the primary melanoma and pathologic information about the regional lymph nodes after partial or complete lymphadenectomy. Pathologic Stage 0 or Stage IA patients are the exception; they do not require pathologic evaluation of their lymph nodes.

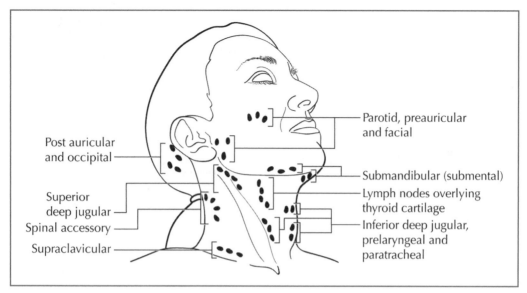

FIGURE 31.1. *Regional lymph nodes for skin sites of the head and neck.*

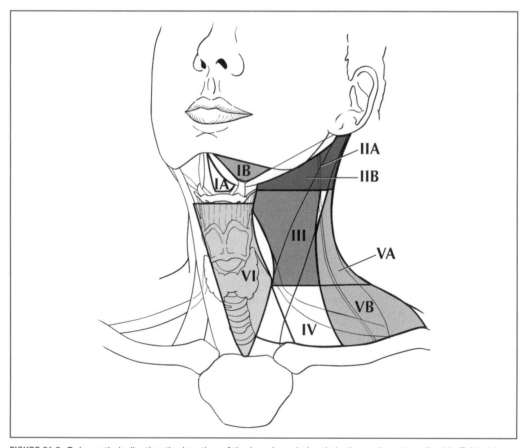

FIGURE 31.2. *Schematic indicating the location of the lymph node levels in the neck as described in Table 31.1.*

TABLE 31.1. *Anatomical Structures Defining the Boundaries of the Neck Levels and Sublevels*

Level	Superior	Inferior	Anterior (Medial)	Posterior (Lateral)
IA	Symphysis of mandible	Body of hyoid	Anterior belly of contralateral digastric muscle	Anterior belly of ipsilateral digastric muscle
IB	Body of mandible	Posterior belly of muscle	Anterior belly of digastric muscle	Stylomyoid muscle
IIA	Skull base	Horizontal plane defined by the inferior body of the hyoid bone	Vertical plane defined by the spinal accessory nerve	Lateral border of the sternocleidomastoid muscle
III	Horizontal planes defined by the inferior body of hyoid	Horizontal plane defined by the inferior border of the cricoid cartilage	Lateral border of the sternohuoid muscle	Lateral border of the sternocleidomastoid or sensory branches of cervical plexus
IV	Horizontal plane defined by the inferior border of the cricoid cartilage	Clavicle	Lateral border of the sternohyoid muscle	Lateral border of the sternocleidomastoid or sensory branches of cervical plexus
VA	Apex of the convergence of the sternocleidomastoid and trapezius muscles	Horizontal plane defined by the lower border of the cricoid cartilage	Posterior border of the sternocleidomastoid muscle or sensory branches of cervical plexus	Anterior border of the the trapezius muscle
VI	Hyoid bone	Suprasternal notch	Common carotid artery	Common carotid artery
VII	Suprasternal notch	Innominate artery	Sternum	Trachea, esophagus, and prevertebral fascia

Modified from Robbins KT, Clayman G, Levine PA, et al.; American Head and Neck Society; American Academy of Otolaryngology–Head and Neck Surgery. Neck dissection classification update: revisions proposed by the American Head and Neck Society and the American Academy of Otolaryngology-Head and Neck Surgery. Arch Otolaryngol Head Neck Surg. 2002 Jul;128(7):751-8, with permission of the American Medical Association.

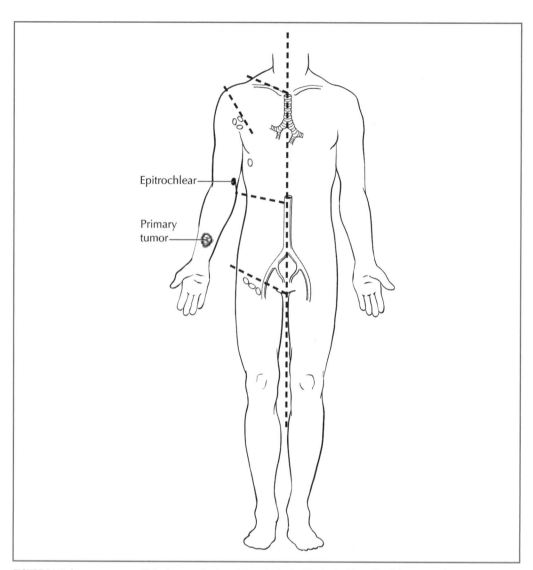

FIGURE 31.3. *Less common clinical or sentinel nodal metastasis. Illustrated is a distal forearm primary tumor with involvement of the epitrochlear node.*

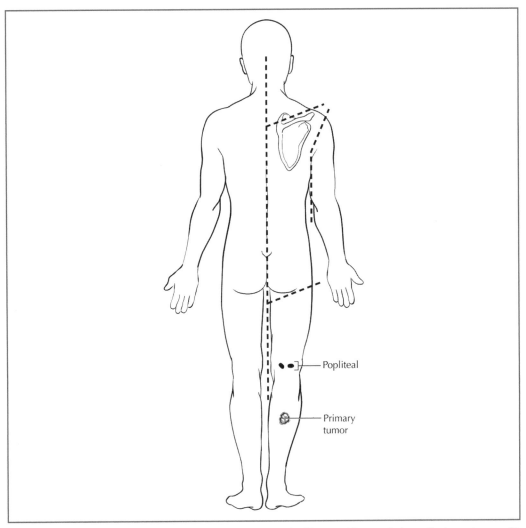

FIGURE 31.4. *Less common clinical or sentinel nodal metastasis. Illustrated is a posterior calf primary tumor with involvement of the popliteal nodes.*

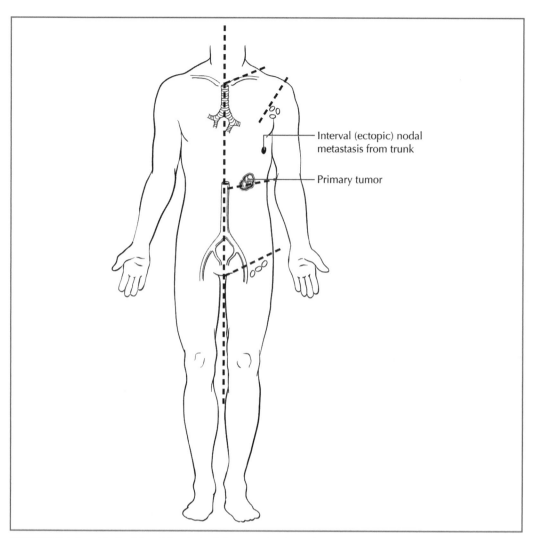

Interval (ectopic) nodal metastasis from trunk

Primary tumor

FIGURE 31.5. *Interval (ectopic) nodal metastasis from trunk primary tumor.*

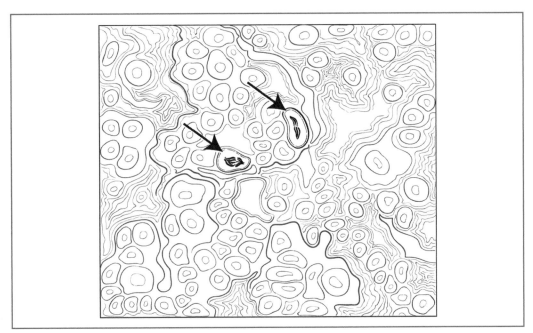

FIGURE 31.6. *Two mitotic figures in a melanoma (arrow heads). Assessment of the number of mitoses per square millimeter used to determine the prognostically relevant "mitotic rate."*

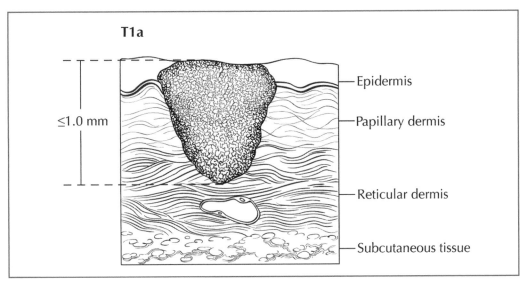

FIGURE 31.7. *T1a is defined as melanoma ≤1.0 mm in thickness, with no ulceration, and mitotic rate <1 mm².*

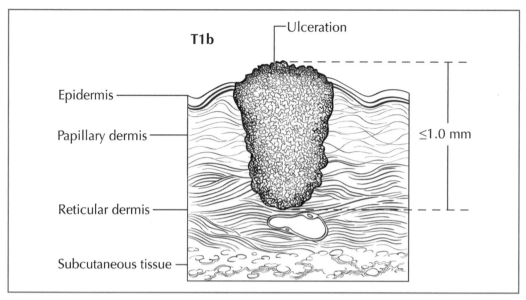

FIGURE 31.8. *T1b is defined as melanoma ≤1.0 mm in thickness with ulceration or mitotic rate ≥1 mm².*

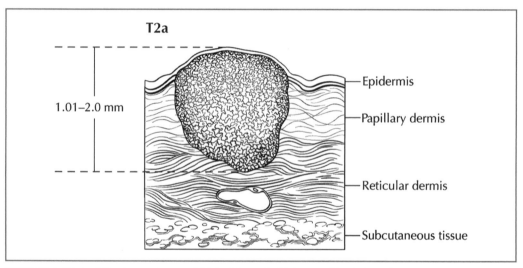

FIGURE 31.9. *T2a is defined as melanoma 1.01 to 2.0 mm in thickness without ulceration.*

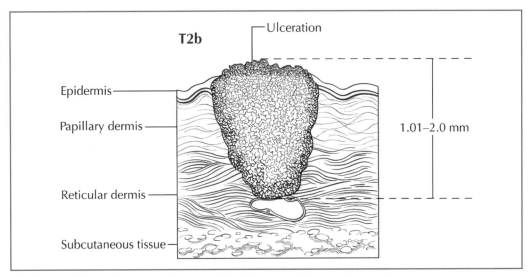

FIGURE 31.10. *T2b is defined as melanoma 1.01 to 2.0 mm in thickness with ulceration.*

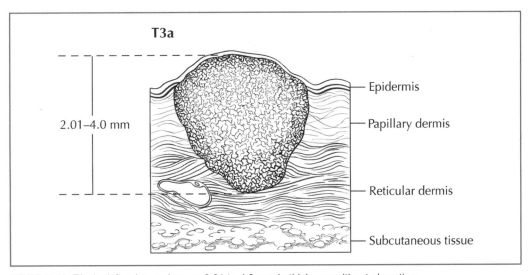

FIGURE 31.11. *T3a is defined as melanoma 2.01 to 4.0 mm in thickness without ulceration.*

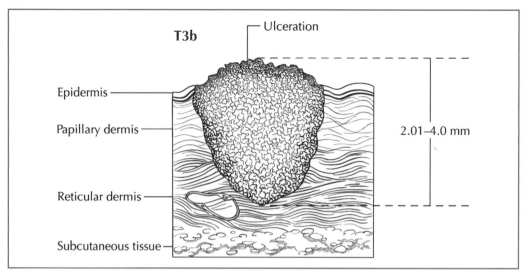

FIGURE 31.12. *T3b is defined as melanoma 2.01 to 4.0 mm in thickness with ulceration.*

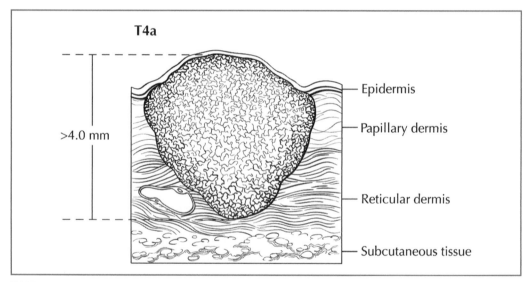

FIGURE 31.13. *T4a is defined as melanoma more than 4.0 mm in thickness without ulceration.*

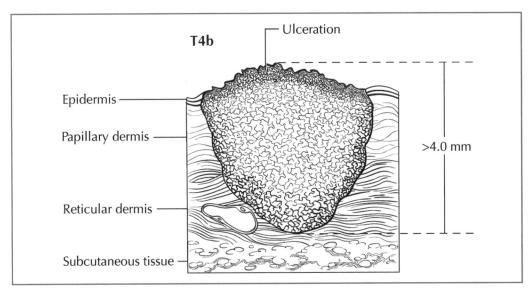

FIGURE 31.14. *T4b is defined as melanoma more than 4.0 mm in thickness with ulceration.*

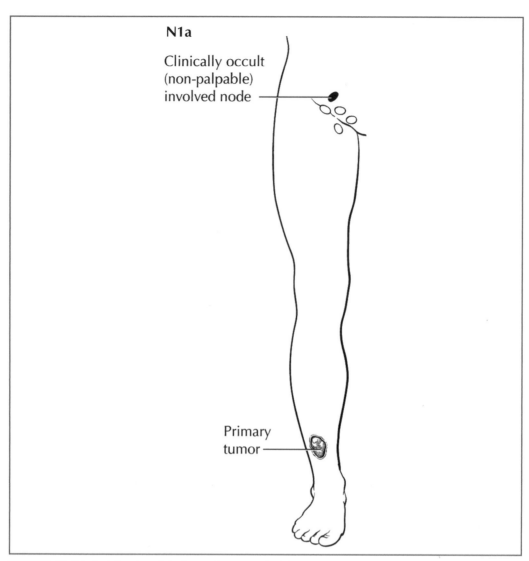

N1a

Clinically occult
(non-palpable)
involved node

Primary
tumor

FIGURE 31.15. *N1a is defined as clinically occult metastasis (micrometastasis) in one lymph node.*

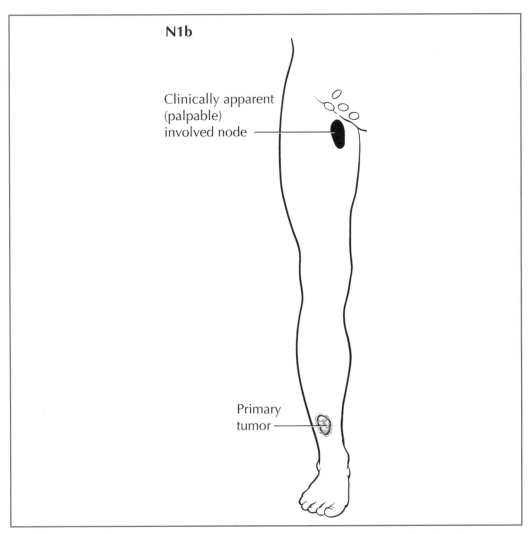

N1b

Clinically apparent (palpable) involved node

Primary tumor

FIGURE 31.16. *N1b is defined as clinically apparent metastasis (macrometastasis) in one lymph node.*

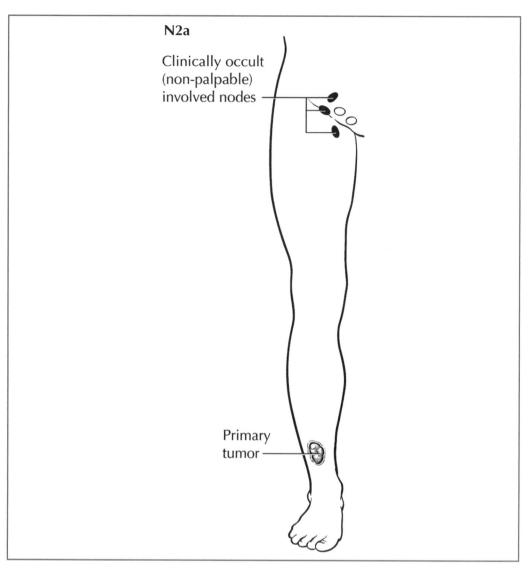

N2a

Clinically occult
(non-palpable)
involved nodes

Primary
tumor

FIGURE 31.17. *N2a is defined as clinically occult metastases (micrometastases) in 2-3 regional nodes.*

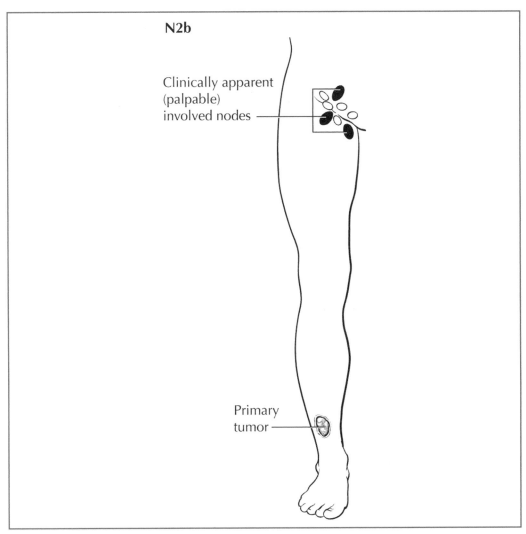

N2b

Clinically apparent
(palpable)
involved nodes

Primary
tumor

FIGURE 31.18. *N2b is defined as clinically apparent metastases (macrometastases) in 2-3 regional nodes.*

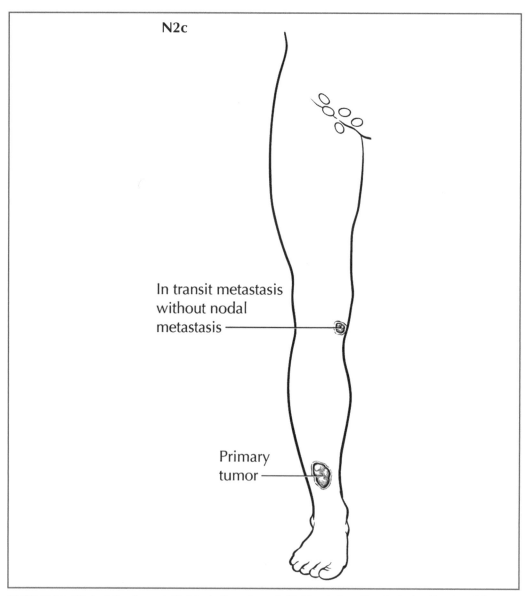

N2c

In transit metastasis
without nodal
metastasis

Primary
tumor

FIGURE 31.19. *N2c is defined as satellite* (including microsatellite**) or in transit metastasis without nodal metastasis. This figure illustrates an in transit metastasis, which is defined as clinically evident cutaneous and/or subcutaneous metastases identified at a distance greater than 2 cm from the primary melanoma in the region between the primary and the first echelon of regional lymph nodes.*

*Satellites are defined as grossly visible cutaneous and/or subcutaneous metastases occurring within 2 cm of the primary melanoma.
**Microsatellites are defined as any discontinuous nest of intralymphatic metastatic cells >0.05 mm in diameter that are clearly separated by normal dermis (not fibrosis or inflammation) from the main invasive component of melanoma by a distance of at least 0.3 mm.

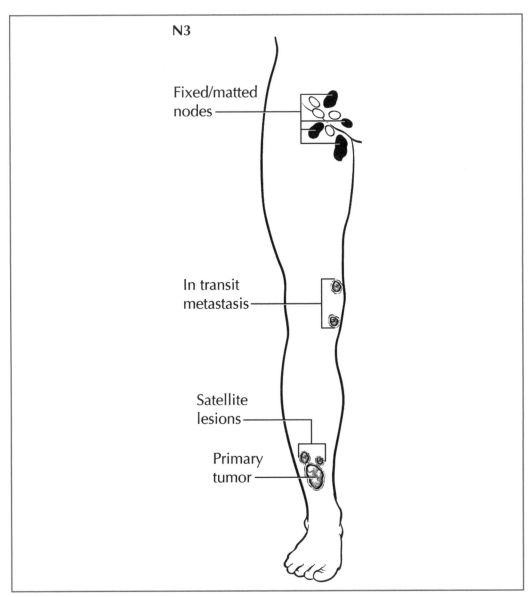

FIGURE 31.20. *N3 may be defined as 4 or more metastatic nodes, or matted nodes, or in transit met(s)/satellite(s) with metastatic node(s).*

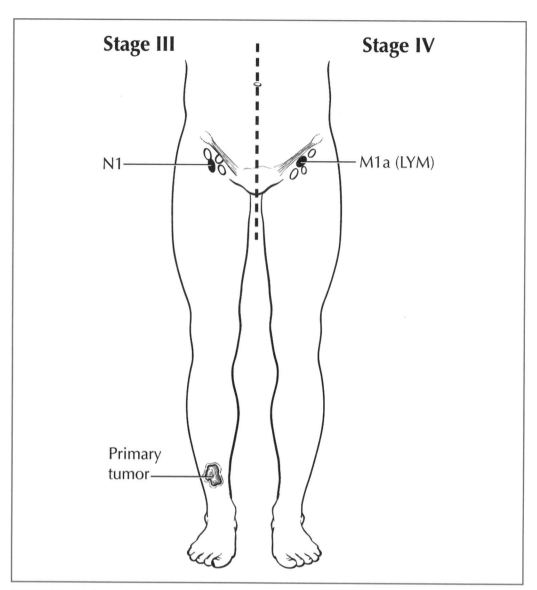

FIGURE 31.21. *N1 disease is defined as regional lymph node metastasis while M1a disease involves distant metastasis to lymph nodes beyond the region of the primary tumor.*

Figure 31.21 illustrates the designation of N1 (Stage III disease) based on metastasis to regional lymph nodes vs. the designation of M1a (Stage IV disease) defined by distant metastasis, in this case to lymph nodes outside the region the primary tumor. Figures 31.22, 31.23, 31.24, and 31.25 illustrate N1 (Stage III) or M1a (Stage IV) disease based upon whether affected lymph nodes fall within or beyond the regional nodal chain of the primary tumor. The shaded areas in the figures indicate disease spread to regional lymph nodes for a classification of N1 (Stage III).

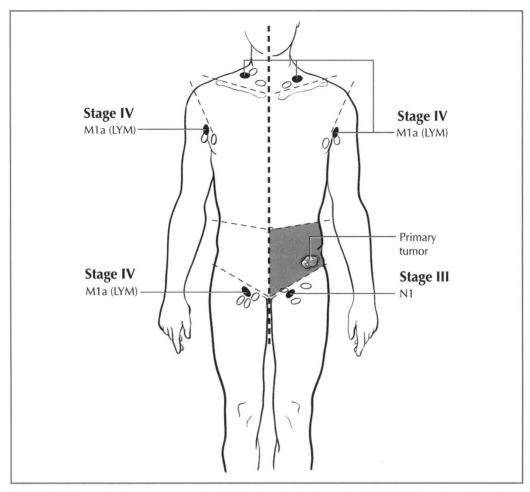

FIGURE 31.22. *Stage of disease as determined by lymph node involvement relative to the location of the primary tumor. The shaded areas indicate involvement of regional lymph nodes or N1 disease (Stage III). Nonshaded areas indicate distant metastasis to lymph nodes outside the primary tumor or M1a disease (Stage IV).*

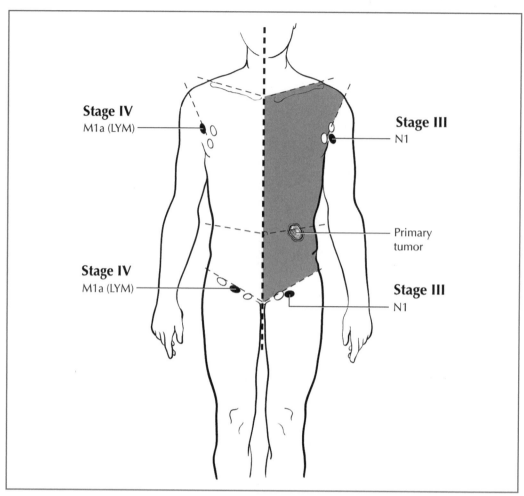

FIGURE 31.23. *Stage of disease as determined by lymph node involvement relative to the location of the primary tumor. The shaded areas indicate involvement of regional lymph nodes or N1 disease (Stage III). Nonshaded areas indicate distant metastasis to lymph nodes outside the primary tumor or M1a disease (Stage IV).*

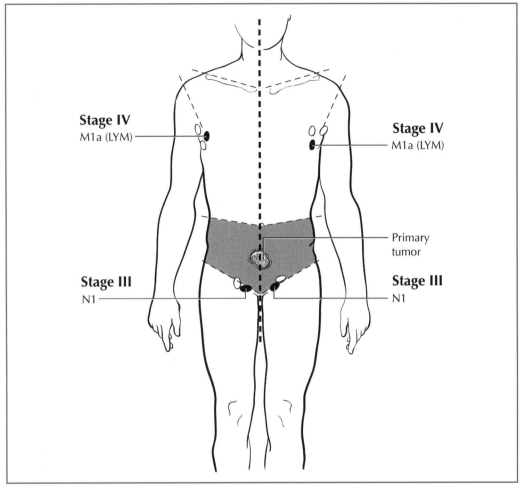

FIGURE 31.24. *Stage of disease as determined by lymph node involvement relative to the location of the primary tumor. The shaded areas indicate involvement of regional lymph nodes or N1 disease (Stage III). Nonshaded areas indicate distant metastasis to lymph nodes outside the primary tumor or M1a disease (Stage IV).*

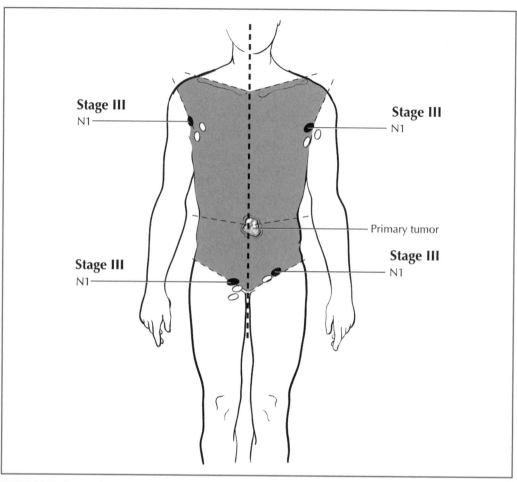

FIGURE 31.25. *Stage of disease as determined by lymph node involvement relative to the location of the primary tumor. The shaded areas indicate involvement of regional lymph nodes or N1 disease (Stage III). Metastasis to either the axillary or inguinal lymph nodes are both considered N1 (Stage III) disease due to the location of the primary tumor directly in the center of the torso.*

PROGNOSTIC FACTORS (SITE-SPECIFIC FACTORS)
(Recommended for Collection)

Required for staging	None
Clinically significant	Measured thickness
	Ulceration
	Serum lactate dehydrogenase (LDH)
	Mitotic rate
	Tumor infiltrating lymphocytes (TIL)
	Level of invasion
	Vertical growth phase
	Regression

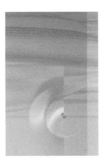

PART VII
Breast

Breast

32

SUMMARY OF CHANGES

Tumor (T)

- Identified specific imaging modalities that can be used to estimate clinical tumor size, including mammography, ultrasound, and magnetic resonance imaging (MRI)
- Made specific recommendations that (1) the microscopic measurement is the most accurate and preferred method to determine pT with a small invasive cancer that can be entirely submitted in one paraffin block, and (2) the gross measurement is the most accurate and preferred method to determine pT with larger invasive cancers that must be submitted in multiple paraffin blocks
- Made the specific recommendation to use the clinical measurement thought to be most accurate to determine the clinical T of breast cancers treated with neoadjuvant therapy. Pathologic (posttreatment) size should be estimated based on the best combination of gross and microscopic histological findings
- Made the specific recommendation to estimate the size of invasive cancers that are unapparent to any clinical modalities or gross pathologic examination by carefully measuring and recording the relative positions of tissue samples submitted for microscopic evaluation and determining which contain tumor
- Acknowledged "ductal intraepithelial neoplasia" (DIN) as uncommon, and still not widely accepted, terminology encompassing both DCIS and ADH, and clarification that only cases referred to as DIN containing DCIS (±ADH) are classified as Tis (DCIS)
- Acknowledged "lobular intraepithelial neoplasia" (LIN) as uncommon, and still not widely accepted, terminology encompassing both LCIS and ALH, and clarification that only cases referred to as LIN containing LCIS (±ALH) are classified as Tis (LCIS)
- Clarification that only Paget's disease NOT associated with an underlying noninvasive (i.e., DCIS and/or LCIS) or invasive breast cancer should be classified as Tis (Paget's) and that Paget's disease associated with an underlying cancer be classified according to the underlying cancer (Tis, T1, etc.)
- Made the recommendation to estimate the size of noninvasive carcinomas (DCIS and LCIS), even though it does not currently change their T classification, because noninvasive cancer size may influence therapeutic decisions, acknowledging that providing a precise size for LCIS may be difficult
- Acknowledged that the prognosis of microinvasive carcinoma is generally thought to be quite favorable, although the clinical impact of multifocal microinvasive disease is not well understood at this time
- Acknowledged that it is not necessary for tumors to be in separate quadrants to be classified as multiple simultaneous ipsilateral carcinomas, providing that they can be unambiguously demonstrated to be macroscopically distinct and measurable using available clinical and pathologic techniques

(continued)

C.C. Compton et al. (eds.), *AJCC Cancer Staging Atlas: A Companion to the Seventh Editions of the AJCC Cancer Staging Manual and Handbook*, DOI 10.1007/978-1-4614-2080-4_32, © 2012 American Joint Committee on Cancer

- Maintained that the term "inflammatory carcinoma" be restricted to cases with typical skin changes involving a third or more of the skin of the breast. While the histologic presence of invasive carcinoma invading dermal lymphatics is supportive of the diagnosis, it is not required, nor is dermal lymphatic invasion without typical clinical findings sufficient for a diagnosis of inflammatory breast cancer
- Recommend that all invasive cancer should be graded using the Nottingham combined histologic grade (Elston-Ellis modification of Scarff– Bloom– Richardson grading system)

Nodes (N)

- Classification of isolated tumor cell clusters and single cells is more stringent. Small clusters of cells not greater than 0.2 mm, or nonconfluent or nearly confluent clusters of cells not exceeding 200 cells in a single histologic lymph node cross section are classified as isolated tumor cells
- Use of the (sn) modifier has been clarified and restricted. When six or more sentinel nodes are identified on gross examination of pathology specimens the (sn) modifier should be omitted
- Stage I breast tumors have been subdivided into Stage IA and Stage IB; Stage IB includes small tumors (T1) with exclusively micrometastases in lymph nodes (N1mi)

Metastases (M)

- Created new M0(i+) category, defined by presence of either disseminated tumor cells detectable in bone marrow or circulating tumor cells or found incidentally in other tissues (such as ovaries removed prophylactically) if not exceeding 0.2 mm. However, this category does not change the Stage Grouping. Assuming that they do not have clinically and/or radiographically detectable metastases, patients with M0(i+) are staged according to T and N

Postneoadjuvant Therapy (yc or ypTNM)

- In the setting of patients who received neoadjuvant therapy, pretreatment clinical T (cT) should be based on clinical or imaging findings
- Postneoadjuvant therapy T should be based on clinical or imaging (ycT) or pathologic findings (ypT)
- A subscript will be added to the clinical N for both node negative and node positive patients to indicate whether the N was derived from clinical examination, fine needle aspiration, core needle biopsy, or sentinel lymph node biopsy
- The posttreatment ypT will be defined as the largest contiguous focus of invasive cancer as defined histopathologically with a subscript to indicate the presence of multiple tumor foci. Note: definition of posttreatment ypT remains controversial and an area in transition
- Posttreatment nodal metastases no greater than 0.2 mm are classified as ypN0(i+) as in patients who have not received neoadjuvant systemic therapy. However, patients with this finding are not considered to have achieved a pathologic complete response (pCR)
- A description of the degree of response to neoadjuvant therapy (complete, partial, no response) will be collected by the registrar with the posttreatment ypTNM. The registrars are requested to describe how they defined response [by physical examination, imaging techniques (mammogram, ultrasound, magnetic resonance imaging (MRI)) or pathologically]
- Patients will be considered to have M1 (and therefore Stage IV) breast cancer if they have had clinically or radiographically detectable metastases, with or without biopsy, prior to neoadjuvant systemic therapy, regardless of their status after neoadjuvant systemic therapy

PROGNOSTIC FEATURES

New biomarkers are added and recommended for collection in addition to hormone receptors (estrogen receptor, ER; progesterone receptor, PgR). These are HER2 (also designated as erbB2 and c-neu) status and multigene signature "score" or classifications.

ICD-O-3 TOPOGRAPHY CODES

C50.0   Nipple
C50.1   Central portion of breast
C50.2   Upper inner quadrant of breast
C50.3   Lower inner quadrant of breast
C50.4   Upper outer quadrant of breast
C50.5   Lower outer quadrant of breast
C50.6   Axillary tail of breast
C50.8   Overlapping lesion of breast
C50.9   Breast, NOS

ICD-O-3 HISTOLOGY CODE RANGES

8000–8576, 8940–8950, 8980–8981, 9020

ANATOMY

Primary Site. The mammary gland (Figure 32.1), situated on the anterior chest wall, is composed of glandular tissue with a dense fibrous stroma. The glandular tissue consists of lobules that group together into 8–15 lobes, occasionally more, arranged approximately in a spoke-like pattern. Multiple major and minor ducts connect the milk-secreting lobular units to the nipple. Small milk ducts course throughout the breast, converging into larger collecting ducts that open into the lactiferous sinus at the base of the nipple. Each duct system has unique anatomy: the smallest systems may comprise only a portion of a quadrant whereas the largest systems may comprise more than a quadrant. The periphery of each system overlaps along their radial boundaries. Most cancers form initially in the terminal duct lobular units of the breast. Carcinoma spreads along the duct system in the radial axis of the lobe; invasive carcinoma is more likely to spread in a centripetal orientation in the breast stroma from the initial locus of invasion, although opportunistic intraductal spread may be enhanced along the radial axes. Glandular tissue is more abundant in the upper outer portion of the breast; as a result, half of all breast cancers occur in this area.

Chest Wall. The chest wall includes ribs, intercostal muscles, and serratus anterior muscle, but not the pectoral muscles. Therefore, involvement of the pectoral muscle does not constitute chest wall invasion.

Regional Lymph Nodes. The breast lymphatics drain by way of three major routes: axillary, transpectoral, and internal mammary. Intramammary lymph nodes reside within breast tissue and are coded as axillary lymph nodes for staging purposes. Supraclavicular lymph nodes are classified as regional lymph nodes for staging purposes. Metastases to any other lymph node, including cervical or contralateral internal mammary or axillary lymph nodes, are classified as distant (M1) (Figure 32.2.)

The regional lymph nodes are as follows:

1. Axillary (ipsilateral): interpectoral (Rotter's) nodes and lymph nodes along the axillary vein and its tributaries that may be (but are not required to be) divided into the following levels:

   a. Level I (low-axilla): lymph nodes lateral to the lateral border of pectoralis minor muscle.
   b. Level II (mid-axilla): lymph nodes between the medial and lateral borders of the pectoralis minor muscle and the interpectoral (Rotter's) lymph nodes.
   c. Level III (apical axilla): lymph nodes medial to the medial margin of the pectoralis minor muscle and inferior to the clavicle. These are also known as apical or infraclavicular nodes. Metastases to these nodes portend a worse prognosis. Therefore, the infraclavicular designation will be used hereafter to differentiate these nodes from the remaining (level I, II) axillary nodes.

2. Internal mammary (ipsilateral): lymph nodes in the intercostal spaces along the edge of the sternum in the endothoracic fascia.

3. Supraclavicular: lymph nodes in the supraclavicular fossa, a triangle defined by the omohyoid muscle and tendon (lateral and superior border), the internal jugular vein (medial border), and the clavicle and subclavian vein (lower border). Adjacent lymph nodes outside of this triangle are considered to be lower cervical nodes (M1).

4. Intramammary: lymph nodes within the breast; these are considered axillary lymph nodes for purposes of N classification and staging.

Metastatic Sites. Tumor cells may be disseminated by either the lymphatic or the blood vascular system. The four major sites of involvement are bone, lung, brain, and liver, but tumor cells are also capable of metastasizing to many other sites. Bone marrow micrometastases, circulating tumor cells, and tumor deposits no larger than 0.2 mm detected inadvertently, such as in prophylactically removed ovarian tissue, are collectively known as microscopic disseminated tumor cells (DTCs). These deposits do not alone define or constitute metastatic disease, although there are data that demonstrate that, in early stage disease, DTCs correlate with recurrence and mortality risk, and in patients with established M1 disease, circulating tumor cells (CTCs) are prognostic for shorter survival.

DEFINITIONS OF TNM

The increasing use of neoadjuvant therapy in breast cancer and the documented prognostic impact of postneoadjuvant extent of disease and response to therapy warrant clear definitions of the use of the "yp" prefix and response to therapy. The use of neoadjuvant therapy does not change the clinical (pretreatment) stage. As per TNM rules, the clinical stage is identified with the prefix "c". In addition, the use of fine needle aspiration and sentinel lymph node biopsy before neoadjuvant therapy is denoted with the subscripts "f" and "sn," respectively. Nodal metastases detected by FNA or core biopsy are classified as macrometastases (N1) regardless of the size of the tumor focus in the final pathologic specimen. For example, if, prior to neoadjuvant systemic therapy, a patient has no palpable nodes but has an ultrasound-guided FNA biopsy of an axillary lymph node that is positive, the patient will be categorized as cN1 (f) for her clinical (pretreatment) staging and would be considered as stage IIA. Likewise, if the patient has a positive axillary sentinel node identified prior to neoadjuvant systemic therapy, the patient will be categorized as cN1 (sn) (Stage IIA).

As per TNM rules, with the absence of pathologic T evaluation (removal of the primary tumor), microscopic evaluation of nodes before neoadjuvant therapy is still classified as clinical "c."

Primary Tumor (T)

The T classification of the primary tumor is the same regardless of whether it is based on clinical or pathologic criteria, or both. Size should be measured to the nearest millimeter. If the tumor size is slightly less than or greater than a cutoff for a given T classification, it is recommended that the size be rounded to the millimeter reading that is closest to the cutoff. For example, a reported size of 1.1 mm is reported as 1 mm, or a size of 2.01 cm is reported as 2.0 cm. Designation should be made with the subscript "c" or "p" modifier to indicate whether the T classification was determined by clinical (physical examination or radiologic) or pathologic measurements, respectively. In general, pathologic determination should take precedence over clinical determination of T size.

TX	Primary tumor cannot be assessed
T0	No evidence of primary tumor
Tis	Carcinoma in situ (Figure 32.3)
Tis (DCIS)	Ductal carcinoma in situ
Tis (LCIS)	Lobular carcinoma in situ
Tis (Paget's)	Paget's disease of the nipple NOT associated with invasive carcinoma and/or carcinoma in situ (DCIS and/or LCIS) in the underlying breast parenchyma. Carcinomas in the breast parenchyma associated with Paget's disease are categorized based on the size and characteristics of the parenchymal disease, although the presence of Paget's disease should still be noted (Figure 32.3)
T1	Tumor ≤20 mm in greatest dimension
T1mi	Tumor ≤1 mm in greatest dimension (Figure 32.4)
T1a	Tumor > 1 mm but ≤5 mm in greatest dimension (Figure 32.5)
T1b	Tumor >5 mm but ≤10 mm in greatest dimension (Figure 32.5)
T1c	Tumor > 10 mm but ≤20 mm in greatest dimension (Figure 32.5)
T2	Tumor >20 mm but ≤50 mm in greatest dimension (Figure 32.6)
T3	Tumor >50 mm in greatest dimension (Figure 32.6)
T4	Tumor of any size with direct extension to the chest wall and/or to the skin (ulceration or skin nodules).

Note: Invasion of the dermis alone does not qualify as T4

T4a	Extension to the chest wall, not including only pectoralis muscle adherence/invasion (Figure 32.7)
T4b	Ulceration and/or ipsilateral satellite nodules and/or edema (including peau d'orange) of the skin, which do not meet the criteria for inflammatory carcinoma (Figure 32.8A, B)
T4c	Both T4a and T4b (Figure 32.9)
T4d	Inflammatory carcinoma (Figure 32.10)

Posttreatment ypT. Clinical (pretreatment) T will be defined by clinical and radiographic findings, while y pathologic (posttreatment) T will be determined by pathologic size and extension. The ypT will be measured as the largest single focus of invasive tumor, with the modifier "m" indicating multiple foci. The measurement of the largest tumor focus should not include areas of fibrosis within the tumor bed. The inclusion of additional information in the pathology report such as the distance over which tumor foci extend, the number of tumor foci present, or the number of slides/blocks in which tumor appears may assist the clinician in estimating the extent of disease. A comparison of the cellularity in the initial biopsy to that in the posttreatment specimen may also aid in the assessment of response.

Note: If a cancer was designated as inflammatory before neoadjuvant chemotherapy, the patient will be designated to have inflammatory breast cancer throughout, even if the patient has complete resolution of inflammatory findings.

Regional Lymph Nodes (N)

Clinical

NX	Regional lymph nodes cannot be assessed (e.g., previously removed)
N0	No regional lymph node metastases
N1	Metastases to movable ipsilateral level I, II axillary lymph node(s) (Figure 32.11)
N2	Metastases in ipsilateral level I, II axillary lymph nodes that are clinically fixed or matted; or in clinically detected* ipsilateral internal mammary nodes in the *absence* of clinically evident axillary lymph node metastases
N2a	Metastases in ipsilateral level I, II axillary lymph nodes fixed to one another (matted) or to other structures (Figure 32.12)
N2b	Metastases only in clinically detected* ipsilateral internal mammary nodes and in the *absence* of clinically evident axillary lymph node metastases (Figure 32.13)
N3	Metastases in ipsilateral infraclavicular (level III axillary) lymph node(s) with or without level I, II axillary lymph node involvement; or in clinically detected* ipsilateral internal mammary lymph node(s) with clinically evident level I, II axillary lymph node metastases; or metastases in ipsilateral supraclavicular lymph node(s) with or without axillary or internal mammary lymph node involvement
N3a	Metastases in ipsilateral infraclavicular lymph node(s) (Figure 32.14)
N3b	Metastases in ipsilateral internal mammary lymph node(s) and axillary lymph node(s) (Figure 32.15)
N3c	Metastases in ipsilateral supraclavicular lymph node(s) (Figure 32.16)

*Note: *Clinically detected* is defined as detected by imaging studies (excluding lymphoscintigraphy) or by clinical examination and having characteristics highly suspicious for malignancy or a presumed pathologic macrometastasis based on fine needle aspiration biopsy with cytologic examination. Confirmation of clinically detected metastatic disease by fine needle aspiration without excision biopsy is designated with an (f) suffix, for example, cN3a(f). Excisional biopsy of a lymph node or biopsy of a sentinel node, in the absence of assignment of a pT, is classified as a clinical N, for example, cN1. Information regarding the confirmation of the nodal status will be designated in site-specific factors as clinical, fine needle aspiration, core biopsy, or sentinel lymph node biopsy. Pathologic classification (pN) is used for excision or sentinel lymph node biopsy only in conjunction with a pathologic T assignment.

Pathologic (pN)*

pNX	Regional lymph nodes cannot be assessed (e.g., previously removed, or not removed for pathologic study)
pN0	No regional lymph node metastasis identified histologically

Note: Isolated tumor cell clusters (ITC) are defined as small clusters of cells not greater than 0.2 mm, or single tumor cells, or a cluster of fewer than 200 cells in a single histologic cross-section. ITCs may be detected by routine histology or by immunohistochemical (IHC) methods. Nodes containing only ITCs are excluded from the total positive node count for purposes of N classification but should be included in the total number of nodes evaluated.

pN0(I–)	No regional lymph node metastases histologically, negative IHC
pN0(i+)	Malignant cells in regional lymph node(s) no greater than 0.2 mm (detected by H&E or IHC including ITC) (Figure 32.17)
pN0(mol–)	No regional lymph node metastases histologically, negative molecular findings (RT-PCR)
pN0(mol+)	Positive molecular findings (RT-PCR),** but no regional lymph node metastases detected by histology or IHC
pN1	Micrometastases; or metastases in 1–3 axillary lymph nodes; and/or in internal mammary nodes with metastases detected by sentinel lymph node biopsy but not clinically detected ***
pN1mi	Micrometastases (greater than 0.2 mm and/or more than 200 cells, but none greater than 2.0 mm) (Figure 32.18)
pN1a	Metastases in 1–3 axillary lymph nodes, at least one metastasis greater than 2.0 mm (Figure 32.18)
pN1b	Metastases in internal mammary nodes with micrometastases or macrometastases detected by sentinel lymph node biopsy but not clinically detected *** (Figure 32.19)
pN1c	Metastases in 1–3 axillary lymph nodes and in internal mammary lymph nodes with micrometastases or macrometastases detected by sentinel lymph node biopsy but not clinically detected*** (Figure 32.20)
pN2	Metastases in 4–9 axillary lymph nodes; or in clinically detected**** internal mammary lymph nodes in the *absence* of axillary lymph node metastases
pN2a	Metastases in 4–9 axillary lymph nodes (at least one tumor deposit greater than 2.0 mm) (Figure 32.18)
pN2b	Metastases in clinically detected**** internal mammary lymph nodes in the *absence* of axillary lymph node metastases (Figure 32.21)
pN3	Metastases in ten or more axillary lymph nodes; or in infraclavicular (level III axillary) lymph nodes; or in clinically detected**** ipsilateral internal mammary lymph nodes in the *presence* of one or more positive level I, II axillary lymph nodes; or in more than three axillary lymph nodes and in internal mammary lymph nodes with micrometastases or macrometastases detected by sentinel lymph node biopsy but not clinically detected***; or in ipsilateral supraclavicular lymph nodes
pN3a	Metastases in ten or more axillary lymph nodes (at least one tumor deposit greater than 2.0 mm); or metastases to the infraclavicular (level III axillary lymph) nodes (Figure 32.18)
pN3b	Metastases in clinically detected**** ipsilateral internal mammary lymph nodes in the *presence* of one or more positive axillary lymph nodes; or in more than three axillary lymph nodes and in internal mammary lymph nodes with micrometastases or macrometastases detected by sentinel lymph node biopsy but not clinically detected*** (Figure 32.22A, B)
pN3c	Metastases in ipsilateral supraclavicular lymph nodes (Figure 32.23)

Notes:

*Classification is based on axillary lymph node dissection with or without sentinel lymph node biopsy. Classification based solely on sentinel lymph node biopsy without subsequent axillary lymph node dissection is designated (sn) for "sentinel node," for example, pN0(sn).

**RT-PCR: reverse transcriptase/polymerase chain reaction.

*** "Not clinically detected" is defined as not detected by imaging studies (excluding lymphoscintigraphy) or not detected by clinical examination.

**** "Clinically detected" is defined as detected by imaging studies (excluding lymphoscintigraphy) or by clinical examination and having characteristics highly suspicious for malignancy or a presumed pathologic macrometastasis based on fine needle aspiration biopsy with cytologic examination.

Posttreatment ypN

- Post-treatment yp "N" should be evaluated as for clinical (pretreatment) "N" methods above. The modifier "sn" is used only if a sentinel node evaluation was performed after treatment. If no subscript is attached, it is assumed that the axillary nodal evaluation was by axillary node dissection (AND).
- The X classification will be used (ypNX) if no yp posttreatment SN or AND was performed.
- N categories are the same as those used for pN.

Distant Metastases (M)

M0	No clinical or radiographic evidence of distant metastases
cM0(i+)	No clinical or radiographic evidence of distant metastases, but deposits of molecularly or microscopically detected tumor cells in circulating blood, bone marrow, or other nonregional nodal tissue that are no larger than 0.2 mm in a patient without symptoms or signs of metastases
M1	Distant detectable metastases as determined by classic clinical and radiographic means and/or histologically proven larger than 0.2 mm

Posttreatment yp M classification. The M category for patients treated with neoadjuvant therapy is the category assigned in the clinical stage, prior to initiation of neoadjuvant therapy. Identification of distant metastases after the start of therapy in cases where pretherapy evaluation showed no metastases is considered progression of disease. If a patient was designated to have detectable distant metastases (M1) before chemotherapy, the patient will be designated as M1 throughout.

ANATOMIC STAGE/PROGNOSTIC GROUPS

Stage 0	Tis	N0	M0
Stage IA	T1*	N0	M0
Stage IB	T0	N1mi	M0
	T1*	N1mi	M0
Stage IIA	T0	N1**	M0
	T1*	N1**	M0
	T2	N0	M0
Stage IIB	T2	N1	M0
	T3	N0	M0
Stage IIIA	T0	N2	M0
	T1*	N2	M0
	T2	N2	M0
	T3	N1	M0
	T3	N2	M0
Stage IIIB	T4	N0	M0
	T4	N1	M0
	T4	N2	M0
Stage IIIC	Any T	N3	M0
Stage IV	Any T	Any N	M1

Notes:
*T1 includes T1mi.
**T0 and T1 tumors with nodal micrometastases only are excluded from Stage IIA and are classified Stage IB.

- M0 includes M0(i+).
- The designation pM0 is not valid; any M0 should be clinical.
- If a patient presents with M1 prior to neoadjuvant systemic therapy, the stage is considered Stage IV and remains Stage IV regardless of response to neoadjuvant therapy. Stage designation may be changed if postsurgical imaging studies reveal the presence of distant metastases, provided that the studies are carried out within 4 months of diagnosis in the absence of disease progression and provided that the patient has not received neoadjuvant therapy.
- Postneoadjuvant therapy is designated with "yc" or "yp" prefix. Of note, no stage group is assigned if there is a complete pathologic response (CR) to neoadjuvant therapy, for example, ypT0ypN0cM0.

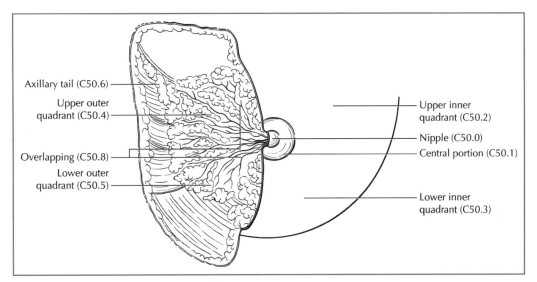

FIGURE 32.1. *Anatomic sites and subsites of the breast.*

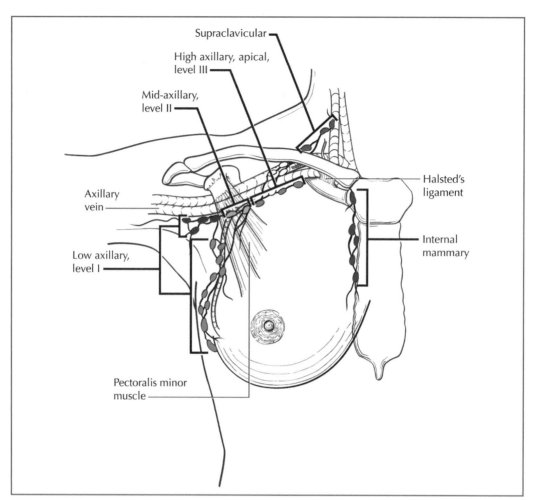

FIGURE 32.2. *Schematic diagram of the breast and regional lymph nodes.*

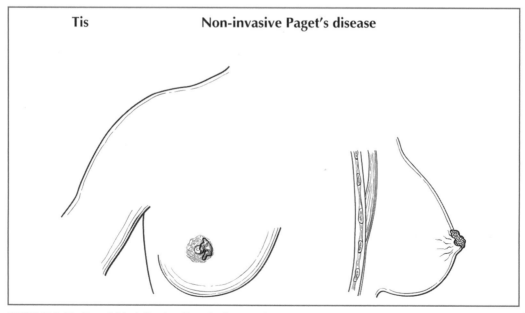

FIGURE 32.3. *Tis (Paget's) is defined as Paget's disease of the nipple with no tumor.*

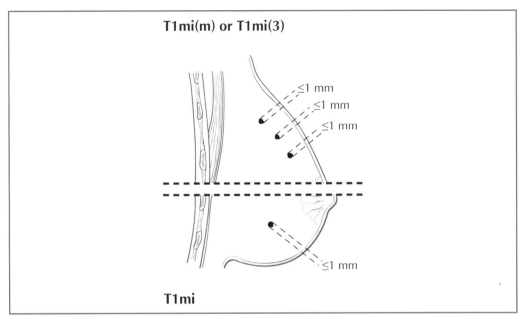

FIGURE 32.4. *T1mi is defined as microinvasion 1 mm or less in greatest dimension. The presence of multiple tumor foci of microinvasion (top of diagram) should be noted in parentheses.*

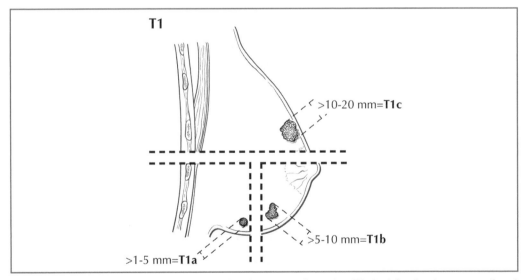

FIGURE 32.5. *T1 is defined as a tumor 20 mm or less in greatest dimension. T1a is defined as tumor more than 1 mm but not more than 5 mm in greatest dimension; T1b is defined as tumor more than 5 mm but not more than 10 mm in greatest dimension; T1c is defined as tumor more than 10 mm but not more than 20 mm in greatest dimension.*

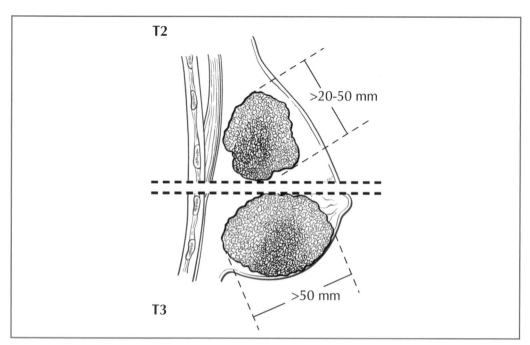

FIGURE 32.6. *T2 (above dotted line) is defined as tumor more than 20 mm but not more than 50 mm in greatest dimension, and T3 (below dotted line) is defined as tumor more than 50 mm in greatest dimension.*

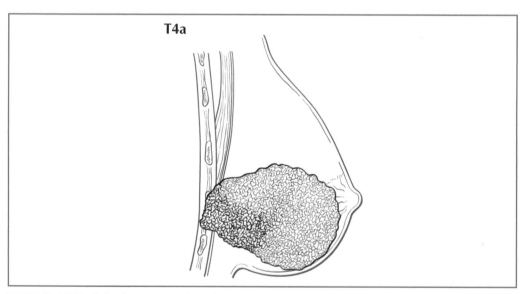

FIGURE 32.7. *T4 is defined as a tumor of any size with direct extension to chest wall and/or to the skin (ulceration or skin nodules). T4a (illustrated here) is extension to the chest wall, not including only pectoralis muscle adherence/invasion.*

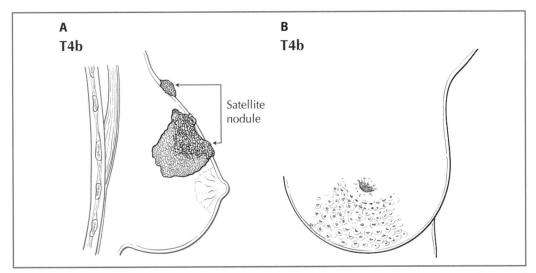

FIGURE 32.8. *(A) T4b, illustrated here as satellite skin nodules, is defined as edema (including peau d'orange) of the skin, or ulceration of the skin of the breast, or satellite skin nodules confined to the same breast. These do not meet the criteria for inflammatory carcinoma. (B) T4b illustrated here as edema (including peau d'orange) of the skin.*

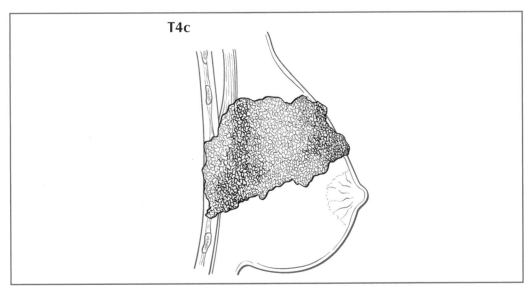

FIGURE 32.9. *T4c is defined as both T4a and T4b.*

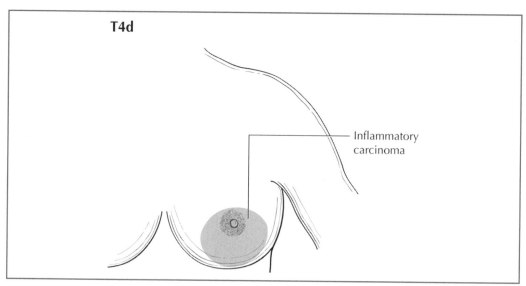

FIGURE 32.10. *T4d is inflammatory carcinoma.*

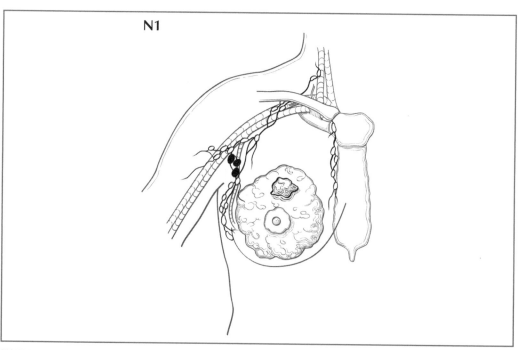

FIGURE 32.11. *N1 is defined as metastasis in movable ipsilateral level I, II axillary lymph node(s).*

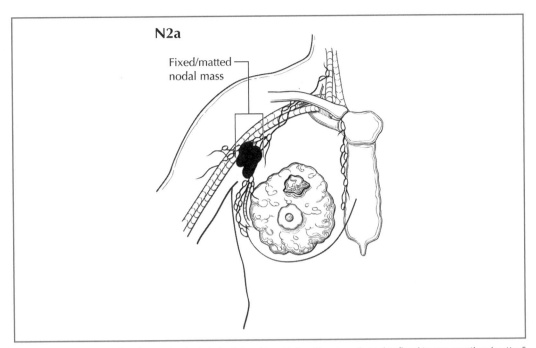

FIGURE 32.12. *N2a is defined as metastasis in ipsilateral level I, II axillary lymph nodes fixed to one another (matted) or to other structures.*

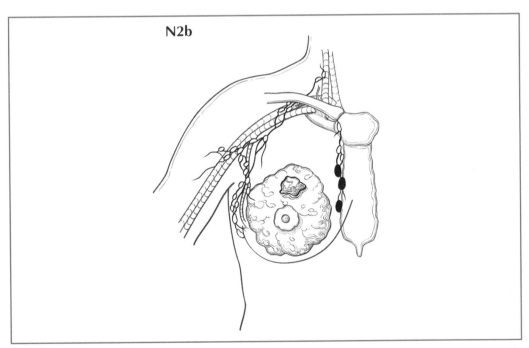

FIGURE 32.13. *N2b is defined as metastasis only in clinically detected ipsilateral internal mammary nodes and in the absence of clinically evident level I, II axillary lymph node metastasis.*

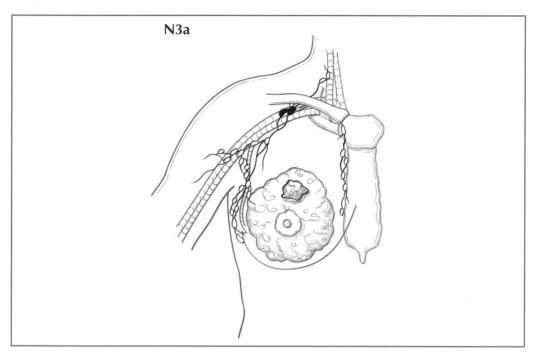

FIGURE 32.14. N3a is defined as metastasis in ipsilateral infraclavicular (level III axillary) lymph node(s) with or without level I, II axillary lymph node involvement.

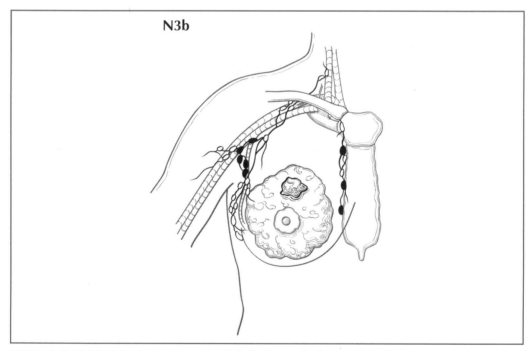

FIGURE 32.15. N3b is defined as metastasis in clinically detected ipsilateral internal mammary lymph node(s) and clinically evident axillary lymph node(s).

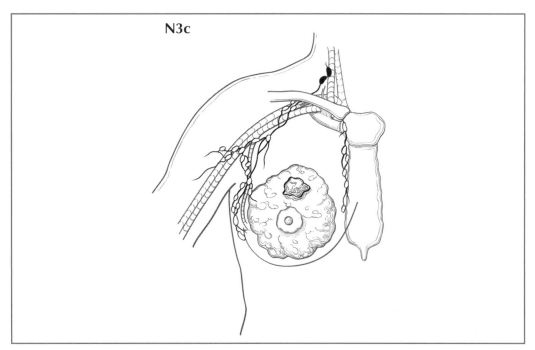

FIGURE 32.16. N3c is defined as metastasis in ipsilateral supraclavicular lymph node(s) with or without axillary or internal mammary lymph node involvement.

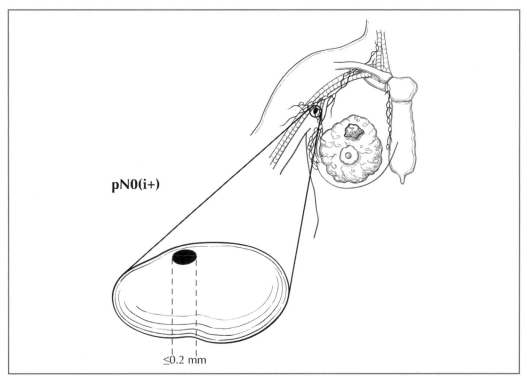

FIGURE 32.17. pN0(i+) is defined as malignant cells in regional lymph node(s) no greater than 0.2 mm (detected by H&E or IHC including ITC).

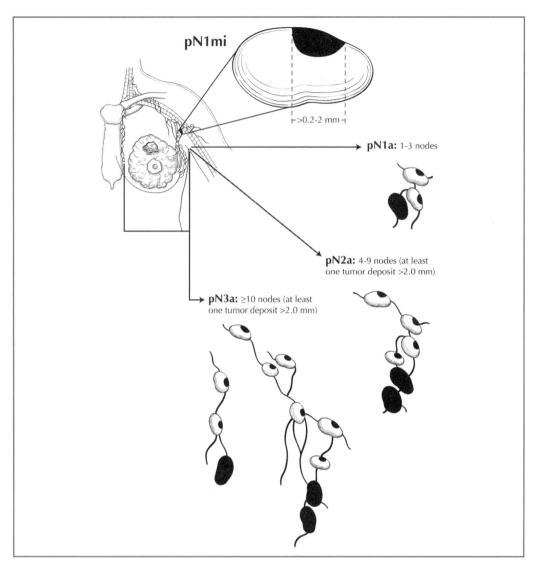

FIGURE 32.18. *Illustrated definition of pN1mi, defined as micrometastasis greater than 0.2 mm and/or more than 200 cells, but none greater than 2.0 mm. Also illustrated are pN1a defined as metastases in 1-3 axillary lymph nodes, at least one metastasis greater than 2.0 mm; pN2a defined as metastases in 4-9 axillary lymph nodes (at least one tumor deposit greater than 2.0 mm); and pN3a defined as metastases in ten or more axillary lymph nodes (at least one tumor deposit greater than 2.0 mm).*

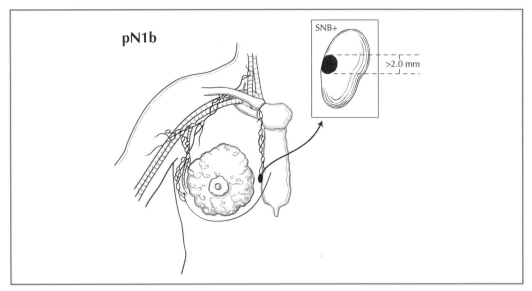

FIGURE 32.19. *pN1b metastases in internal mammary nodes detected by sentinel lymph node biopsy but not clinically detected.*

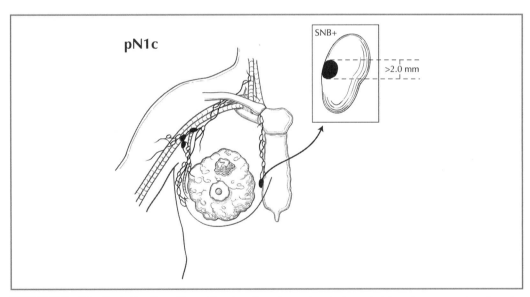

FIGURE 32.20. *pN1c illustrating 3 positive axillary lymph nodes and metastases in internal mammary lymph nodes detected by sentinel lymph node biopsy but not clinically detected.*

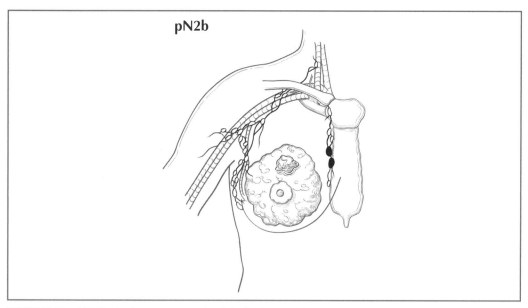

FIGURE 32.21. *pN2b illustrating metastases in clinically detected internal mammary nodes with no axillary lymph node involvement.*

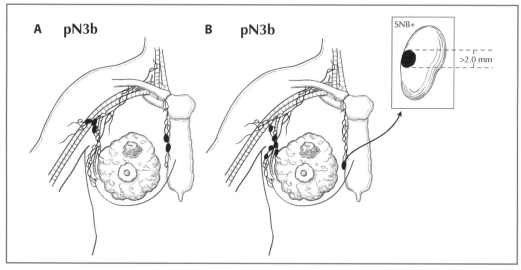

FIGURE 32.22. *(A) pN3b illustrated as metastases in clinically detected internal mammary nodes in the presence of 3 positive axillary lymph nodes. (B) pN3b illustrated as metastases in 6 positive axillary lymph nodes and in one internal mammary lymph node with micrometastases or macrometastases detected by sentinel lymph node biopsy but not clinically detected.*

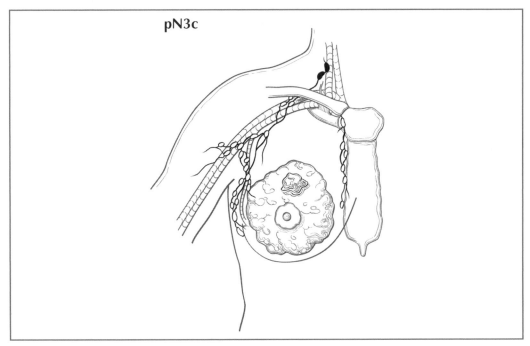

FIGURE 32.23. *pN3c illustrated as metastases in ipsilateral supraclavicular lymph nodes.*

PROGNOSTIC FACTORS (SITE-SPECIFIC FACTORS)
(Recommended for Collection)

Required for staging	None
Clinically significant	Paget's disease
	Tumor grade (Scarff–Bloom–Richardson system)
	Estrogen receptor and test method (IHC, RT-PCR, other)
	Progesterone receptor and test method (IHC, RT-PCR, other)
	HER2 status and test method (IHC, FISH, CISH, RT-PCR, other)
	Method of lymph node assessment (e.g., clinical, fine needle aspiration; core biopsy; sentinel lymph node biopsy)
	IHC of regional lymph nodes
	Molecular studies regional lymph nodes
	Distant metastases method of detection (clinical, radiographic, biopsy)
	Circulating tumor cells (CTC) and method of detection (RT-PCR, immunomagnetic separation, other)
	Disseminated tumor cells (DTC; bone marrow micrometastases) and method of detection (RT-PCR, immunohistochemical, other)
	Multigene signature score
Response to neoadjuvant therapy	Will be collected in the registry but does not affect the postneoadjuvant stage

PROGNOSTIC FACTORS (SITE-SPECIFIC FACTORS) (continued)

Complete response (CR)	Pathologic complete response can only be deter- mined by histopathologic evaluation and is defined by the absence of invasive carcinoma in the breast and lymph nodes. Residual in situ cancer, in the absence of invasive disease, constitutes a pCR. Patients with isolated tumor foci in lymph nodes are not classified as having a CR. The presence of axillary nodal tumor deposits of any size, including cell clusters less than or equal to 0.2 mm, excludes a complete response. These patients will be categorized as ypN0(i+).
Partial response (PR)	A decrease in either or both the T or N category compared to the pretreatment T or N, and no increase in either T or N. After chemotherapy, one should use the method that most clearly defined tumor dimensions at baseline for this comparison, although prechemotherapy pT cannot be measured. Clinical (pretreatment) T will be defined by clinical and radiographic findings. y pathologic (posttreatment) T will be determined by pathologic size and extension. Nodal response should be determined by physical examination or radiologic evaluation, if the nodes are palpable or visible before chemotherapy. If prechemotherapy pathologic lymph node involvement is demonstrated by fine needle aspiration, core biopsy, or sentinel node biopsy, it should be recorded as such. Absence of posttreatment pathologic nodal involvement should be used to document pathologic complete response, and should be recorded, but does not necessarily represent a true "response" since one does not know whether lymph nodes removed surgically postchemotherapy were involved prior to chemotherapy.
No response (NR)	No apparent change in either the T or N categories compared to the clinical (pretreatment) assignment or an increase in the T or N category at the time of y pathologic evaluation. Clinical (pretreatment) T will be defined by clinical and radiographic findings. yp (posttreatment) T will be determined by pathologic size. The response category will be appended to the y stage description. For example: • ypTisypN0cM0CR; ypT1ypN0cM0PR; ypT2ypN1cM0NR

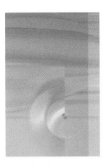

PART VIII
Gynecologic Sites

Cervix uteri, corpus uteri, ovary, vagina, vulva, fallopian tube, and gestational trophoblastic tumors are the sites included in this section. Cervix uteri and corpus uteri were among the first sites to be classified by the TNM system. The League of Nations stages for carcinoma of the cervix were first introduced more than 70 years ago, and since 1937 the Fédération Internationale de Gynécologie et d'Obstétrique (FIGO) has continued to modify these staging systems and collect outcomes data from throughout the world. The TNM categories have therefore been defined to correspond to the FIGO stages. Some amendments have been made in collaboration with FIGO, and the classifications now published have the approval of FIGO, the American Joint Committee on Cancer (AJCC), and all other national TNM committees of the International Union Against Cancer (UICC).

Vulva

(Mucosal malignant melanoma is not included)

33

ICD-O-3 TOPOGRAPHY CODES

C51.0 Labium majus
C51.1 Labium minus
C51.2 Clitoris
C51.8 Overlapping lesion of vulva
C51.9 Vulva, NOS

ICD-O-3 HISTOLOGY CODE RANGES

8000–8246, 8248–8576, 8940–8950, 8980–8981

ANATOMY

Primary Site. The vulva is the anatomic area immediately external to the vagina (Figure 33.1). It includes the labia and the perineum. The tumor may extend to involve the vagina, urethra, or anus. It may be fixed to the pubic bone. Changes to the staging classification reflect a belief that tumor size independent of other factors (spread to adjacent structures, nodal metastases) is less important in predicting survival.

Regional Lymph Nodes. The femoral and inguinal nodes are the sites of regional spread (Figure 33.2). For pN, histologic examination of regional lymphadenectomy specimens will ordinarily include six or more lymph nodes. For TNM staging, cases with fewer than six resected nodes should be classified using the TNM pathologic classification according to the status of those nodes (e.g., pN0; pN1) as per the general rules of TNM. The number of resected and positive nodes should be recorded (note that FIGO classifies cases with less than six nodes resected as pNX). The concept of sentinel lymph node mapping where only one or two key nodes are removed is currently being investigated. In most cases, a surgical assessment of regional lymph nodes (inguinal-femoral lymphadenectomy) is performed. Rarely, assessment of lymph nodes will be made by radiologic guided fine-needle aspiration or use of imaging techniques [computerized tomography (CT), magnetic resonance imaging (MRI), or positron emission tomography (PET)]. The current revisions to staging adopted reflect a recognition that the number and size of lymph node metastases more accurately reflect prognosis.

Metastatic Sites. The metastatic sites include any site beyond the area of the regional lymph nodes. Tumor involvement of pelvic lymph nodes, including internal iliac, external iliac, and common iliac lymph nodes, is considered distant metastasis.

C.C. Compton et al. (eds.), *AJCC Cancer Staging Atlas: A Companion to the Seventh Editions of the AJCC Cancer Staging Manual and Handbook*, DOI 10.1007/978-1-4614-2080-4_33,
© 2012 American Joint Committee on Cancer

PROGNOSTIC FEATURES

Vulvar cancer is a surgically staged malignancy. Surgical-pathologic staging provides specific information about primary tumor size and lymph node status, which are the most important prognostic factors in vulvar cancer. Other commonly evaluated items, such as histologic type, differentiation, DNA ploidy, and S-phase fraction analysis, as well as age, are not uniformly identified as important prognostic factors in vulvar cancer.

DEFINITIONS OF TNM

The definitions of the T categories correspond to the stages accepted by the Fédération Internationale de Gynécologie et d'Obstétrique (FIGO). Both systems are included for comparison.

Primary Tumor (T)

TNM Categories	FIGO Stages	
TX		Primary tumor cannot be assessed
T0		No evidence of primary tumor
Tis*		Carcinoma in situ (preinvasive carcinoma)
T1a	IA	Lesions 2 cm or less in size, confined to the vulva or perineum and with stromal invasion 1.0 mm or less** (Figures 33.3, 33.4A)
T1b	IB	Lesions more than 2 cm in size *or* any size with stromal invasion more than 1.0 mm, confined to the vulva or perineum (Figures 33.4B, 33.5)
T2***	II	Tumor of any size with extension to adjacent perineal structures (lower/distal 1/3 urethra, lower/distal 1/3 vagina, anal involvement) (Figures 33.6A, 33.6B)
T3****	IVA	Tumor of any size with extension to any of the following: upper/proximal 2/3 of urethra, upper/proximal 2/3 vagina, bladder mucosa, rectal mucosa, or fixed to pelvic bone (Figure 33.7)

*Note: FIGO no longer includes Stage 0 (Tis).

**Note: The depth of invasion is defined as the measurement of the tumor from the epithelial–stromal junction of the adjacent most superficial dermal papilla to the deepest point of invasion.

***FIGO uses the classification T2/T3. This is defined as T2 in TNM.

****FIGO uses the classification T4. This is defined as T3 in TNM.

Regional Lymph Nodes (N)

TNM Categories	FIGO Stages	
NX		Regional lymph nodes cannot be assessed
N0		No regional lymph node metastasis
N1		One or two regional lymph nodes with the following features
N1a	IIIA	One or two lymph node metastases each less than 5 mm (Figure 33.8A)
N1b	IIIA	One lymph node metastasis 5 mm or greater (Figure 33.8B)

N2	IIIB	Regional lymph node metastasis with the following features
N2a	IIIB	Three or more lymph node metastases each less than 5 mm (Figure 33.9A)
N2b	IIIB	Two or more lymph node metastases 5 mm or greater (Figure 33.9B)
N2c	IIIC	Lymph node metastasis with extracapsular spread (Figure 33.9C)
N3	IVA	Fixed or ulcerated regional lymph node metastasis (Figure 33.10)

An effort should be made to describe the site and laterality of lymph node metastases.

Distant Metastasis (M)

TNM Categories	FIGO Stages	
M0		No distant metastasis
M1	IVB	Distant metastasis (including pelvic lymph node metastasis) (Figure 33.11)

ANATOMIC STAGE/PROGNOSTIC GROUPS

Stage 0*	Tis	N0	M0
Stage I	T1	N0	M0
Stage IA	T1a	N0	M0
Stage IB	T1b	N0	M0
Stage II	T2	N0	M0
Stage IIIA	T1, T2	N1a, N1b	M0
Stage IIIB	T1, T2	N2a, N2b	M0
Stage IIIC	T1, T2	N2c	M0
Stage IVA	T1, T2	N3	M0
	T3	Any N	M0
Stage IVB	Any T	Any N	M1

*Note: FIGO no longer includes Stage 0 (Tis).

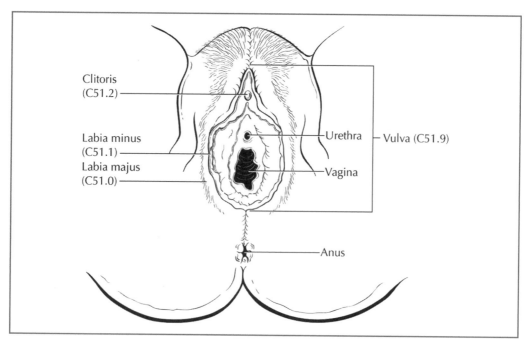

FIGURE 33.1. Anatomic sites and subsites of the vulva.

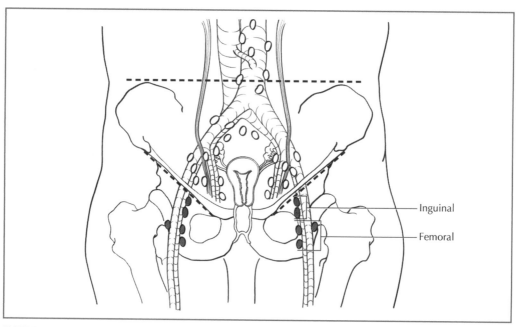

FIGURE 33.2. Regional lymph nodes of the vulva.

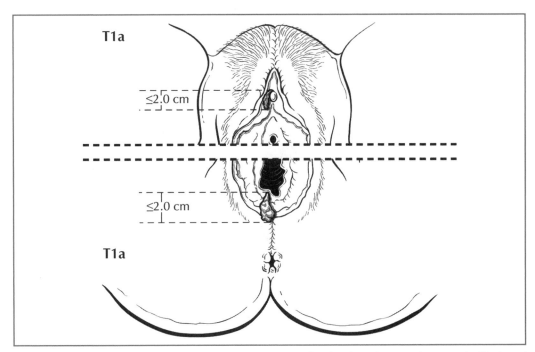

FIGURE 33.3. *T1a is defined as lesions 2 cm or less in size, confined to the vulva or perineum and with stromal invasion 1.0 mm or less.*

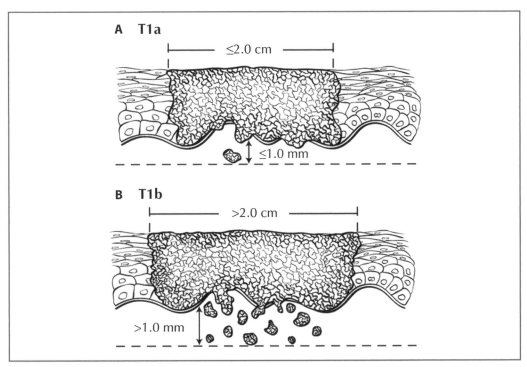

FIGURE 33.4. *(A) T1a is defined as lesions 2 cm or less in size, confined to the vulva or perineum and with stromal invasion 1.0 mm or less. (B) T1b is defined as lesions more than 2 cm in size or any size with stromal invasion more than 1.0 mm, confined to the vulva or perineum.*

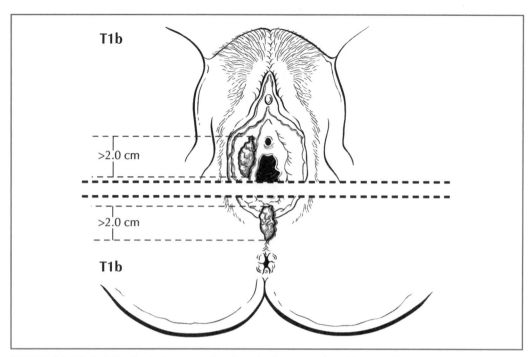

FIGURE 33.5. *T1b is defined as lesions more than 2 cm in size or any size with stromal invasion more than 1.0 mm, confined to the vulva or perineum.*

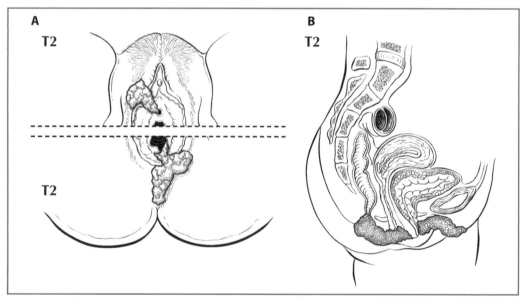

FIGURE 33.6. *(A) T2 is defined as tumor of any size with extension to adjacent perineal structures (lower/distal third of urethra, lower/distal third of vagina, anal involvement). (B) Cross-sectional diagram showing spread of tumor into anus, lower vagina, and lower urethra. T2 is defined as tumor of any size with extension to adjacent perineal structures (lower/distal third of urethra, lower/distal third of vagina, anal involvement).*

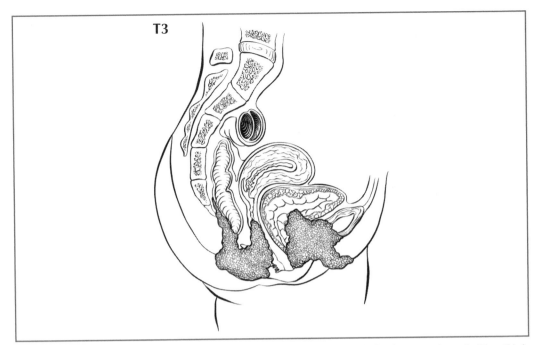

FIGURE 33.7. *T3 is defined as tumor of any size with extension to any of the following: upper/promixal two-thirds of urethra, upper/proximal two-thirds of vagina, bladder mucosa, rectal mucosa, or fixed to pelvic bone.*

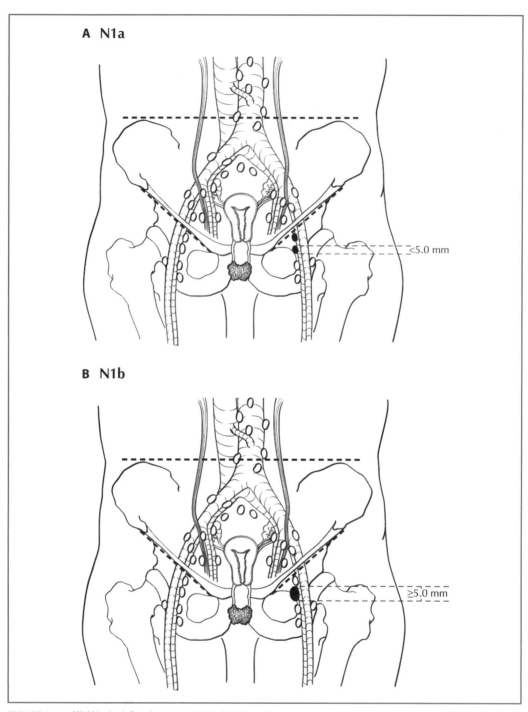

FIGURE 33.8. *(A) N1a is defined as one or two lymph nodes metastasis each less than 5 mm. (B) N1b is defined as one lymph node metastasis 5 mm or greater.*

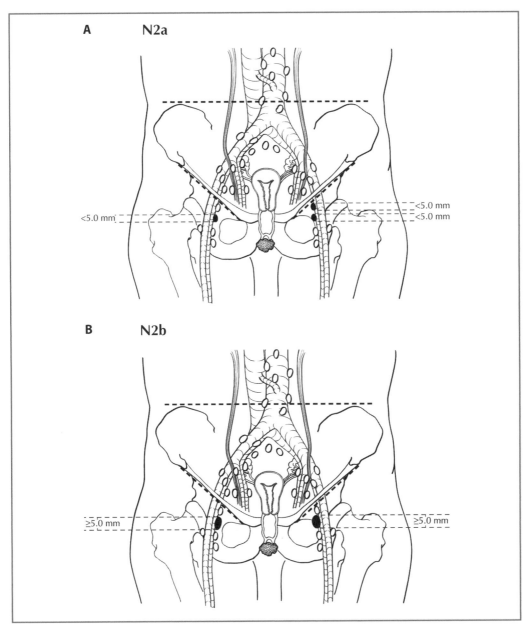

FIGURE 33.9. *(A) N2a is defined as three or more lymph node metastases each less than 5 mm. (B) N2b is defined as two or more lymph node metastases 5 mm or greater.*

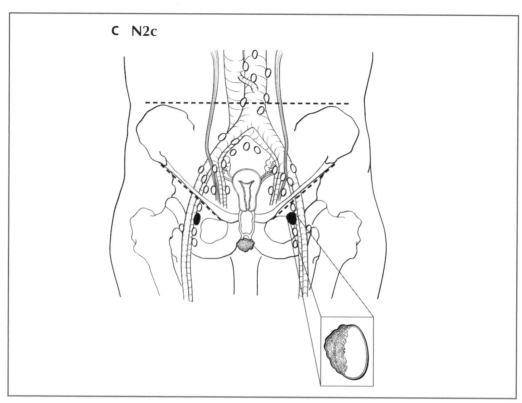

FIGURE 33.9. (continued) (C) N2c is defined as lymph node metastasis with extracapsular spread.

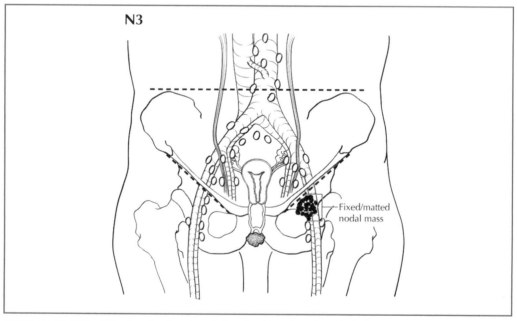

FIGURE 33.10. N3 is defined as fixed or ulcerated regional lymph node metastasis.

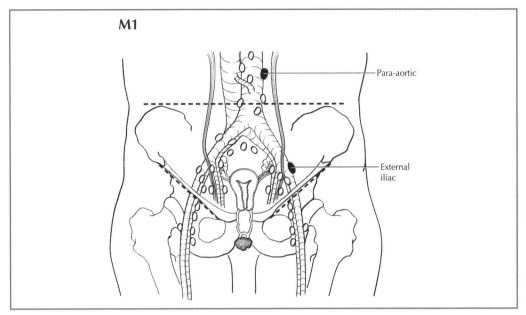

FIGURE 33.11. *These nodal metastases are considered M1.*

PROGNOSTIC FACTORS (SITE-SPECIFIC FACTORS)

(Recommended for Collection)

Required for staging	None
Clinically significant	FIGO Stage
	Pelvic nodal status and method of assessment
	Femoral-inguinal nodal status and method of assessment

Vagina

ICD-O-3 TOPOGRAPHY CODE

C52.9   Vagina, NOS

ICD-O-3 HISTOLOGY CODE RANGES

8000–8576, 8800–8801, 8940–8950, 8980–8981

ANATOMY

Primary Site. The vagina extends from the vulva upward to the uterine cervix (Figure 34.1). It is lined by squamous epithelium with only rare glandular structures. The vagina is drained by lymphatics toward the pelvic nodes in its upper two-thirds and toward the inguinal nodes in its lower third.

Regional Lymph Nodes. The upper two-thirds of the vagina is drained by lymphatics to the pelvic nodes, including the following (Figure 34.2):

Obturator
Internal iliac (hypogastric)
External iliac
Pelvic, NOS

The lower third of the vagina is drained to the groin nodes, including the following:

Inguinal
Femoral

Metastatic Sites. The most common sites of distant spread include the aortic lymph nodes, lungs, and skeleton.

PROGNOSTIC FEATURES

The most significant prognostic factor is anatomic staging, which reflects the extent of invasion into the surrounding tissue or of metastatic spread.

C.C. Compton et al. (eds.), *AJCC Cancer Staging Atlas: A Companion to the Seventh Editions of the AJCC Cancer Staging Manual and Handbook*, DOI 10.1007/978-1-4614-2080-4_34,
© 2012 American Joint Committee on Cancer

DEFINITIONS OF TNM

The definitions of the T categories correspond to the stages accepted by the Fédération Internationale de Gynécologie et d'Obstétrique (FIGO). Both systems are included for comparison.

Primary Tumor (T)

TNM Categories	FIGO Stages	
TX		Primary tumor cannot be assessed
T0		No evidence of primary tumor
Tis*		Carcinoma in situ (preinvasive carcinoma)
T1	I	Tumor confined to vagina (Figure 34.3)
T2	II	Tumor invades paravaginal tissues but not to pelvic wall (Figure 34.4)
T3	III	Tumor extends to pelvic wall** (Figure 34.5)
T4	IVA	Tumor invades mucosa of the bladder or rectum and/or extends beyond the true pelvis (bullous edema is not sufficient evidence to classify a tumor as T4) (Figure 34.6)

*Note: FIGO no longer includes Stage 0 (Tis).
**Note: Pelvic wall is defined as muscle, fascia, neurovascular structures, or skeletal portions of the bony pelvis. On rectal examination, there is no cancer-free space between the tumor and pelvic walls.

Regional Lymph Nodes (N)

TNM Categories	FIGO Stages	
NX		Regional lymph nodes cannot be assessed
N0		No regional lymph node metastasis
N1	III	Pelvic or inguinal lymph node metastasis (Figure 34.7)

Distant Metastasis (M)

TNM Categories	FIGO Stages	
M0		No distant metastasis
M1	IVB	Distant metastasis

ANATOMIC STAGE/PROGNOSTIC GROUPS

Stage 0*	Tis	N0	M0
Stage I	T1	N0	M0
Stage II	T2	N0	M0
Stage III	T1–T3	N1	M0
	T3	N0	M0
Stage IVA	T4	Any N	M0
Stage IVB	Any T	Any N	M1

*Note: FIGO no longer includes Stage 0 (Tis).

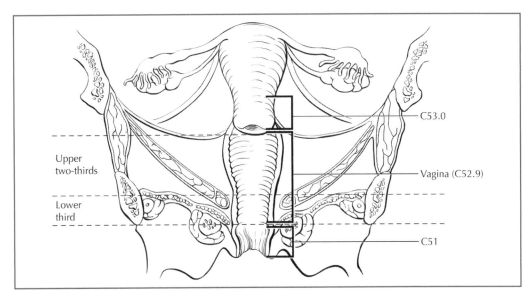

FIGURE 34.1. Anatomic site and subsites of the vagina.

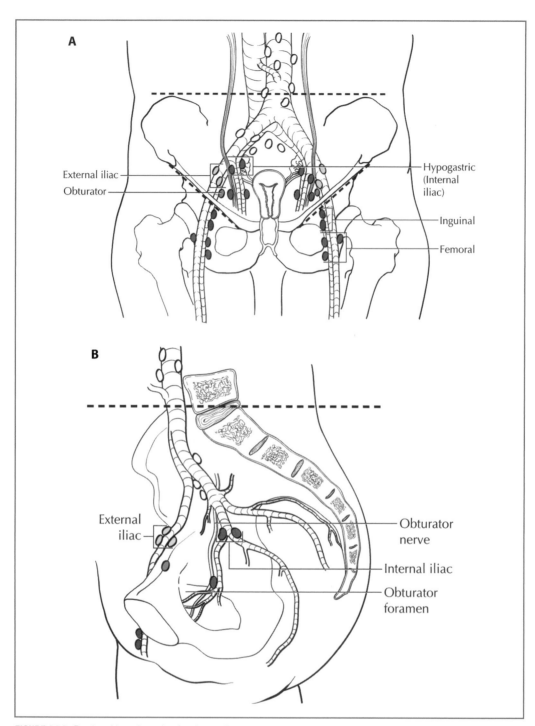

FIGURE 34.2. *Regional lymph nodes for the vagina.*

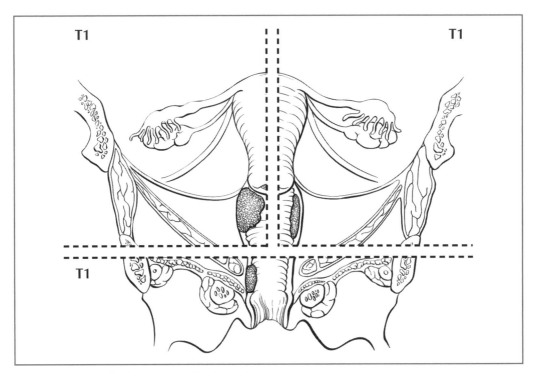

FIGURE 34.3. *T1 is defined as tumor confined to vagina.*

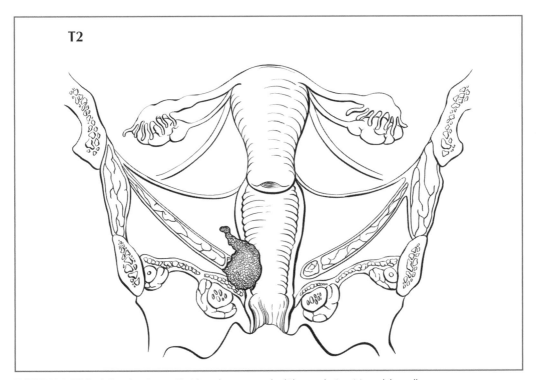

FIGURE 34.4. *T2 is defined as tumor that invades paravaginal tissues but not to pelvic wall.*

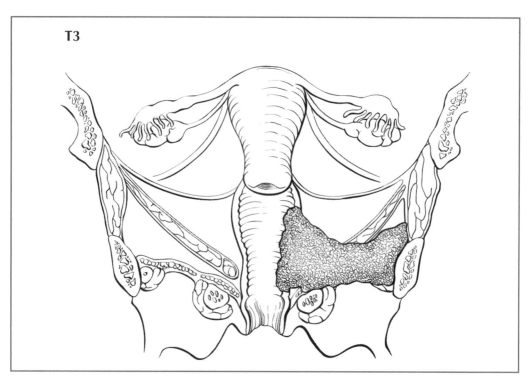

FIGURE 34.5. *T3 is defined as tumor extending to pelvic wall.*

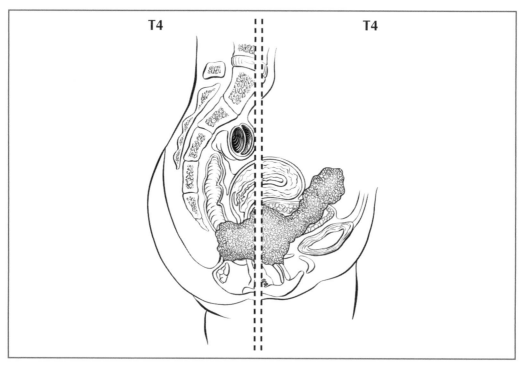

FIGURE 34.6. *T4 is defined as tumor that invades mucosa of the bladder or rectum and/or extends beyond the true pelvis (bullous edema (of the bladder) is not sufficient evidence to classify a tumor as T4).*

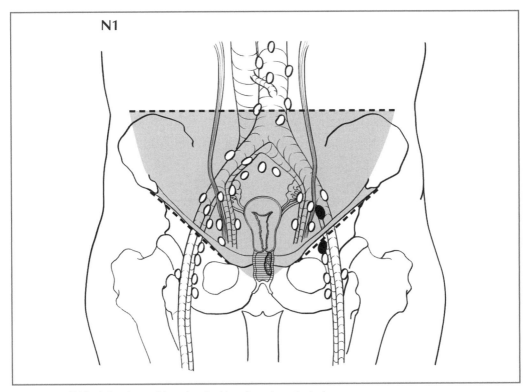

FIGURE 34.7. *N1 is defined as pelvic or inguinal lymph node metastasis.*

PROGNOSTIC FACTORS (SITE-SPECIFIC FACTORS)
(Recommended for Collection)

Required for staging	None
Clinically significant	FIGO Stage
	Pelvic nodal status and method of assessment
	Para-aortic nodal status and method of assessment
	Distant (mediastinal, scalene) nodal status and method of assessment

Cervix Uteri

35

SUMMARY OF CHANGES

- The definition of TNM and the Stage Grouping for this chapter have changed from the Sixth Edition and reflect new staging adopted by the International Federation of Gynecology and Obstetrics (FIGO) (2008)

ICD-O-3 TOPOGRAPHY CODES

C53.0   Endocervix
C53.1   Exocervix
C53.8   Overlapping lesion of cervix uteri
C53.9   Cervix uteri

ICD-O-3 HISTOLOGY CODE RANGES

8000–8576, 8940–8950, 8980–8981

ANATOMY

Primary Site. The cervix is the lower third of the uterus (Figure 35.1). It is roughly cylindrical in shape and projects into the upper vagina. The endocervical canal is lined by glandular or columnar epithelium. Through the cervix runs the endocervical canal, which is the passageway connecting the vagina with the uterine cavity. The vaginal portion of the cervix, known as the exocervix, is covered by squamous epithelium. The squamocolumnar junction is usually located at the external cervical os, where the endocervical canal begins. Cancer of the cervix may originate from the squamous epithelium of the exocervix or the glandular epithelium of the canal.

Regional Lymph Nodes. The cervix is drained by parametrial, cardinal, and uterosacral ligament routes into the following regional lymph nodes (Figure 35.2):

Parametrial
Obturator
Internal iliac (hypogastric)
External iliac
Common iliac
Sacral
Presacral

For pN, histologic examination of regional lymphadenectomy specimens will ordinarily include six or more lymph nodes. For TNM staging, cases with fewer than six resected nodes should be

---

classified using the TNM pathologic classification according to the status of those nodes (e.g., pN0; pN1) as per the general rules of TNM. The number of resected and positive nodes should be recorded (note that FIGO classifies cases with less than six nodes resected as pNX).

Metastatic Sites. The most common sites of distant spread include the paraaortic and mediastinal nodes, lungs, peritoneal cavity, and skeleton. Mediastinal or supraclavicular node involvement is considered distant metastasis and is coded M1.

PROGNOSTIC FEATURES

Current data suggest that more than 90% of squamous cervical cancer contains human papilloma virus (HPV) DNA, most frequently types 16 and 18. In addition to extent or stage of disease, prognostic factors include histology and tumor differentiation. Small cell, neuroendocrine, and clear cell lesions have a worse prognosis, as do poorly differentiated cancers. Women with cervical cancer who are infected with human immunodeficiency virus (HIV) are defined as having autoimmune deficiency syndrome (AIDS), and they have a very poor prognosis, often with rapidly progressive cancer.

DEFINITIONS OF TNM

The definitions of the T categories correspond to the stages accepted by the Fédération Internationale de Gynécologie et d'Obstétrique (FIGO). Both systems are included for comparison.

Primary Tumor (T)		
TNM Categories	*FIGO Stages*	
TX		Primary tumor cannot be assessed
T0		No evidence of primary tumor
Tis*		Carcinoma in situ (preinvasive carcinoma)
T1	I	Cervical carcinoma confined to uterus (extension to corpus should be disregarded)
T1a**	IA	Invasive carcinoma diagnosed only by microscopy. Stromal invasion with a maximum depth of 5.0 mm measured from the base of the epithelium and a horizontal spread of 7.0 mm or less. Vascular space involvement, venous or lymphatic, does not affect classification (Figure 35.3)
T1a1	IA1	Measured stromal invasion 3.0 mm or less in depth and 7.0 mm or less in horizontal spread (Figure 35.4)
T1a2	IA2	Measured stromal invasion more than 3.0 mm and not more than 5.0 mm with a horizontal spread 7.0 mm or less (Figure 35.5)
T1b	IB	Clinically visible lesion confined to the cervix or microscopic lesion greater than T1a/IA2 (Figure 35.6)
T1b1	IB1	Clinically visible lesion 4.0 cm or less in greatest dimension (Figure 35.7)
T1b2	IB2	Clinically visible lesion more than 4.0 cm in greatest dimension (Figure 35.8)
T2	II	Cervical carcinoma invades beyond uterus but not to pelvic wall or to lower third of vagina

(continued)

Primary Tumor (T) *(continued)*

T2a	IIA	Tumor without parametrial invasion
T2a1	IIA1	Clinically visible lesion 4.0 cm or less in greatest dimension (Figure 35.9A)
T2a2	IIA2	Clinically visible lesion more than 4.0 cm in greatest dimension (Figure 35.9B)
T2b	IIB	Tumor with parametrial invasion (Figure 35.10)
T3	III	Tumor extends to pelvic wall and/or involves lower third of vagina, and/or causes hydronephrosis or nonfunctioning kidney
T3a	IIIA	Tumor involves lower third of vagina, no extension to pelvic wall (Figure 35.11A)
T3b	IIIB	Tumor extends to pelvic wall and/or causes hydronephrosis or nonfunctioning kidney (Figure 35.11B)
T4	IVA	Tumor invades mucosa of bladder or rectum, and/or extends beyond true pelvis (bullous edema is not sufficient to classify a tumor as T4) (Figure 35.12)

*Note: FIGO no longer includes Stage 0 (Tis).
**Note: All macroscopically visible lesions, even with superficial invasion, are T1b/IB.

Regional Lymph Nodes (N)

TNM Categories	FIGO Stages	
NX		Regional lymph nodes cannot be assessed
N0		No regional lymph node metastasis
N1	IIIB	Regional lymph node metastasis (Figure 35.13)

Distant Metastasis (M)

TNM Categories	FIGO Stages	
M0		No distant metastasis
M1	IVB	Distant metastasis (including peritoneal spread, involvement of supraclavicular, mediastinal, or paraaortic lymph nodes, lung, liver, or bone)

ANATOMIC STAGE/PROGNOSTIC GROUPS

Stage 0*	Tis	N0	M0
Stage I	T1	N0	M0
Stage IA	T1a	N0	M0
Stage IA1	T1a1	N0	M0
Stage IA2	T1a2	N0	M0
Stage IB	T1b	N0	M0
Stage IB1	T1b1	N0	M0
Stage IB2	T1b2	N0	M0
Stage II	T2	N0	M0
Stage IIA	T2a	N0	M0
Stage IIA1	T2a1	N0	M0
Stage IIA2	T2a2	N0	M0
Stage IIB	T2b	N0	M0
Stage III	T3	N0	M0
Stage IIIA	T3a	N0	M0
Stage IIIB	T3b	Any N	M0
	T1-3	N1	M0
Stage IVA	T4	Any N	M0
Stage IVB	Any T	Any N	M1

*Note: FIGO no longer includes Stage 0 (Tis).

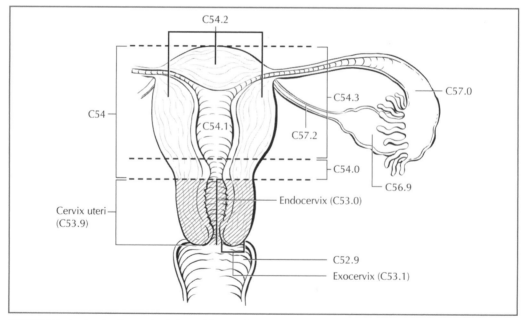

FIGURE 35.1. *Anatomic sites and subsites of the cervix uteri.*

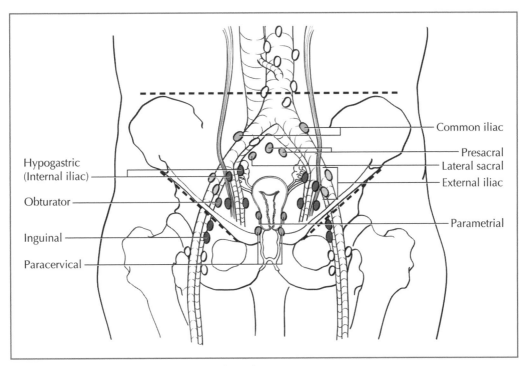

FIGURE 35.2. *Regional lymph nodes for the cervix uteri.*

Common iliac
Presacral
Lateral sacral
External iliac
Parametrial
Hypogastric (Internal iliac)
Obturator
Inguinal
Paracervical

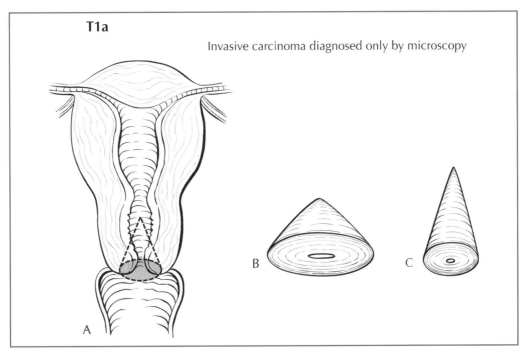

T1a

Invasive carcinoma diagnosed only by microscopy

A

B

C

FIGURE 35.3. *(A-C) T1a is defined as invasive carcinoma diagnosed only by microscopy. Stromal invasion with a maximum depth of 5.0 mm measured from the base of the epithelium and a horizontal spread of 7.0 mm or less. Vascular space involvement, venous or lymphatic, does not affect classification.*

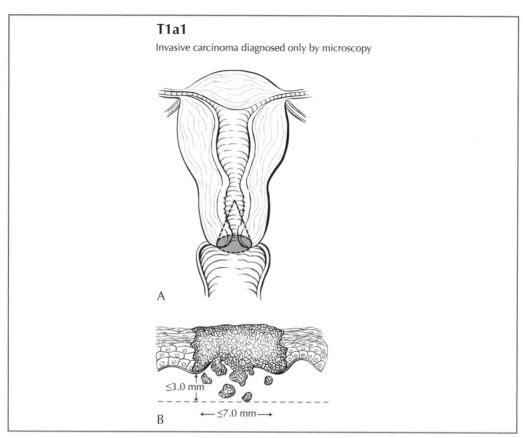

T1a1

Invasive carcinoma diagnosed only by microscopy

A

≤3.0 mm

B ←— ≤7.0 mm —→

FIGURE 35.4. *T1a1 is defined as measured stromal invasion 3.0 mm or less in depth and 7.0 mm or less in horizontal spread (B).*

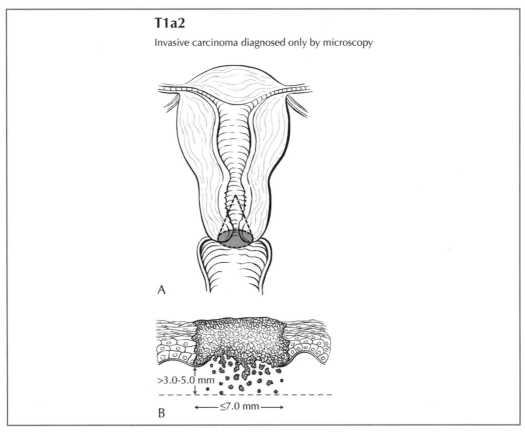

T1a2

Invasive carcinoma diagnosed only by microscopy

A

>3.0-5.0 mm

≤7.0 mm

B

FIGURE 35.5. *T1a2 is defined as measured stromal invasion more than 3.0 mm and not more than 5.0 mm with a horizontal spread 7.0 mm or less (B).*

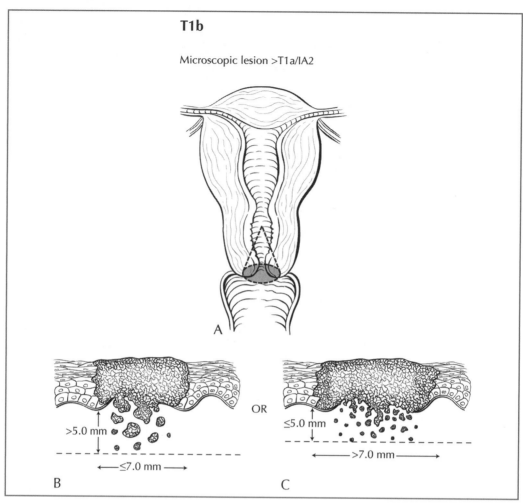

T1b

Microscopic lesion >T1a/IA2

>5.0 mm

≤7.0 mm

OR

≤5.0 mm

>7.0 mm

A

B

C

FIGURE 35.6. *T1b is defined as clinically visible lesion confined to the cervix or microscopic lesion greater than T1a (B and C).*

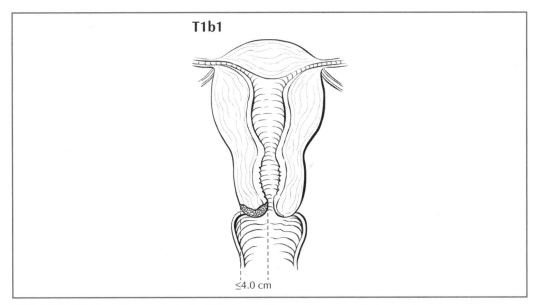

FIGURE 35.7. *T1b1 is defined as clinically visible lesion 4.0 cm or less in greatest dimension.*

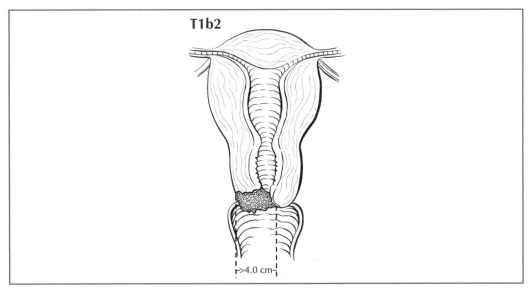

FIGURE 35.8. *T1b2 is defined as clinically visible lesion more than 4.0 cm in greatest dimension.*

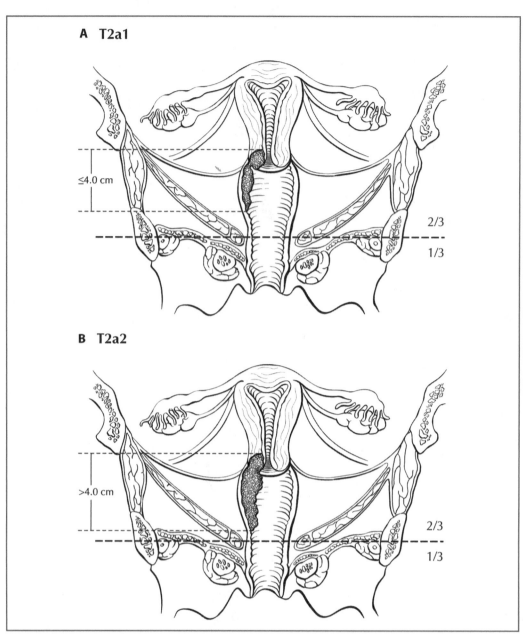

A T2a1

≤4.0 cm

2/3

1/3

B T2a2

>4.0 cm

2/3

1/3

FIGURE 35.9. *(A) T2a is defined as tumor without parametrial invasion. T2a1 is defined as clinically visible lesion 4.0 cm or less in greatest dimension. (B) T2a2 is defined as clinically visible lesion more than 4.0 cm in greatest dimension.*

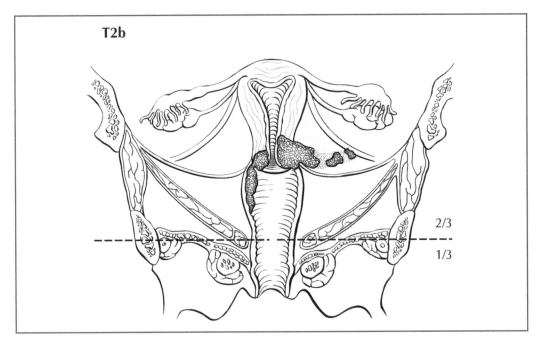

FIGURE 35.10. *T2b is defined as tumor with parametrial invasion.*

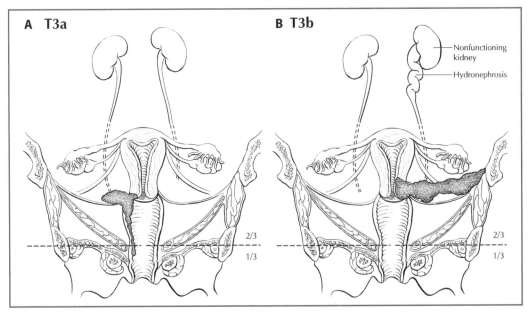

FIGURE 35.11. *(A) T3a is defined as tumor that involves lower third of vagina, no extension to pelvic wall. (B) T3b is defined as tumor that extends to pelvic wall and/or causes hydronephrosis or nonfunctioning kidney.*

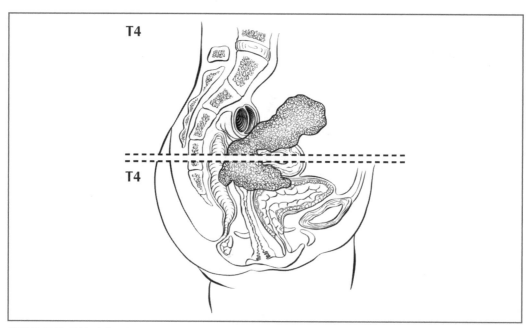

FIGURE 35.12. *T4 is defined as tumor that invades mucosa of bladder or rectum, and/or extends beyond true pelvis (bullous edema (of the bladder) is not sufficient to classify a tumor as T4).*

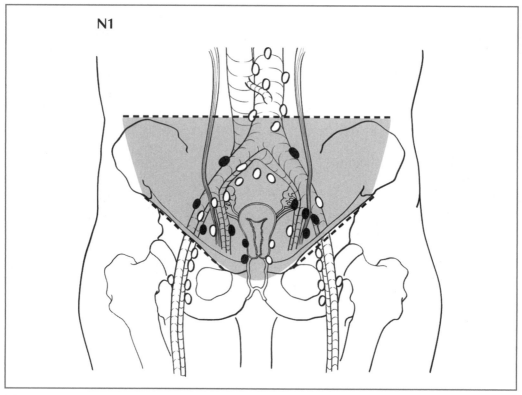

FIGURE 35.13. *N1 is defined as regional lymph node metastasis.*

PROGNOSTIC FACTORS (SITE-SPECIFIC FACTORS)
(Recommended for Collection)

Required for staging	None
Clinically significant	FIGO Stage
	Pelvic nodal status and method of assessment
	Distant (paraaortic) nodal status and method of assessment
	Distant (mediastinal, scalene) nodal status and method of assessment

Corpus Uteri

36

SUMMARY OF CHANGES

- The definition of TNM and the Stage Grouping for this chapter have changed from the Sixth Edition and reflect new staging adopted by the International Federation of Gynecology and Obstetrics (FIGO) (2008)
- A separate staging schema adopted by FIGO for uterine sarcoma has been added

---

ICD-O-3 TOPOGRAPHY CODES

C54.0 Isthmus uteri
C54.1 Endometrium
C54.2 Myometrium
C54.3 Fundus uteri
C54.8 Overlapping lesion of corpus uteri
C54.9 Corpus uteri
C55.9 Uterus, NOS

ICD-O-3 HISTOLOGY CODE RANGES

8000-8790, 8950-8951, 8980-8981 (Carcinoma) 8800, 8890-8898, 8900-8921, 8930-8931, 8935 (Leiomyosarcoma and Endometrial Stromal Sarcoma) 8933 (Adenosarcoma)

ANATOMY

Primary Site. The upper two-thirds of the uterus above the level of the internal cervical os is referred to as the uterine corpus (Figure 36.1). The oviducts (fallopian tubes) and the round ligaments enter the uterus at the upper and outer corners (cornu) of the pear-shaped organ. The portion of the uterus that is above a line connecting the tubo-uterine orifices is referred to as the uterine fundus. The lower third of the uterus is called the cervix and lower uterine segment. Tumor involvement of the cervical stroma is prognostically important and affects staging (T2). The new staging system no longer distinguishes endocervical mucosal/glandular involvement (formerly stage IIA). The location of the tumor must be carefully evaluated and recorded by the pathologist. The depth of tumor invasion into the myometrium is also of prognostic significance and should be included in the pathology report. Involvement of the ovaries by direct extension or metastases, or penetration of tumor to the uterine serosa is important to identify and classify the tumor as T3a.

Malignant cells in peritoneal cytology samples have been documented in approximately 10% of cases of presumed uterine confined endometrial cancer cases. The prognostic importance of positive cytology has been debated. Depth of myometrial invasion, tumor grade, and presence of extrauterine disease are felt to be more prognostically significant, and as such the 2008 FIGO staging system will no longer use peritoneal cytology for the purposes of staging (formerly T3a, FIGO stage IIIA). T3b lesions reflect regional extension of disease and include extension of the tumor through the myometrial wall of the uterus into the parametrium and/or extension/metastatic involvement of the vagina.

C.C. Compton et al. (eds.), *AJCC Cancer Staging Atlas: A Companion to the Seventh Editions of the AJCC Cancer Staging Manual and Handbook*, DOI 10.1007/978-1-4614-2080-4_36,
© 2012 American Joint Committee on Cancer

Regional Lymph Nodes. The regional lymph nodes are paired and each of the paired sites should be examined. The regional nodes are as follows (Figure 36.2):

Obturator
Internal iliac (hypogastric)
External iliac
Common iliac
Para-aortic
Presacral
Parametrial

For adequate evaluation of the regional lymph nodes, a representative evaluation of bilateral para-aortic and pelvic lymph nodes (including external iliac, internal iliac, and obturator nodes) should be documented in the operative and surgical pathology reports. Parametrial nodes are not commonly detected unless a radical hysterectomy is performed for cases with gross cervical stromal invasion.

For pN, histologic examination of regional lymphadenectomy specimens will ordinarily include six or more lymph nodes. For TNM staging, cases with fewer than six resected nodes should be classified using the TNM pathologic classification according to the status of those nodes (e.g., pN0; pN1) as per the general rules of TNM. The number of resected and positive nodes should be recorded (note that FIGO classifies cases with less than six nodes resected as pNX).

Metastatic Sites. The vagina and lung are the common metastatic sites. Intra-abdominal metastases to peritoneal surfaces or the omentum are seen particularly with serous and clear cell tumors.

PROGNOSTIC FEATURES

The presence or absence of metastatic disease in the regional lymph nodes is the most important prognostic factor in carcinomas clinically confined to the uterus. The AJCC strongly advocates the use of surgical/pathologic assessment of nodal status whenever possible. Palpation of regional nodes is well recognized to be much less accurate than pathologic evaluation of the nodes.

Historically, the factors of grade of the tumor and depth of myometrial invasion have been recognized as important prognostic factors. In surgically staged patients, using multivariate analysis, these factors are surrogates for the probability of nodal metastasis. Preoperative endometrial biopsy does not accurately correlate with tumor grade and depth of myometrial invasion.

The presence or absence of lymphovascular space involvement of the myometrium is important in most, but not all, series. When present, lymphovascular space involvement increases the probability of metastatic involvement of the regional lymph nodes. The presence or absence of lymphovascular space involvement should be recorded in the pathology report.

The importance of tumor cells in peritoneal "washings" and the presence of metastatic foci in adnexal structures may have an adverse impact on prognosis, but they remain controversial and require further study. The newly adopted staging system (FIGO 2008) no longer utilizes positive cytology to alter stage. When collected, cytology results should be recorded.

Serous papillary and clear cell adenocarcinomas have a higher incidence of extrauterine disease at detection than endometrioid adenocarcinomas. The risk of extrauterine disease does not correlate with the depth of myometrial invasion, because nodal or intraperitoneal mestastases can be found even when there is no myometrial invasion. For this reason, they are classified as Grade 3 tumors.

In malignancies with squamous elements, the aggressiveness of the tumor seems to be related to the degree of differentiation of the glandular component rather than the squamous element. Clinicopathologic and immunohistochemical studies support classifying malignant mixed mesodermal tumors as high-grade (G3) malignancies of epithelial origin rather than as sarcomas with mixed epithelial and mesenchymal differentiation, as in earlier classification systems.

The data regarding the impact of DNA ploidy, estrogen and progesterone receptor status, and tumor suppressor gene and oncogene expression are not sufficiently mature to incorporate into the stage grouping at this time.

DEFINITIONS OF TNM

The definitions of the T categories correspond to the stages accepted by FIGO.

UTERINE CARCINOMAS

Carcinosarcomas should be staged as carcinoma.

FIGO stages are further subdivided by histologic grade of tumor – for example, Stage IC G2. Both systems are included for comparison.

Primary Tumor (T)

TNM Categories	FIGO Stages	
TX		Primary tumor cannot be assessed
T0		No evidence of primary tumor
Tis*		Carcinoma in situ (preinvasive carcinoma)
T1	I	Tumor confined to corpus uteri
T1a	IA	Tumor limited to endometrium or invades less than one-half of the myometrium (Figure 36.3A)
T1b	IB	Tumor invades one-half or more of the myometrium (Figure 36.3B)
T2	II	Tumor invades stromal connective tissue of the cervix but does not extend beyond uterus** (Figure 36.4)
T3a	IIIA	Tumor involves serosa and/or adnexa (direct extension or metastasis) (Figure 36.5)
T3b	IIIB	Vaginal involvement (direct extension or metastasis) or parametrial involvement (Figure 36.5)
T4	IVA	Tumor invades bladder mucosa and/or bowel mucosa (bullous edema is not sufficient to classify a tumor as T4) (Figure 36.6)

*Note: FIGO no longer includes Stage 0 (Tis).

**Endocervical glandular involvement only should be considered as Stage I and not as Stage II.

Regional Lymph Nodes (N)

TNM Categories	FIGO Stages	
NX		Regional lymph nodes cannot be assessed
N0		No regional lymph node metastasis
N1	IIIC1	Regional lymph node metastasis to pelvic lymph nodes (Figure 36.7)
N2	IIIC2	Regional lymph node metastasis to para-aortic lymph nodes, with or without positive pelvic lymph nodes (Figure 36.8)

Distant Metastasis (M)

TNM Categories	FIGO Stages	
M0		No distant metastasis
M1	IVB	Distant metastasis (includes metastasis to inguinal lymph nodes intraperitoneal disease, or lung, liver, or bone. It excludes metastasis to para-aortic lymph nodes, vagina, pelvic serosa, or adnexa) (Figure 36.9)

ANATOMIC STAGE/PROGNOSTIC GROUPS

Carcinomas*

Stage 0**	Tis	N0	M0
Stage I	T1	N0	M0
Stage IA	T1a	N0	M0
Stage IB	T1b	N0	M0
Stage II	T2	N0	M0
Stage III	T3	N0	M0
Stage IIIA	T3a	N0	M0
Stage IIIB	T3b	N0	M0
Stage IIIC1	T1-T3	N1	M0
Stage IIIC2	T1-T3	N2	M0
Stage IVA	T4	Any N	M0
Stage IVB	Any T	Any N	M1

*Carcinosarcomas should be staged as carcinoma.

**Note: FIGO no longer includes Stage 0 (Tis).

UTERINE SARCOMAS

(Includes Leiomyosarcoma, Endometrial Stromal Sarcoma, and Adenosarcoma)

LEIOMYOSARCOMA AND ENDOMETRIAL STROMAL SARCOMA

Primary Tumor (T)

TNM Categories	FIGO Stages	
TX		Primary tumor cannot be assessed
T0		No evidence of primary tumor
T1	I	Tumor limited to the uterus
T1a	IA	Tumor 5 cm or less in greatest dimension (Figure 36.10)
T1b	IB	Tumor more than 5 cm (Figure 36.11)
T2	II	Tumor extends beyond the uterus, within the pelvis
T2a	IIA	Tumor involves adnexa (Figure 36.12)
T2b	IIB	Tumor involves other pelvic tissues (Figure 36.13)
T3	III*	Tumor infiltrates abdominal tissues
T3a	IIIA	One site (Figure 36.14)
T3b	IIIB	More than one site (Figure 36.15)
T4	IVA	Tumor invades bladder or rectum (Figure 36.16)

Note: Simultaneous tumors of the uterine corpus and ovary/pelvis in association with ovarian/pelvic endometriosis should be classified as independent primary tumors.

*In this stage lesions must infiltrate abdominal tissues and not just protrude into the abdominal cavity.

Regional Lymph Nodes (N)

TNM Categories	FIGO Stages	
NX		Regional lymph nodes cannot be assessed
N0		No regional lymph node metastasis
N1	IIIC	Regional lymph node metastasis (Figure 36.17)

Distant Metastasis (M)

TNM Categories	FIGO Stages	
M0		No distant metastasis
M1	IVB	Distant metastasis (excluding adnexa, pelvic, and abdominal tissues)

Primary Tumor (T)

TNM Categories	FIGO Stages	
TX		Primary tumor cannot be assessed
T0		No evidence of primary tumor
T1	I	Tumor limited to the uterus
T1a	IA	Tumor limited to the endometrium/endocervix (Figure 36.18)
T1b	IB	Tumor invades to less than half of the myometrium (Figure 36.19)
T1c	IC	Tumor invades more than half of the myometrium (Figure 36.20)
T2	II	Tumor extends beyond the uterus, within the pelvis
T2a	IIA	Tumor involves adnexa (Figure 36.12)
T2b	IIB	Tumor involves other pelvic tissues (Figure 36.13)
T3	III*	Tumor involves abdominal tissues
T3a	IIIA	One site (Figure 36.14)
T3b	IIIB	More than one site (Figure 36.15)
T4	IVA	Tumor invades bladder or rectum (Figure 36.16)

Note: Simultaneous tumors of the uterine corpus and ovary/pelvis in association with ovarian/pelvic endometriosis should be classified as independent primary tumors.

*In this stage lesions must infiltrate abdominal tissues and not just protrude into the abdominal cavity.

Regional Lymph Nodes (N)

TNM Categories	FIGO Stages	
NX		Regional lymph nodes cannot be assessed
N0		No regional lymph node metastasis
N1	IIIC	Regional lymph node metastasis (Figure 36.17)

Distant Metastasis (M)

TNM Categories	FIGO Stages	
M0		No distant metastasis
M1	IVB	Distant metastasis (excluding adnexa, pelvic and abdominal tissues)

ANATOMIC STAGE/PROGNOSTIC GROUPS

Uterine Sarcomas

Stage I	T1	N0	M0
Stage IA*	T1a	N0	M0
Stage IB*	T1b	N0	M0
Stage IC**	T1c	N0	M0
Stage II	T2	N0	M0
Stage IIIA	T3a	N0	M0
Stage IIIB	T3b	N0	M0
Stage IIIC	T1, T2, T3	N1	M0
Stage IVA	T4	Any N	M0
Stage IVB	Any T	Any N	M1

*Stage IA and IB differ from those applied for leiomyosarcoma and endometrial stromal sarcoma
**Note: Stage IC does not apply for leiomyosarcoma and endometrial stromal sarcoma.

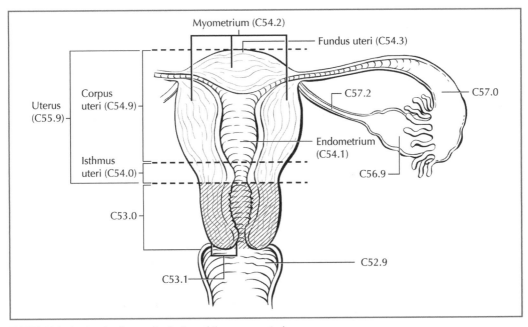

FIGURE 36.1. Anatomic sites and subsites of the corpus uteri.

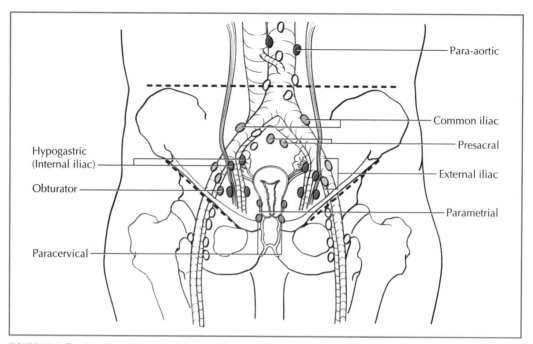

FIGURE 36.2. *Regional lymph nodes of the corpus uteri.*

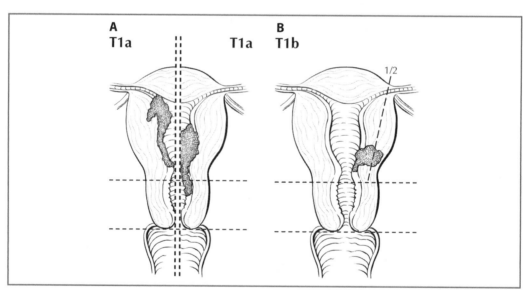

FIGURE 36.3. *(A) For carcinomas T1a is defined as tumor limited to endometrium or that invades less than one-half of the myometrium. (B) For carcinomas T1b is defined as tumor that invades one-half or more of the myometrium.*

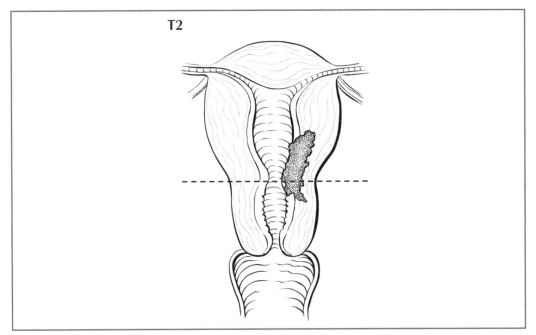

FIGURE 36.4. *For carcinomas T2 is defined as tumor that invades stromal connective tissue of the cervix but does not extend beyond uterus.*

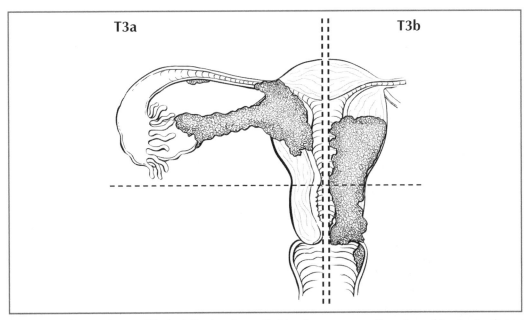

FIGURE 36.5. *For carcinomas T3a is defined as tumor that involves serosa and/or adnexa (direct extension or metastasis). T3b is defined as vaginal involvement (direct extension or metastasis) or parametrial involvement.*

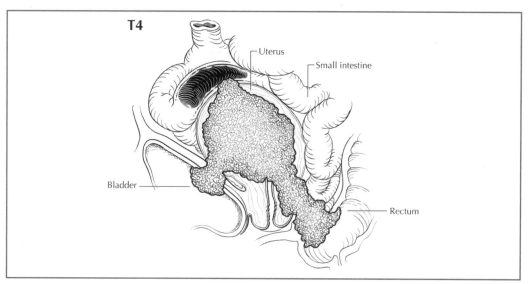

FIGURE 36.6. *For carcinomas T4 is defined as tumor that invades bladder mucosa and/or bowel mucosa (bullous edema (of the bladder) is not sufficient to classify a tumor as T4).*

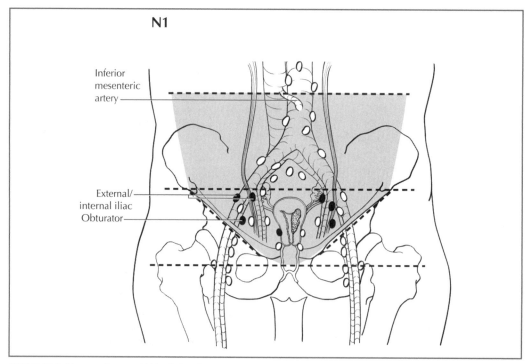

FIGURE 36.7. *For carcinomas N1 is defined as regional lymph node metastasis to pelvic lymph nodes.*

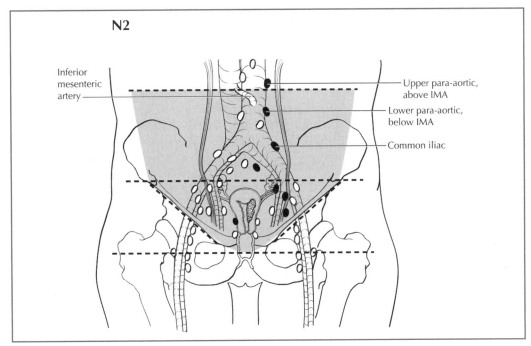

FIGURE 36.8. *For carcinomas N2 is defined as regional lymph node metastasis to para-aortic lymph nodes, with or without positive pelvic lymph nodes.*

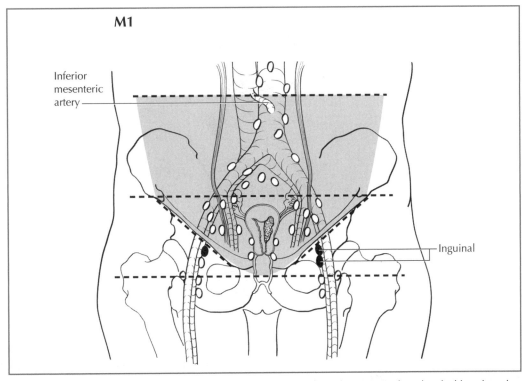

FIGURE 36.9. *For carcinomas M1 is defined as distant metastasis (includes metastasis to inguinal lymph nodes, intraperitoneal disease, or lung, liver, or bone. It excludes metastasis to para-aortic lymph nodes, vagina, pelvic serosa, or adnexa).*

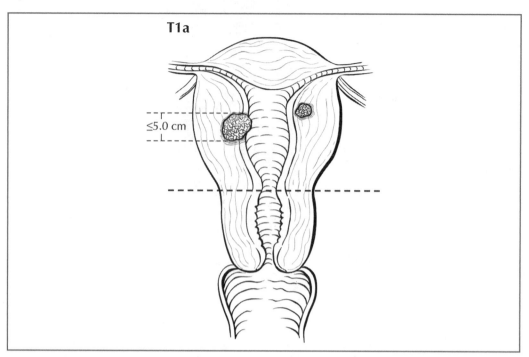

FIGURE 36.10. *T1 for leiomyosarcoma and endometrial stromal sarcoma is defined as tumor limited to the uterus. T1a is defined as tumor 5 cm or less in greatest dimension.*

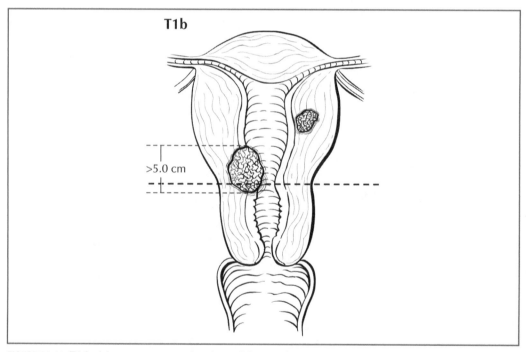

FIGURE 36.11. *T1 for leiomyosarcoma and endometrial stromal sarcoma is defined as tumor limited to the uterus. T1b is defined as tumor more than 5 cm.*

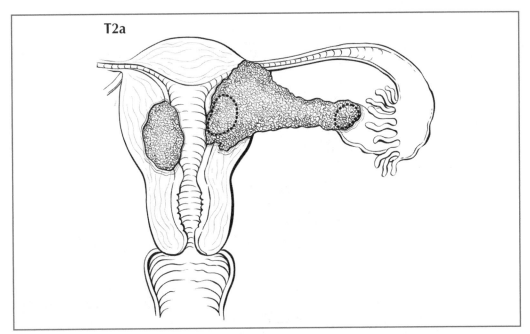

FIGURE 36.12. *T2 for leiomyosarcoma, endometrial stromal sarcoma, and adenosarcoma is defined as tumor that extends beyond the uterus, within the pelvis. T2a for sarcomas is defined as tumor that involves adnexa.*

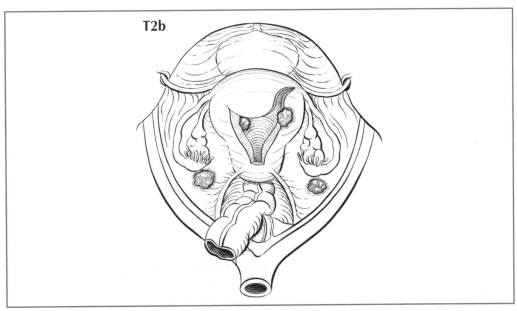

FIGURE 36.13. *T2b for leiomyosarcoma, endometrial stromal sarcoma, and adenosarcoma is defined as tumor that involves other pelvic tissues.*

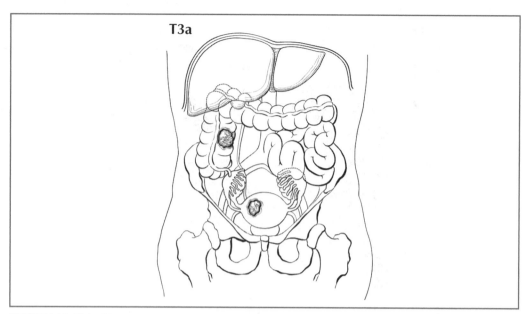

FIGURE 36.14. *T3 for leiomyosarcoma, endometrial stromal sarcoma, and adenosarcoma is defined as tumor that infiltrates abdominal tissues. T3a for sarcomas is defined as one site.*

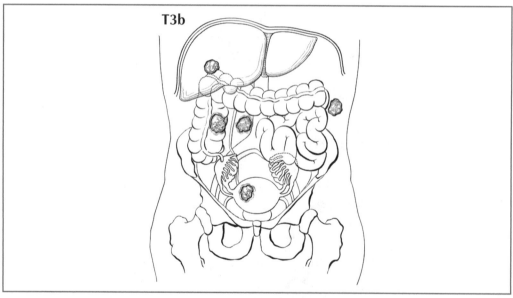

FIGURE 36.15. *T3 for leiomyosarcoma, endometrial stromal sarcoma, and adenosarcoma is defined as tumor that infiltrates abdominal tissues. T3b for sarcomas is defined as more than one site.*

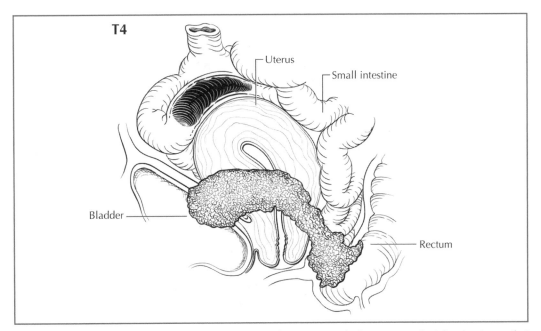

FIGURE 36.16. *T4 for leiomyosarcoma, endometrial stromal sarcoma, and adenosarcoma is defined as tumor that invades bladder or rectum.*

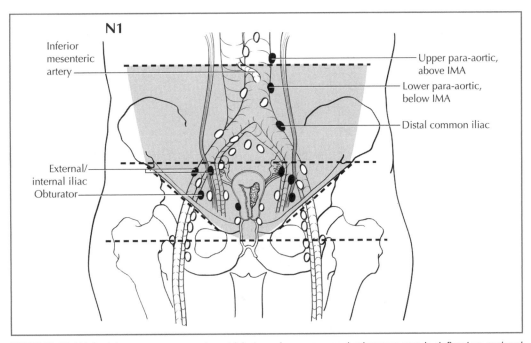

FIGURE 36.17. *N1 for leiomyosarcoma, endometrial stromal sarcoma, and adenosarcoma is defined as regional lymph node metastasis.*

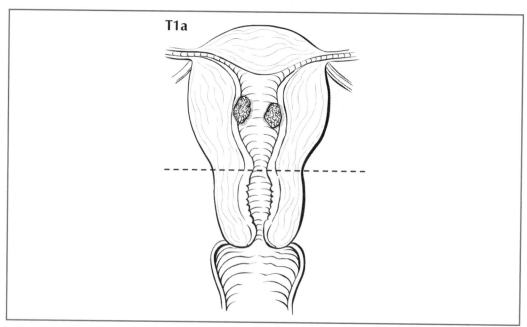

FIGURE 36.18. *T1 for adenosarcoma is defined as tumor limited to the uterus. T1a is defined as tumor limited to the endometrium/endocervix.*

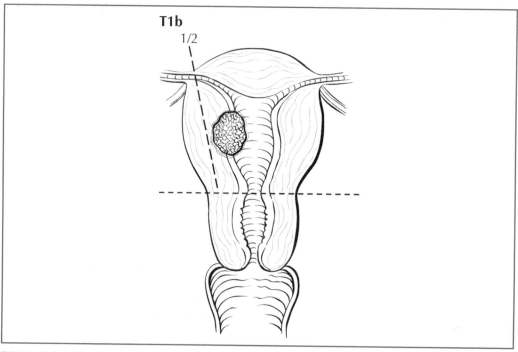

FIGURE 36.19. *T1 for adenosarcoma is defined as tumor limited to the uterus. T1b is defined as tumor that invades to less than half of the myometrium.*

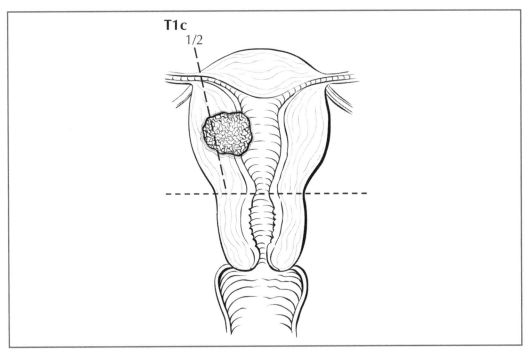

FIGURE 36.20. *T1 for adenosarcoma is defined as tumor limited to the uterus. T1c is defined as tumor that invades more than half of the myometrium.*

PROGNOSTIC FACTORS (SITE-SPECIFIC FACTORS)	
(Recommended for Collection for Carcinomas and Sarcomas)	
Required for staging	None
Clinically significant	FIGO Stage
	Peritoneal cytology results
	Pelvic nodal dissection with number of nodes positive/examined
	Para-aortic nodal dissection with number of nodes positive/examined
	Percentage of nonendometrioid cell type in mixed histology tumors
	Omentectomy performed

Ovary and Primary Peritoneal Carcinoma

37

ICD-O-3 TOPOGRAPHY CODES

C56.9 Ovary
C48.1 Specified parts of peritoneum (female only)
C48.2 Peritoneum (female only)
C48.8 Overlapping lesion of retroperito-neum and peritoneum (female only)

ICD-O-3 HISTOLOGY CODE RANGES

8000–8576, 8590–8671, 8930–9110 (C56.9 only)
8000–8576, 8590–8671, 8930–8934, 8940–9110 (C48.1–C48.8 only)

ANATOMY

Primary Site. The ovaries are a pair of solid, flattened ovoids 2–4 cm in diameter that are connected by a peritoneal fold to the broad ligament and by the infundibulopelvic ligament to the lateral wall of the pelvis (Figure 37.1). They are attached medially to the uterus by the utero-ovarian ligament.

In some cases, an adenocarcinoma is primary in the peritoneum (Figure 37.1). The ovaries are not involved or are only involved with minimal surface implants. The clinical presentation, surgical therapy, chemotherapy, and prognosis of these peritoneal tumors mirror those of papillary serous carcinoma of the ovary. Patients who undergo prophylactic oophorectomy for a familial history of ovarian cancer appear to retain a 1–2% chance of developing peritoneal adenocarcinoma, which is histopathologically and clinically similar to primary ovarian cancer.

Regional Lymph Nodes. The lymphatic drainage occurs by the infundibulopelvic and round ligament trunks and an external iliac accessory route into the following regional nodes (Figure 37.2):

External iliac
Internal iliac (hypogastric)
Obturator
Common iliac
Para-aortic
Inguinal
Pelvic, NOS
Retroperitoneal, NOS
For pN0, histologic examination should include both pelvic and para-aortic lymph nodes.

C.C. Compton et al. (eds.), *AJCC Cancer Staging Atlas: A Companion to the Seventh Editions of the AJCC Cancer Staging Manual and Handbook*, DOI 10.1007/978-1-4614-2080-4_37,
© 2012 American Joint Committee on Cancer

Metastatic Sites. The peritoneum, including the omentum and the pelvic and abdominal visceral and parietal peritoneum, comprises common sites for seeding. Diaphragmatic and liver surface involvement are also common. However, to be consistent with FIGO staging, these implants within the abdominal cavity (T3) are not considered distant metastases. Extraperitoneal sites, including parenchymal liver, lung, skeletal metastases, and supraclavicular and axillary nodes, are M1.

PROGNOSTIC FEATURES

Histology and grade are important prognostic factors. Women with borderline tumors (low malignant potential) have an excellent prognosis, even when extraovarian disease is found. In patients with invasive ovarian cancer, well-differentiated lesions have a better prognosis than poorly differentiated tumors, stage for stage. Histologic type is also extremely important, because some stromal tumors (theca cell, granulosa) have an excellent prognosis, whereas epithelial tumors in general have a less favorable outcome. For this reason, epithelial cell types are generally reported together, and sex-cord stromal tumors and germ cell tumors are reported separately. Tumor cell type also helps to guide the type of chemotherapy that is recommended.

In advanced disease, the most important prognostic factor is the residual disease after the initial surgical management. Even with advanced stage, patients with no gross residual after the surgical debulking have a considerably better prognosis than those with minimal or extensive residual. Not only is the size of the residual important, but the number of sites of residual tumor also appears to be important (tumor volume).

The tumor marker CA-125 is useful for following the response to therapy in patients with epithelial ovarian cancer who have elevated levels of this marker. The rate of regression during chemotherapy treatment may have prognostic significance. Women with germ cell tumors may also have elevated serum tumor markers – alpha fetoprotein (AFP) or human chorionic gonadotropin (β-hCG). Other factors, such as growth factors and oncogene amplification, are currently under investigation.

DEFINITIONS OF TNM

The definitions of the T categories correspond to the stages accepted by the Fédération Internationale de Gynécologie et d'Obstétrique (FIGO). Both systems are included for comparison.

Primary Tumor (T)		
TNM Categories	*FIGO Stages*	
TX		Primary tumor cannot be assessed
T0		No evidence of primary tumor
T1	I	Tumor limited to ovaries (one or both)
T1a	IA	Tumor limited to one ovary; capsule intact, no tumor on ovarian surface. No malignant cells in ascites or peritoneal washings (Figure 37.3)
T1b	IB	Tumor limited to both ovaries; capsules intact, no tumor on ovarian surface. No malignant cells in ascites or peritoneal washings (Figure 37.4)

(continued)

Primary Tumor (T) *(continued)*

T1c	IC	Tumor limited to one or both ovaries with any of the following: capsule ruptured, tumor on ovarian surface, malignant cells in ascites or peritoneal washings (Figure 37.5)
T2	II	Tumor involves one or both ovaries with pelvic extension
T2a	IIA	Extension and/or implants on uterus and/or tube(s). No malignant cells in ascites or peritoneal washings (Figure 37.6)
T2b	IIB	Extension to and/or implants on other pelvic tissues. No malignant cells in ascites or peritoneal washings (Figure 37.7)
T2c	IIC	Pelvic extension and/or implants (T2a or T2b) with malignant cells in ascites or peritoneal washings (Figure 37.8)
T3	III	Tumor involves one or both ovaries with microscopically confirmed peritoneal metastasis outside the pelvis (Figures 37.9, 37.10)
T3a	IIIA	Microscopic peritoneal metastasis beyond pelvis (no macroscopic tumor) (Figure 37.9)
T3b	IIIB	Macroscopic peritoneal metastasis beyond pelvis 2 cm or less in greatest dimension (Figure 37.9)
T3c	IIIC	Peritoneal metastasis beyond pelvis more than 2 cm in greatest dimension and/or regional lymph node metastasis (Figure 37.9, Figure 37.10)

Note: Liver capsule metastasis T3/Stage III; liver parenchymal metastasis M1/Stage IV (Figure 37.11). Pleural effusion must have positive cytology for M1/Stage IV.

Regional Lymph Nodes (N)

TNM Categories	*FIGO Stages*	
NX		Regional lymph nodes cannot be assessed
N0		No regional lymph node metastasis
N1	IIIC	Regional lymph node metastasis (Figure 37.12)

Distant Metastasis (M)

TNM Categories	*FIGO Stages*	
M0		No distant metastasis
M1	IV	Distant metastasis (excludes peritoneal metastasis)

pTNM Pathologic Classification. The pT, pN, and pM categories correspond to the T, N, and M categories.

ANATOMIC STAGE/PROGNOSTIC GROUPS

Stage I	T1	N0	M0
Stage IA	T1a	N0	M0
Stage IB	T1b	N0	M0
Stage IC	T1c	N0	M0
Stage II	T2	N0	M0
Stage IIA	T2a	N0	M0
Stage IIB	T2b	N0	M0
Stage IIC	T2c	N0	M0
Stage III	T3	N0	M0
Stage IIIA	T3a	N0	M0
Stage IIIB	T3b	N0	M0
Stage IIIC	T3c	N0	M0
	Any T	N1	M0
Stage IV	Any T	Any N	M1

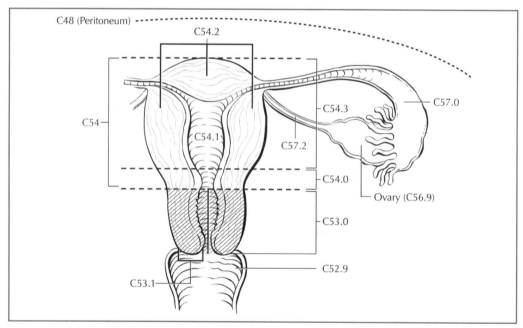

FIGURE 37.1. Anatomic sites of the ovary and peritoneum.

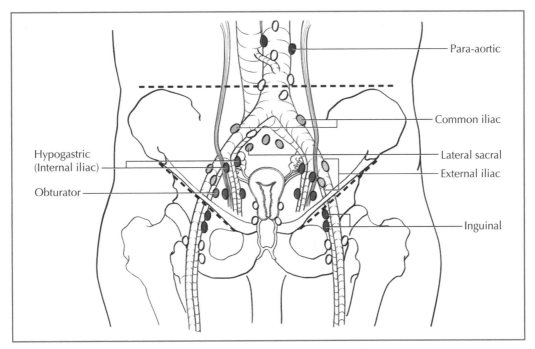

FIGURE 37.2. *Regional lymph nodes of the ovary and primary peritoneal carcinomas.*

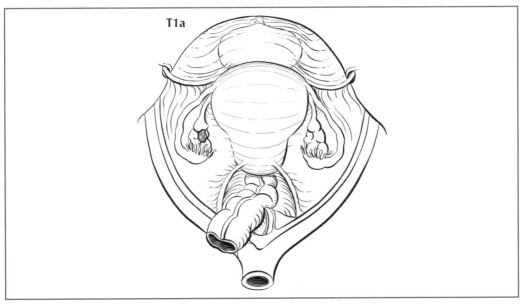

FIGURE 37.3. *T1 is defined as tumor limited to ovaries. T1a is defined as tumor limited to one ovary; capsule intact, no tumor on ovarian surface. No malignant cells in ascites or peritoneal washings.*

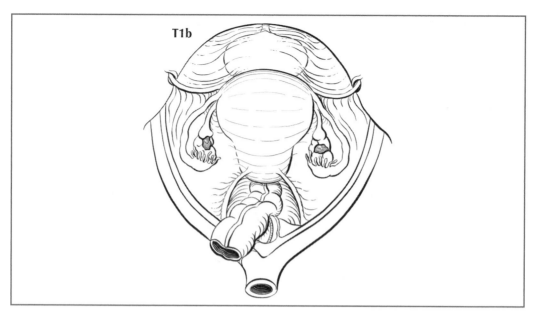

FIGURE 37.4. *T1b is defined as tumor limited to both ovaries; capsules intact, no tumor on ovarian surface. No malignant cells in ascites or peritoneal washings.*

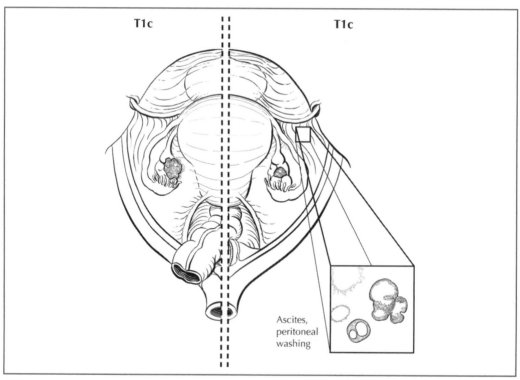

Ascites, peritoneal washing

FIGURE 37.5. *T1c is defined as tumor limited to one or both ovaries with any of the following: capsule ruptured, tumor on ovarian surface, malignant cells in ascites or peritoneal washings.*

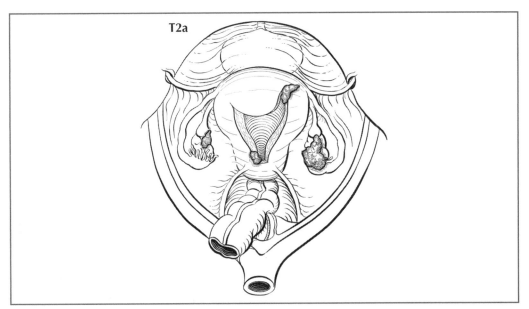

FIGURE 37.6. *T2 is defined as tumor that involves one or both ovaries with pelvic extension. T2a is defined as extension and/or implants on uterus and/or tube(s). No malignant cells in ascites or peritoneal washings.*

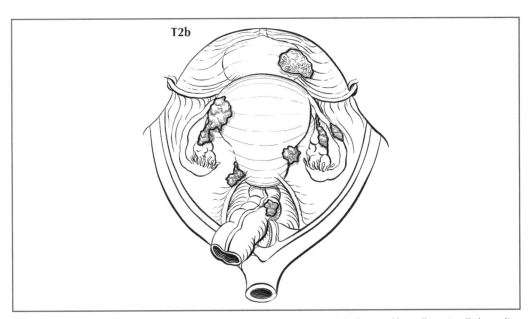

FIGURE 37.7. *T2b is defined as extension to and/or implants on other pelvic tissues. No malignant cells in ascites or peritoneal washings.*

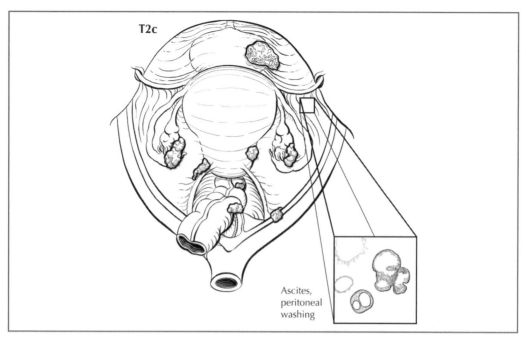

FIGURE 37.8. *T2c is defined as pelvic extension and/or implants (T2a or T2b) with malignant cells in ascites or peritoneal washings.*

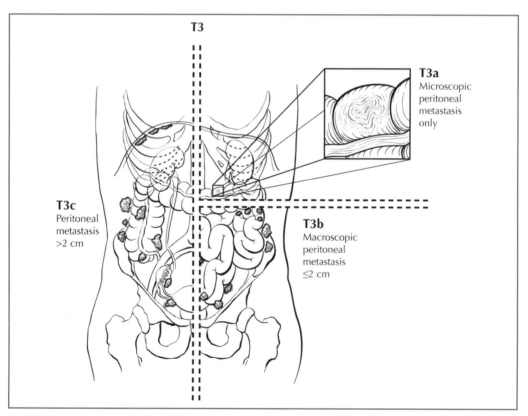

FIGURE 37.9. *T3 is defined as tumor that involves one or both ovaries with microscopically confirmed peritoneal metastasis outside the pelvis. T3a is defined as microscopic peritoneal metastasis beyond pelvis (no macroscopic tumor). T3b is defined as macroscopic peritoneal metastasis beyond pelvis 2 cm or less in greatest dimension. T3c is defined as peritoneal metastasis beyond pelvis more than 2 cm in greatest dimension and/or regional lymph node metastasis.*

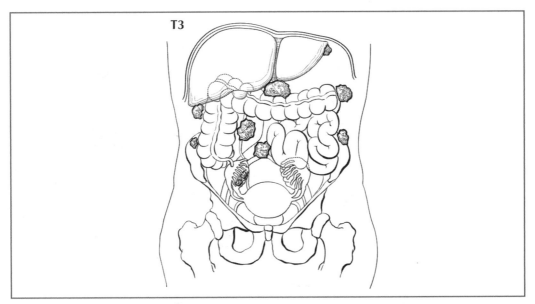

FIGURE 37.10. *T3 for primary peritoneal carcinoma is the same definition as ovary, tumor involves one or both ovaries with microscopically confirmed peritoneal metastasis outside the pelvis. T3a is defined as microscopic peritoneal metastasis beyond pelvis (no macroscopic tumor). T3b is defined as macroscopic peritoneal metastasis beyond pelvis 2 cm or less in greatest dimension. T3c is defined as peritoneal metastasis beyond pelvis more than 2 cm in greatest dimension and/or regional lymph node metastasis. T3c is shown in the illustration.*

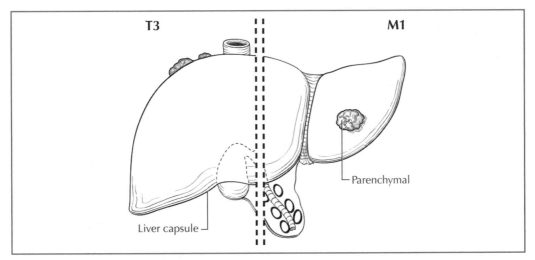

FIGURE 37.11. *Liver capsule metastasis is T3; whereas liver parenchymal metastasis is M1.*

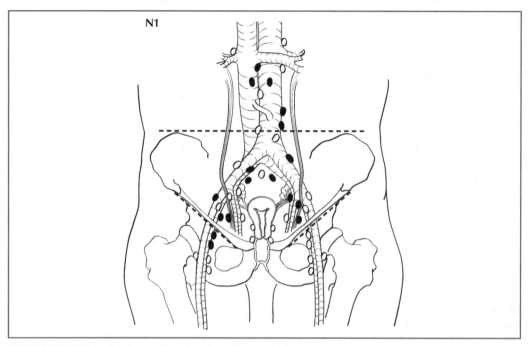

FIGURE 37.12. *N1 is defined as regional lymph node metastasis.*

PROGNOSTIC FACTORS (SITE-SPECIFIC FACTORS)
(Recommended for Collection)

Required for staging	None
Clinically significant	FIGO stage
	Preoperative CA-125
	Gross residual tumor after primary cyto-reductive surgery (present, absent, unknown, "y" meaning patient received chemotherapy prior to surgery)
	Residual tumor volume after primary cyto-reductive surgery (no gross, ≤1 cm, >1 cm, unknown, "y" meaning patient received chemotherapy prior to surgery)
	Residual tumor location following primary cyto-reductive surgery ("y" indicates patient received chemotherapy prior to surgery)
	Malignant ascites volume

Fallopian Tube

38

SUMMARY OF CHANGES

- The definition of TNM and the Stage Grouping for this chapter have not changed from the Sixth Edition

ICD-O-3 TOPOGRAPHY CODE

C57.0   Fallopian tube

ICD-O-3 HISTOLOGY CODE RANGES

8000–8576, 8940–8950, 8980–8981

ANATOMY

Primary Site. The fallopian tube extends from the posterior superior aspect of the uterine fundus laterally and anteriorly to the ovary (Figure 38.1). Its length is approximately 10 cm. The medial end arises in the cornual portion of the uterine cavity, and the lateral end opens to the peritoneal cavity.

Carcinoma of the fallopian tube is almost always an adenocarcinoma arising from an in situ lesion of the tubal mucosa. It invades locally into the muscular wall of the tube and then into the peritubal soft tissue or adjacent organs such as the uterus or ovary, or through the serosa of the tube into the peritoneal cavity. Metastatic tumor implants can be found throughout the peritoneal cavity. The tumor may obstruct the tubal lumen and present as a ruptured or unruptured hydrosalpinx or hematosalpinx.

Regional Nodes. Carcinoma of the fallopian tube can also metastasize to the regional lymph nodes, which include the following (Figure 38.2):

Common iliac
External iliac
Internal iliac (hypogastric)
Obturator
Paraaortic
Inguinal
Pelvic lymph nodes, NOS

Adequate evaluation of the regional lymph nodes usually includes aortic and pelvic nodes.

Distant Metastases. Surface implants within the pelvic cavity and the abdominal cavity are common, but these are classified as T2 and T3 disease, respectively. Parenchymal liver metastases and extraperitoneal sites, including lung and skeletal metastases, are M1.

PROGNOSTIC FEATURES

The surgical-pathologic stage is the most significant prognostic characteristic. Tumor differentiation is an important prognostic characteristic in all stages of disease. In patients with localized tumors, depth of invasion into the tubal musculature and rupture of the tube have prognostic importance. With advanced disease, the volume of residual tumor after surgical debulking appears to be related to prognosis.

DEFINITIONS OF TNM

Primary Tumor (T)

TNM Categories	FIGO Stages	
TX		Primary tumor cannot be assessed
T0		No evidence of primary tumor
Tis*		Carcinoma in situ (limited to tubal mucosa)
T1	I	Tumor limited to the fallopian tube(s)
T1a	IA	Tumor limited to one tube, without penetrating the serosal surface; no ascites (Figure 38.3)
T1b	IB	Tumor limited to both tubes, without penetrating the serosal surface; no ascites (Figure 38.4)
T1c	IC	Tumor limited to one or both tubes with extension onto or through the tubal serosa, or with malignant cells in ascites or peritoneal washings (Figure 38.5)
T2	II	Tumor involves one or both fallopian tubes with pelvic extension
T2a	IIA	Extension and/or metastasis to the uterus and/or ovaries (Figure 38.6)
T2b	IIB	Extension to other pelvic structures (Figure 38.7)
T2c	IIC	Pelvic extension with malignant cells in ascites or peritoneal washings (Figure 38.8)
T3	III	Tumor involves one or both fallopian tubes, with peritoneal implants outside the pelvis
T3a	IIIA	Microscopic peritoneal metastasis outside the pelvis (Figure 38.9)
T3b	IIIB	Macroscopic peritoneal metastasis outside the pelvis 2 cm or less in greatest dimension (Figure 38.9)
T3c	IIIC	Peritoneal metastasis outside the pelvis and more than 2 cm in diameter (Figure 38.9)

*Note: FIGO no longer includes Stage 0 (Tis).
Note: Liver capsule metastasis is T3/Stage III; liver parenchymal metastasis is M1/Stage IV (Figure 38.10). Pleural effusion must have positive cytology for M1/Stage IV.

Regional Lymph Nodes (N)

TNM Categories	FIGO Stages	
NX		Regional lymph nodes cannot be assessed
N0		No regional lymph node metastasis
N1	IIIC	Regional lymph node metastasis (Figure 38.11)

Distant Metastasis (M)

TNM Categories	FIGO Stages	
M0		No distant metastasis
M1	IV	Distant metastasis (excludes metastasis within the peritoneal cavity)

ANATOMIC STAGE/PROGNOSTIC GROUPS

Stage 0*	Tis	N0	M0
Stage I	T1	N0	M0
Stage IA	T1a	N0	M0
Stage IB	T1b	N0	M0
Stage IC	T1c	N0	M0
Stage II	T2	N0	M0
Stage IIA	T2a	N0	M0
Stage IIB	T2b	N0	M0
Stage IIC	T2c	N0	M0
Stage III	T3	N0	M0
Stage IIIA	T3a	N0	M0
Stage IIIB	T3b	N0	M0
Stage IIIC	T3c	N0	M0
	Any T	N1	M0
Stage IV	Any T	Any N	M1

*Note: FIGO no longer includes Stage 0 (Tis).

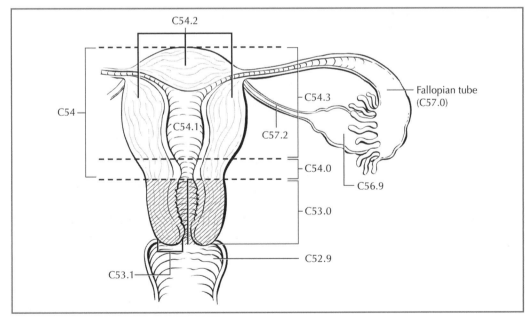

FIGURE 38.1. *Anatomic site of the fallopian tube.*

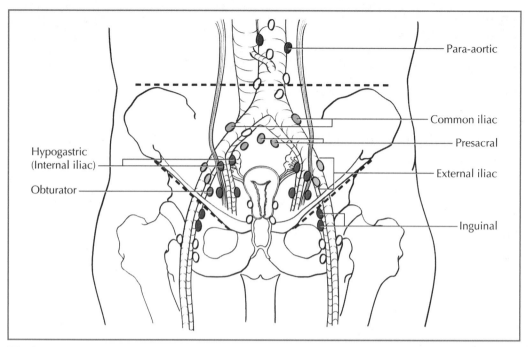

FIGURE 38.2. *Regional lymph nodes of the fallopian tube.*

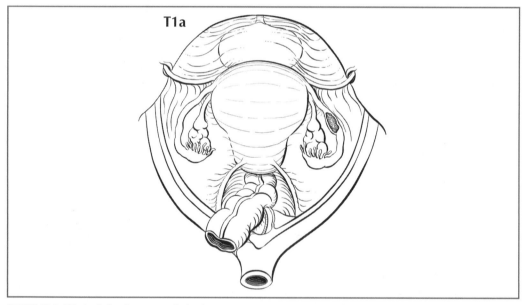

FIGURE 38.3. *T1a is defined as tumor limited to one tube, without penetrating the serosal surface; no ascites.*

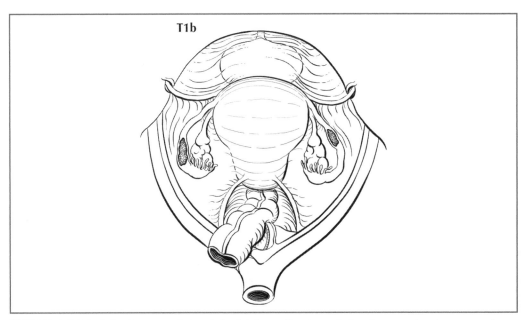

FIGURE 38.4. *T1b is defined as tumor limited to both tubes, without penetrating the serosal surface; no ascites.*

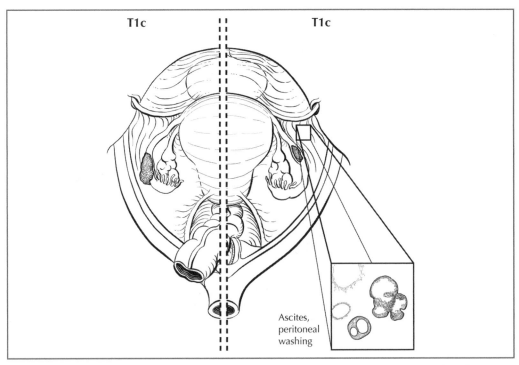

Ascites,
peritoneal
washing

FIGURE 38.5. *T1c is defined as tumor limited to one or both tubes with extension onto or through the tubal serosa, or with malignant cells in ascites or peritoneal washings.*

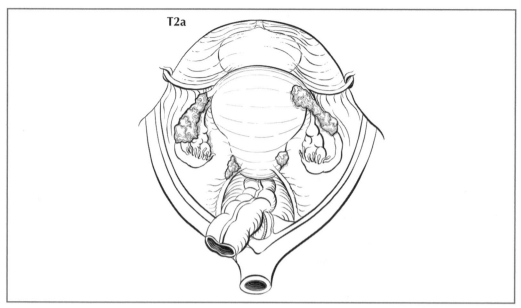

FIGURE 38.6. *T2 is defined as tumor that involves one or both fallopian tubes with pelvic extension. T2a is defined as extension and/or metastasis to the uterus and/or ovaries.*

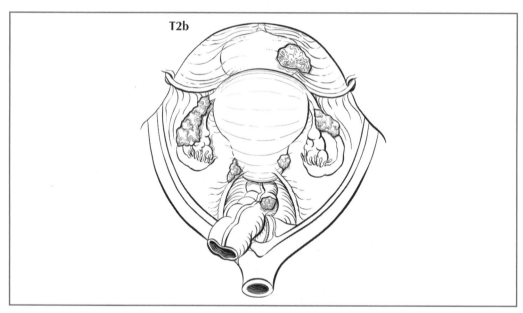

FIGURE 38.7. *T2b is defined as extension to other pelvic structures.*

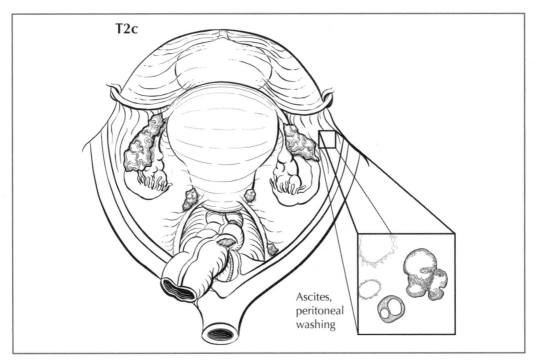

FIGURE 38.8. *T2c is defined as pelvic extension with malignant cells in ascites or peritoneal washings.*

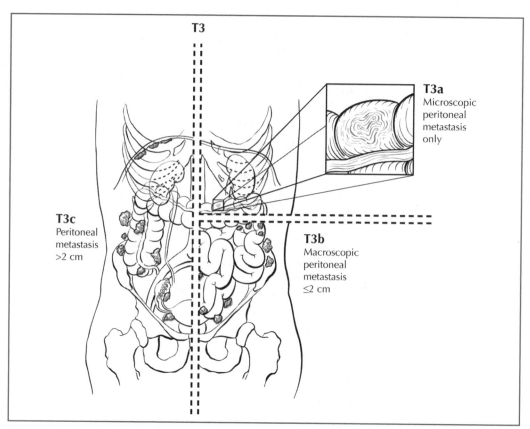

FIGURE 38.9. *T3 is defined as tumor that involves one or both fallopian tubes, with peritoneal implants outside the pelvis. T3a is defined as microscopic peritoneal metastasis outside the pelvis. T3b is defined as macroscopic peritoneal metastasis outside the pelvis 2 cm or less in greatest dimension. T3c is defined as peritoneal metastasis outside the pelvis and more than 2 cm in diameter.*

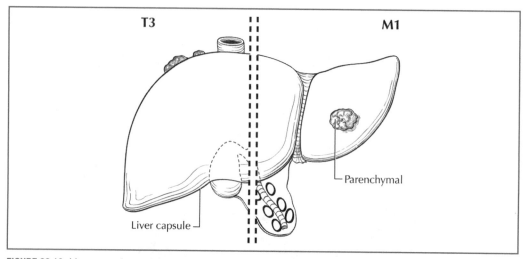

FIGURE 38.10. *Liver capsule metastasis is T3; whereas liver parenchymal metastasis is M1.*

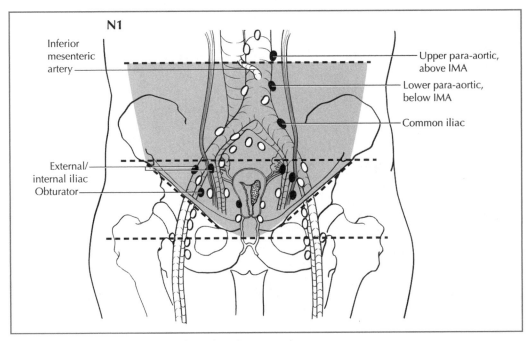

FIGURE 38.11. *N1 is defined as regional lymph node metastasis.*

PROGNOSTIC FACTORS (SITE-SPECIFIC FACTORS)
(Recommended for Collection)

Required for staging	None
Clinically significant	FIGO Stage
	Tumor location, involvement of fimbria
	Pelvic nodal status and method of assessment

Gestational Trophoblastic Tumors

39

SUMMARY OF CHANGES

- The definition of TNM and the Stage Grouping for this chapter have not changed from the Sixth Edition

ICD-O-3 TOPOGRAPHY CODE

C58.9   Placenta

ICD-O-3 HISTOLOGY CODE RANGES

9100–9105

ANATOMY

Because of the responsiveness of this tumor to treatment and the accuracy of the serum tumor marker hCG in reflecting the status of disease, the traditional anatomic staging system used in most solid tumors has little prognostic significance. Trophoblastic tumors not associated with pregnancy (ovarian teratomas) are not included in this classification.

Primary Site. By definition, gestational trophoblastic tumors arise from placental tissue in the uterus (Figure 39.1). Although most of these tumors are noninvasive and are removed by dilatation and suction evacuation, local invasion of the myometrium can occur. When this is diagnosed on a hysterectomy specimen (rarely done these days), it may be reported as an *invasive* hydatidiform mole.

Regional Lymph Nodes. Nodal involvement in gestational trophoblastic tumors is rare but has a very poor prognosis when diagnosed. There is no regional nodal designation in the staging of these tumors. Nodal metastases should be classified as metastatic (M1) disease.

Metastatic Sites. This is a highly vascular tumor that results in frequent, widespread metastases when these lesions become malignant. The cervix and vagina are common pelvic sites of metastases (T2), and the lungs are often involved by distant metastases (M1a). Other, less frequently encountered metastatic sites include kidney, gastrointestinal tract, and spleen (M1b). The liver and brain are occasionally involved and may harbor metastatic sites that are difficult to treat with chemotherapy.

Prognostic Index Scores. The score on the Prognostic Scoring Index is used to substage patients (Table 39.1). Each stage is anatomically defined, but substage A (low risk) and B (high risk) are assigned on the basis of a nonanatomic risk factor scoring system. The prognostic scores are 0, 1, 2, and 4 for the individual risk factors. The current prognostic scoring system eliminates the ABO blood group risk factors that were featured in the WHO scoring system and upgrades the risk factor for liver metastasis from 2 to 4, the highest category. Low risk is a score of 6 or less, and high risk is a score of 7 or greater.

C.C. Compton et al. (eds.), *AJCC Cancer Staging Atlas: A Companion to the Seventh Editions of the AJCC Cancer Staging Manual and Handbook*, DOI 10.1007/978-1-4614-2080-4_39, © 2012 American Joint Committee on Cancer

TABLE 39.1. *Prognostic scoring index for gestational trophoblastic tumors*

Prognostic factor	Risk score			
	0	*1*	*2*	*4*
Age	<40	≥40		
Antecedent pregnancy	Hydatidiform mole	Abortion	Term pregnancy	
Interval months from index pregnancy	<4	4–6	7–12	>12
Pretreatment hCG (IU/ml)	<10^3	10^3 to <10^4	10^4 to <10^5	≥10^5
Largest tumor size, including uterus	<3 cm	3–5 cm	>5 cm	
Site of metastases	Lung	Spleen, kidney	Gastrointestinal tract	Brain, liver
Number of metastases identified		1–4	5–8	>8
Previous failed chemotherapy			Single drug	Two or more drugs
Total Score				

Low risk is a score of 6 or less. High risk is a score of 7 or greater.

PROGNOSTIC FEATURES

Outcomes Results. Gestational trophoblastic tumors may require only uterine evacuation for treatment, but even when chemotherapy is required, cure rates approach 100%. Prognostic factors are listed in the Prognostic Scoring Index. Patients with low-risk disease are usually treated with single-agent chemotherapy, whereas combined, multiple-agent chemotherapy usually results in a cure for high-risk patients.

DEFINITIONS OF TNM

Primary Tumor (T)

TNM Categories	FIGO Stages	
TX		Primary tumor cannot be assessed
T0		No evidence of primary tumor
T1	I	Tumor confined to uterus (Figure 39.2)
T2	II	Tumor extends to other genital structures (ovary, tube, vagina, broad ligaments) by metastasis or direct extension (Figure 39.3)

Distant Metastasis (M)

TNM Categories	FIGO Stages	
M0		No distant metastasis
M1		Distant metastasis
M1a	III	Lung metastasis (Figure 39.4)
M1b	IV	All other distant metastasis (Figure 39.5)

ANATOMIC STAGE/PROGNOSTIC GROUPS

Group	T	M	Risk Factors
Stage I	T1	M0	Unknown
Stage IA	T1	M0	Low risk
Stage IB	T1	M0	High risk
Stage II	T2	M0	Unknown
Stage IIA	T2	M0	Low risk
Stage IIB	T2	M0	High risk
Stage III	Any T	M1a	Unknown
Stage IIIA	Any T	M1a	Low risk
Stage IIIB	Any T	M1a	High risk
Stage IV	Any T	M1b	Unknown
Stage IVA	Any T	M1b	Low risk
Stage IVB	Any T	M1b	High risk

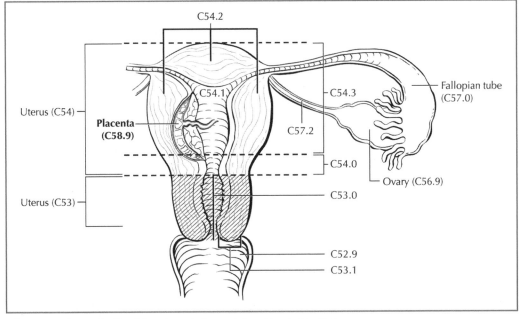

FIGURE 39.1. *Anatomic site of the placenta for gestational trophoblastic tumors.*

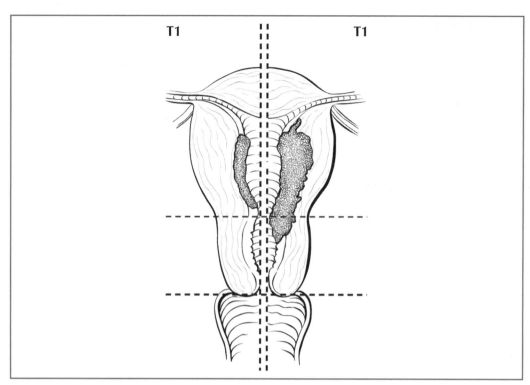

FIGURE 39.2. *T1 is defined as tumor confined to uterus.*

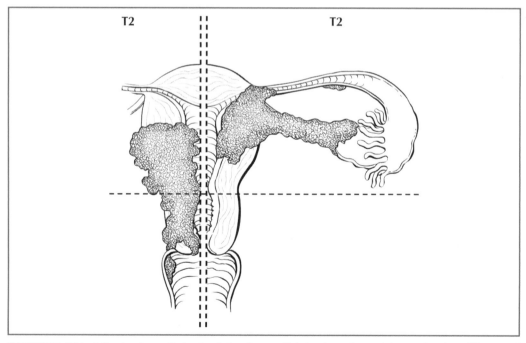

FIGURE 39.3. *T2 is defined as tumor that extends to other genital structures (ovary, tube, vagina, broad ligaments) by metastasis or direct extension.*

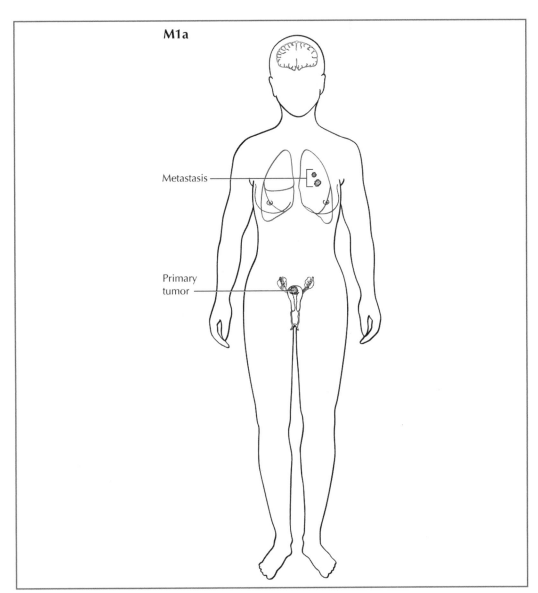

M1a

Metastasis

Primary tumor

FIGURE 39.4. *M1a is defined as lung metastasis.*

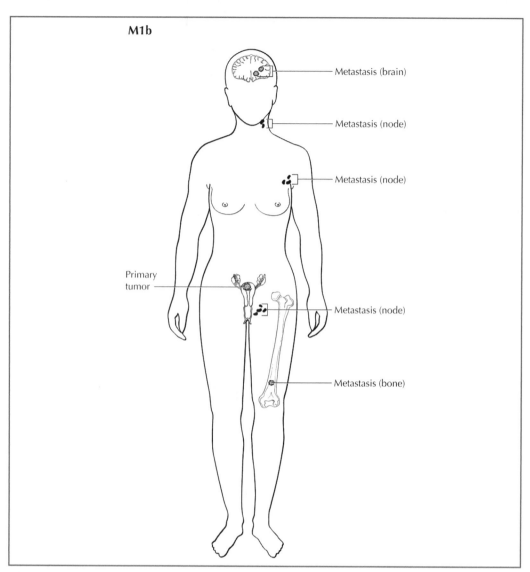

FIGURE 39.5. *M1b is defined as all other distant metastasis.*

PROGNOSTIC FACTORS (SITE-SPECIFIC FACTORS)
(Recommended for Collection)

Required for staging	Risk factors (Table 39.1)
Clinically significant	FIGO Stage

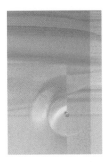

PART IX
Genitourinary Sites

Penis

(Primary urethral carcinomas and melanomas are not included)

40

SUMMARY OF CHANGES

The following changes in the definition of TNM and the Stage Grouping for this chapter have been made since the Sixth Edition

- T1 has been subdivided into T1a and T1b based on the presence or absence of lymphovascular invasion or poorly differentiated cancers
- T3 category is limited to urethral invasion and prostatic invasion is now considered T4
- Nodal staging is divided into both clinical and pathologic categories
- The distinction between superficial and deep inguinal lymph nodes has been eliminated
- Stage II grouping includes T1b N0M0 as well as T2-3 N0M0

ICD-O-3 TOPOGRAPHY CODES

C60.0 Prepuce
C60.1 Glans penis
C60.2 Body of penis
C60.8 Overlapping lesion of penis
C60.9 Penis, NOS

ICD-O-3 HISTOLOGY CODE RANGES

8000–8246, 8248–8576, 8940–8950, 8980–8981

ANATOMY

Primary Site. The penis is composed of three cylindrical masses of cavernous tissue bound together by fibrous tissue (Figure 40.1). Two masses are lateral and are known as the corpora cavernosa penis. The corpus spongiosum penis is a median mass and contains the greater part of the urethra. The distal expansion of the corpus spongoiusum forms the glans penis. The penis is attached to the front and the sides of the pubic arch. The skin covering the penis is thin and loosely connected with the deeper parts of the organ. This skin at the root of the penis is continuous with that over the scrotum and perineum. Distally, the skin becomes folded upon itself to form the prepuce, or foreskin. Circumcision has been associated with a decreased incidence of cancer of the penis.

Regional Lymph Nodes. The regional lymph nodes are as follows (Figure 40.2):

Superficial and deep inguinal (femoral)
External iliac
Internal iliac (hypogastric)
Pelvic nodes, NOS

Metastatic Sites. Lung, liver, and bone are most often involved.

C.C. Compton et al. (eds.), *AJCC Cancer Staging Atlas: A Companion to the Seventh Editions of the AJCC Cancer Staging Manual and Handbook*, DOI 10.1007/978-1-4614-2080-4_40,
© 2012 American Joint Committee on Cancer

DEFINITIONS OF TNM

Primary Tumor (T)

TX	Primary tumor cannot be assessed
T0	No evidence of primary tumor
Tis	Carcinoma in situ
Ta	Noninvasive verrucous carcinoma* (Figure 40.3)
T1a	Tumor invades subepithelial connective tissue without lymph vascular invasion and is not poorly differentiated (i.e., grade 3–4) (Figure 40.4)
T1b	Tumor invades subepithelial connective tissue with lymph vascular invasion or is poorly differentiated (Figure 40.4)
T2	Tumor invades corpus spongiosum or cavernosum (Figure 40.5)
T3	Tumor invades urethra (Figure 40.6)
T4	Tumor invades other adjacent structures (Figures 40.7A, B, C)

*Note: Broad pushing penetration (invasion) is permitted; destructive invasion is against this diagnosis.

Regional Lymph Nodes (N)

Clinical Stage Definition*

cNX	Regional lymph nodes cannot be assessed
cN0	No palpable or visibly enlarged inguinal lymph nodes
cN1	Palpable mobile unilateral inguinal lymph node (Figure 40.8)
cN2	Palpable mobile multiple or bilateral inguinal lymph nodes (Figures 40.9A, B)
cN3	Palpable fixed inguinal nodal mass or pelvic lymphadenopathy unilateral or bilateral (Figure 40.10A, B, C, D)

*Note: Clinical stage definition based on palpation, imaging.

Pathologic Stage Definition*

pNX	Regional lymph nodes cannot be assessed
pN0	No regional lymph node metastasis
pN1	Metastasis in a single inguinal lymph node (Figure 40.11)
pN2	Metastasis in multiple or bilateral inguinal lymph nodes (Figures 40.12A, B)
pN3	Extranodal extension of lymph node metastasis or pelvic lymph node(s) unilateral or bilateral (Figures 40.13A, B, C, D)

*Note: Pathologic stage definition based on biopsy or surgical excision.

Distant Metastasis (M)

M0	No distant metastasis
M1	Distant metastasis*

*Note: Lymph node metastasis outside of the true pelvis in addition to visceral or bone sites.

Additional Descriptor. The m suffix indicates the presence of multiple primary tumors and is recorded in parentheses – e.g., pTa (m) N0M0.

ANATOMIC STAGE/PROGNOSTIC GROUPS

Stage 0	Tis	N0	M0
	Ta	N0	M0
Stage I	T1a	N0	M0
Stage II	T1b	N0	M0
	T2	N0	M0
	T3	N0	M0
Stage IIIa	T1-3	N1	M0
Stage IIIb	T1-3	N2	M0
Stage IV	T4	Any N	M0
	Any T	N3	M0
	Any T	Any N	M1

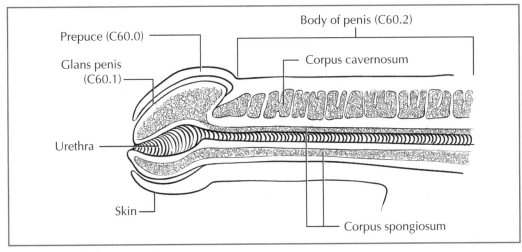

FIGURE 40.1. *Anatomy of the penis.*

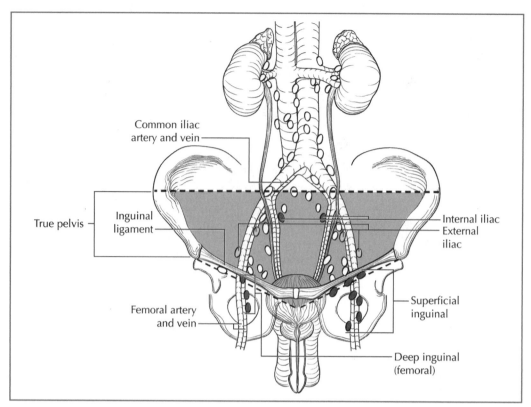

FIGURE 40.2. *Regional lymph nodes of the penis.*

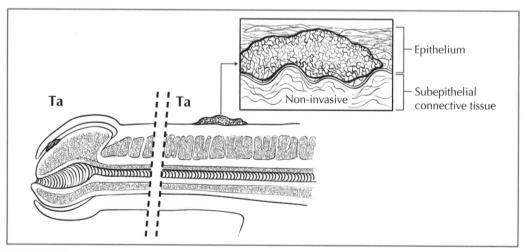

FIGURE 40.3. *Ta is defined as noninvasive verrucous carcinoma.*

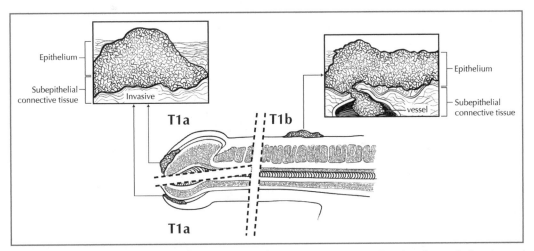

FIGURE 40.4. *T1a is defined as tumor that invades subepithelial connective tissue without lymph vascular invasion and not poorly differentiated. T1b is defined as tumor that invades subepithelial connective tissue with lymph vascular invasion or is poorly differentiated (grade 3-4).*

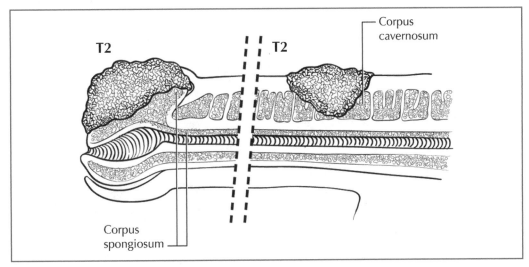

FIGURE 40.5. *T2 is defined as tumor that invades corpus spongiosum or cavernosum.*

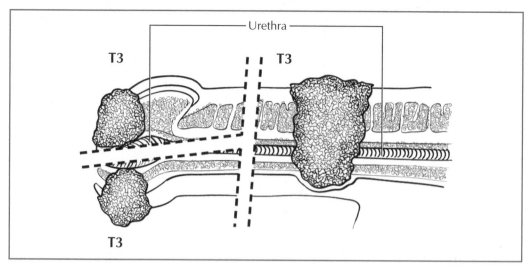

FIGURE 40.6. *T3 is defined as tumor that invades urethra.*

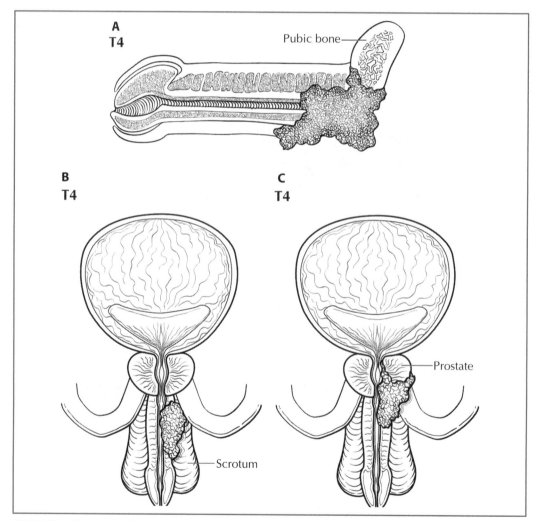

FIGURE 40.7. *T4 is defined as tumor that invades other adjacent structures including prostate. (A) Illustrated is invasion of the pubic bone. (B) Illustrated is invasion of the scrotum. (C) Illustrated is invasion of the prostate.*

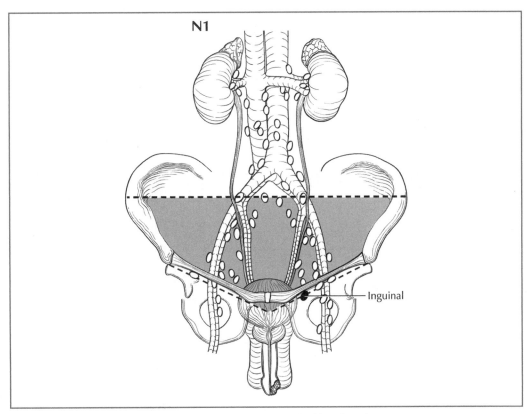

FIGURE 40.8. *cN1 is defined as a palpable mobile unilateral inguinal lymph node.*

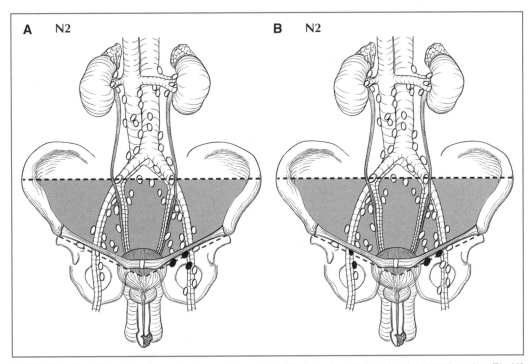

FIGURE 40.9. *(A) cN2 is defined as palpable mobile multiple (illustrated) or bilateral inguinal lymph nodes. (B) cN2 is defined as palpable mobile multiple or bilateral (illustrated) inguinal lymph nodes.*

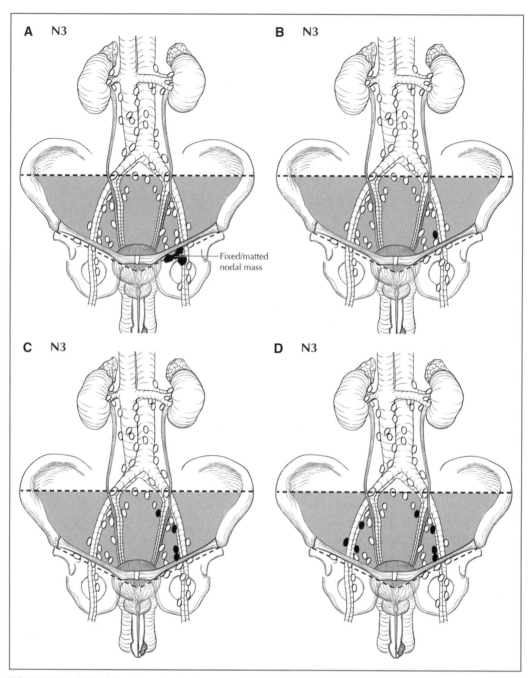

FIGURE 40.10. *cN3 is defined as palpable fixed inguinal nodal mass (A) or pelvic lymphadenopthy unilateral with a single node (B), with multiple nodes (C), or bilateral (D).*

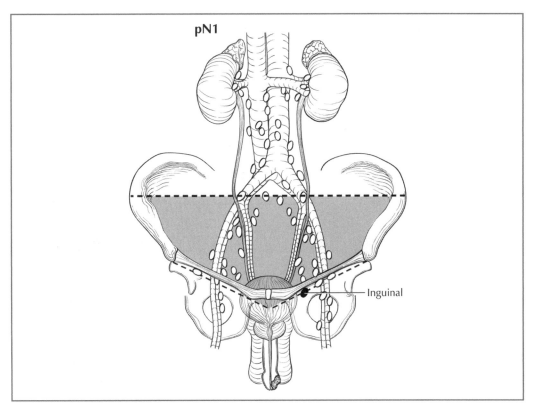

FIGURE 40.11. *pN1 is defined as involvement in a single inguinal lymph node.*

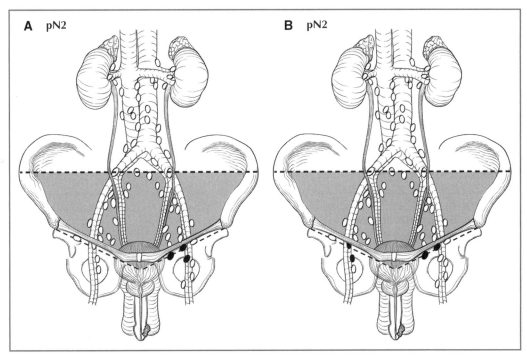

FIGURE 40.12. *(A) pN2 is defined as involvement in multiple (illustrated) or bilateral inguinal lymph nodes. (B) pN2 is defined as involvement in multiple or bilateral (illustrated) inguinal lymph nodes.*

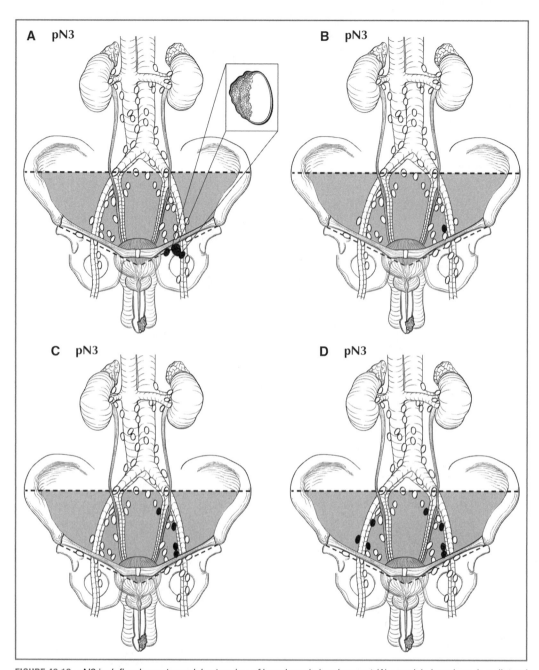

FIGURE 40.13. *pN3 is defined as extranodal extension of lymph node involvement (A) or pelvic lymph node unilateral (B), with multiple nodes (C), or bilateral (D).*

Prostate

(Sarcomas and transitional cell carcinomas are not included)

41

SUMMARY OF CHANGES

- Extraprostatic invasion with microscopic bladder neck invasion (T4) is included with T3a
- Gleason Score now recognized as the preferred grading system
- Prognostic factors have been incorporated in the Anatomic Stage/Prognostic Groups

  - Gleason Score
  - Preoperative prostate-specific antigen (PSA)

ICD-O-3 TOPOGRAPHY CODE

C61.9   Prostate gland

ICD-O-3 HISTOLOGY CODE RANGES

8000–8110, 8140–8576, 8940–8950, 8980–8981

ANATOMY

Primary Site. Adenocarcinoma of the prostate (Figures 41.1 and 41.2A, B, C) most commonly arises within the peripheral zone of the gland, where it may be amenable to detection by DRE. A less common site of origin is the anteromedial prostate, the transition zone, which is remote from the rectal surface and is the site of origin of benign nodular hyperplasia. The central zone, which makes up most of the base of the prostate, seldom is the source of cancer but is often invaded by the spread of larger cancers. Pathologically, cancers of the prostate are often multifocal; 80–85% arise from peripheral zone, 10–15% from transitional zone, and 5–10% from central zone.

The histologic grade of the prostate cancer is important for prognosis. The histopathologic grading of these tumors can be complex because of the morphologic heterogeneity of prostate cancer and its inherent tendency to be multifocal. There have been many grading schemes proposed for prostate cancer. However, the scoring system for assessing this histologic pattern or prostate cancer with the highest reproducibility and best validation in relation to outcome is the Gleason score. This is now considered the grading scheme of choice and should be utilized in assessing all cases of prostate cancer.

Regional Lymph Nodes. The regional lymph nodes are the nodes of the true pelvis, which essentially are the pelvic nodes below the bifurcation of the common iliac arteries (Figure 41.3). They include the following groups:

Pelvic, NOS
Hypogastric
Obturator

C.C. Compton et al. (eds.), *AJCC Cancer Staging Atlas: A Companion to the Seventh Editions of the AJCC Cancer Staging Manual and Handbook*, DOI 10.1007/978-1-4614-2080-4_41,
© 2012 American Joint Committee on Cancer

Iliac (internal, external, or NOS)
Sacral (lateral, presacral, promontory [Gerota's], or NOS)
Laterality does not affect the N classification.

Distant Lymph Nodes. Distant lymph nodes lie outside the confines of the true pelvis. They can be imaged using ultrasound, computed tomography, magnetic resonance imaging, or lymphangiography. Although enlarged lymph nodes can occasionally be visualized on radiographic imaging, fewer patients are initially discovered with clinically evident metastatic disease. In lower risk patients, imaging tests have proven unhelpful. In lieu of imaging, risk tables are many times used to determine individual patient risk of nodal involvement prior to therapy. Involvement of distant lymph nodes is classified as M1a. The distant lymph nodes include the following:

Aortic (para-aortic lumbar)
Common iliac
Inguinal, deep
Superficial inguinal (femoral)
Supraclavicular
Cervical
Scalene
Retroperitoneal, NOS

Metastatic Sites. Osteoblastic metastases are the most common nonnodal site of prostate cancer metastasis. In addition, this tumor can spread to distant lymph nodes. Lung and liver metastases are usually identified late in the course of the disease.

PROGNOSTIC FEATURES

An increasing number of proposed molecular markers (such as ploidy, p53, and bcl-2) as well as other clinical features have been identified that may predict stage at diagnosis and outcomes following therapy. A number of algorithms have been published that enable the merging of these data to predict local stage, risk of positive nodes, or risk of treatment failure. Each of these predictive tools employ common as well as unique variables and vary in their evaluation technique. Within the confines of the TNM staging, the clinical predictors of serum prostate-specific antigen, Gleason score, and tumor stage all have a clear, recognized, and significant impact on prognosis.

Recent studies have demonstrated that Gleason score provides extremely important information about prognosis. In an analysis, conducted by the Radiation Therapy Oncology Group (RTOG), of nearly 1,500 men treated on prospective randomized trials, Gleason score was the single most important predictor of death from prostate cancer. Combined with the AJCC stage, investigators demonstrated that four prognostic subgroups could be identified that allowed disease-specific survival to be predicted at 5, 10, and 15 years. Additional studies conducted by the RTOG also demonstrated that a pretreatment PSA > 20 ng/ml predicts a greater likelihood of distant failure and a greater need for hormonal therapy. A recent validation study confirmed that a PSA > 20 ng/ml was associated with a greater risk of prostate cancer death.

Thus, in addition to the AJCC clinical stage, pretreatment PSA and Gleason score provide important prognostic information that might affect decisions regarding therapy. In an attempt to better stratify these patients compared to the previous stage groups and avoid the large number of patients previously placed in stage group 1, the seventh edition includes a new prognostic staging for clinically localized (T1 and T2) disease that include these clinically based variables. Any type of grouping scheme such as this will not apply equally well to every individual patient situation, and this grouping still is primarily based on anatomic clinical T staging, the crux of the TNM staging historically. Other clinical features as well as pathologic features postprostatectomy, such as the number/percentage of positive biopsies and surgical margin status, likely provide additional prognostic information, and other prognostic tools that go well beyond the TNM structure may be more accurate for an individual patient. As a result, data continue to be collected in the National Cancer Database by registrars to provide long-term confirmatory data on the independent impact of multiple variables on prognosis.

OUTCOMES BY STAGE, GRADE, AND PSA

A number of endpoints are useful in assessing disease outcomes following therapy. Because the vast majority of patients diagnosed with prostate cancer are diagnosed with clinically localized disease, similar to pretreatment tools, multiple predictive models for clinical outcome have been proposed posttherapy. Biochemical (or PSA)-free recurrence indicates the likelihood that a patient treated for prostate cancer remains free of recurrent disease as manifested by a rising PSA. Prostate cancer-specific survival and overall survival are key endpoints that many studies do not evaluate due to the length of follow-up required. Biochemical failure can be a useful surrogate endpoint to predict risk of death from prostate cancer in patients with a prolonged expected survival; however, the natural history of biochemical failure progressing to clinical disease recurrence is highly variable and may depend on multiple variables including TNM characteristics as well as PSA and PSA kinetics, Gleason sum, treatment modality, and timing of biochemical recurrence. Studies continue to evaluate predictors of ultimate outcome for patients following different therapies.

DEFINITIONS OF TNM

Primary Tumor (T)

Clinical (cT)

TX	Primary tumor cannot be assessed
T0	No evidence of primary tumor
T1	Clinically inapparent tumor neither palpable nor visible by imaging
T1a	Tumor incidental histologic finding in 5% or less of tissue resected (Figure 41.4)
T1b	Tumor incidental histologic finding in more than 5% of tissue resected (Figure 41.4)
T1c	Tumor identified by needle biopsy (e.g., because of elevated PSA)
T2	Tumor confined within prostate*
T2a	Tumor involves one-half of one lobe or less (Figure 41.5)
T2b	Tumor involves more than one-half of one lobe but not both lobes (Figure 41.5)
T2c	Tumor involves both lobes (Figure 41.6)
T3	Tumor extends through the prostate capsule**
T3a	Extracapsular extension (unilateral or bilateral) (Figure 41.7A, B)
T3b	Tumor invades seminal vesicle(s) (Figure 41.8)
T4	Tumor is fixed or invades adjacent structures other than seminal vesicles such as external sphincter, rectum, bladder, levator muscles, and/or pelvic wall (Figure 41.9A, B)

*Note: Tumor found in one or both lobes by needle biopsy, but not palpable or reliably visible by imaging, is classified as T1c.

**Note: Invasion into the prostatic apex or into (but not beyond) the prostatic capsule is classified not as T3 but as T2.

Primary Tumor (T) (continued)
Pathologic (pT)*

pT2	Organ confined
pT2a	Unilateral, one-half of one side or less (Figure 41.5)
pT2b	Unilateral, involving more than one-half of side but not both sides (Figure 41.5)
pT2c	Bilateral disease (Figure 41.6)
pT3	Extraprostatic extension
pT3a	Extraprostatic extension or microscopic invasion of bladder neck** (Figure 41.7A, B)
pT3b	Seminal vesicle invasion (Figure 41.8)
pT4	Invasion of rectum, levator muscles, and/or pelvic wall (Figure 41.9A, B)

*Note: There is no pathologic T1 classification.
**Note: Positive surgical margin should be indicated by an R1 descriptor (residual microscopic disease).

Regional Lymph Nodes (N)
Clinical

NX	Regional lymph nodes were not assessed
N0	No regional lymph node metastasis
N1	Metastasis in regional lymph node(s) (Figure 41.10A, B)

Pathologic

pNX	Regional nodes not sampled
pN0	No positive regional nodes
pN1	Metastases in regional node(s) (Figure 41.10A, B)

Distant Metastasis (M)*

M0	No distant metastasis
M1	Distant metastasis
M1a	Nonregional lymph node(s)
M1b	Bone(s)
M1c	Other site(s) with or without bone disease

*Note: When more than one site of metastasis is present, the most advanced category is used. pM1c is most advanced.

ANATOMIC STAGE/PROGNOSTIC GROUPS*

Group	T	N	M	PSA	Gleason
I	T1a – c	N0	M0	PSA < 10	Gleason ≤6
	T2a	N0	M0	PSA < 10	Gleason ≤6
	T1 – 2a	N0	M0	PSA X	Gleason X
IIA	T1a – c	N0	M0	PSA < 20	Gleason 7
	T1a – c	N0	M0	PSA ≥ 10 < 20	Gleason ≤6
	T2a	N0	M0	PSA ≥ 10 < 20	Gleason ≤6
	T2a	N0	M0	PSA < 20	Gleason 7
	T2b	N0	M0	PSA < 20	Gleason ≤7
	T2b	N0	M0	PSA X	Gleason X
IIB	T2c	N0	M0	Any PSA	Any Gleason
	T1 – 2	N0	M0	PSA ≥ 20	Any Gleason
	T1 – 2	N0	M0	Any PSA	Gleason ≥8
III	T3a – b	N0	M0	Any PSA	Any Gleason
IV	T4	N0	M0	Any PSA	Any Gleason
	Any T	N1	M0	Any PSA	Any Gleason
	Any T	Any N	M1	Any PSA	Any Gleason

*When either PSA or Gleason is not available, grouping should be determined by T stage and/or either PSA or Gleason as available.

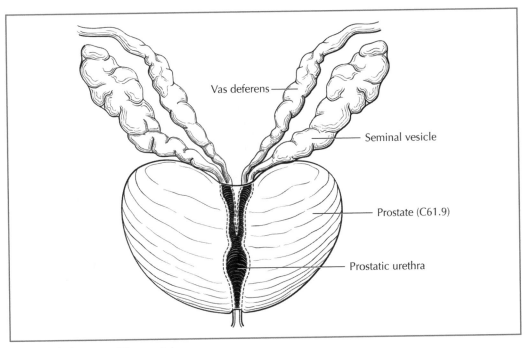

FIGURE 41.1. *Anatomy of the prostate.*

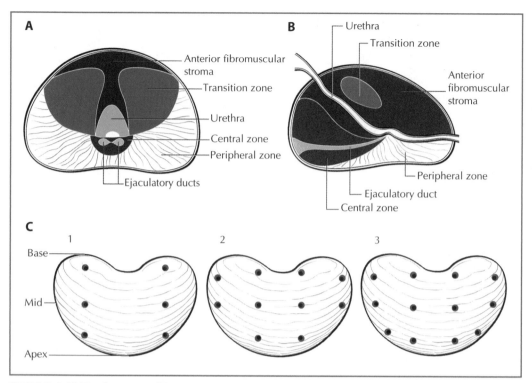

FIGURE 41.2. *(A) Zonal anatomy of the prostate, a transverse view as seen on ultrasound. (B) Zonal anatomy of the prostate, a sagittal view as seen on ultrasound. (C) Locations of the prostate for systematic biopsy schemes.*

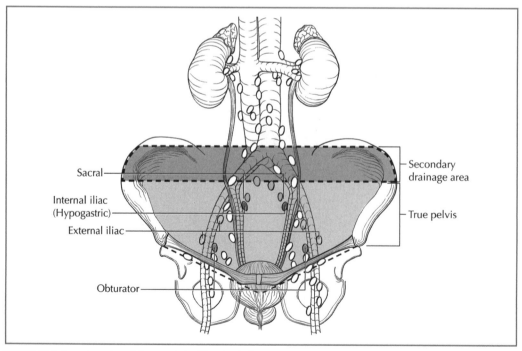

FIGURE 41.3. *Lymph nodes of the prostate. The shaded area represents regional distribution of lymph nodes. The non-shaded area indicates nodes outside of regional distribution.*

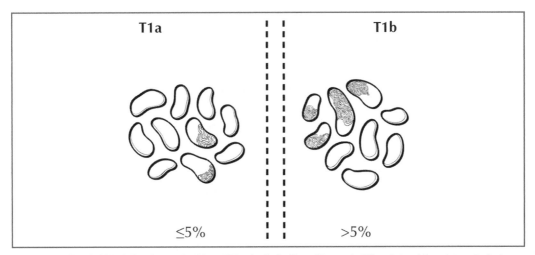

FIGURE 41.4. *T1a (left) is defined as an incidental histologic finding of tumor in 5% or less of tissue resected, shown here as tissue fragments from a transurethral resection. T1b (right) is defined as an incidental histologic finding of tumor in more than 5% of tissue resected.*

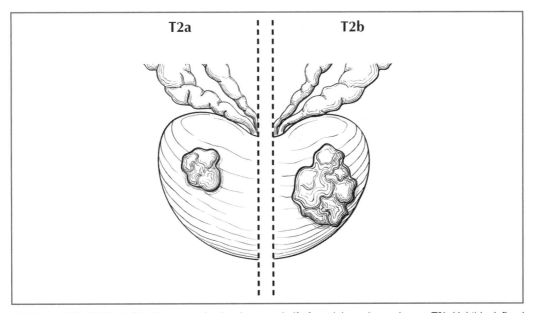

FIGURE 41.5. *T2a (left) is defined as tumor that involves one-half of one lobe or less, whereas T2b (right) is defined as tumor that involves more than one-half of one lobe but not both lobes, without extracapsular extension.*

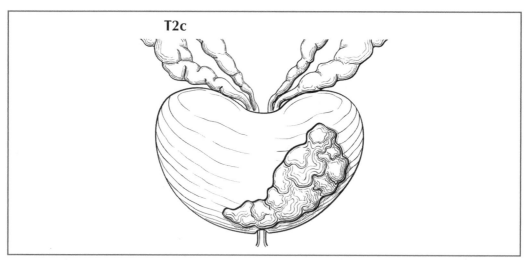

FIGURE 41.6. *T2c is defined as tumor that involves both lobes, without extraprostatic extension.*

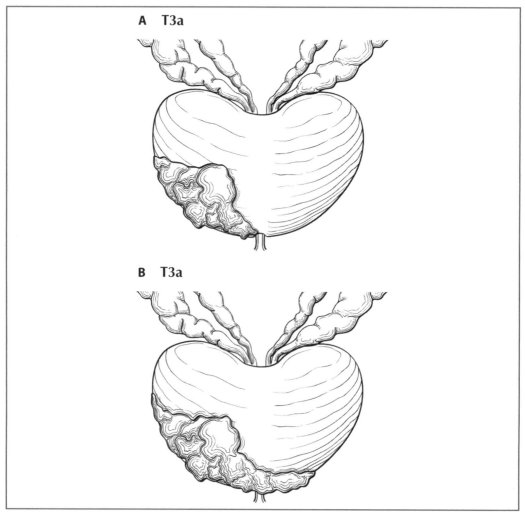

FIGURE 41.7. *(A) T3a is defined as a tumor with unilateral extracapsular extension. (B) T3a is defined as tumor with bilateral extracapsular extension.*

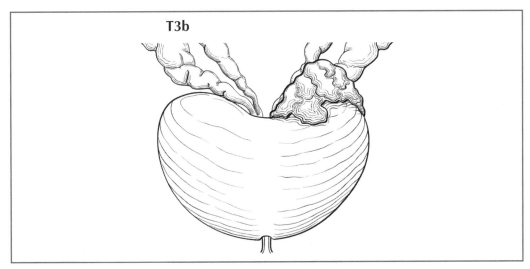

FIGURE 41.8. *T3b is defined as tumor that invades seminal vesicle(s).*

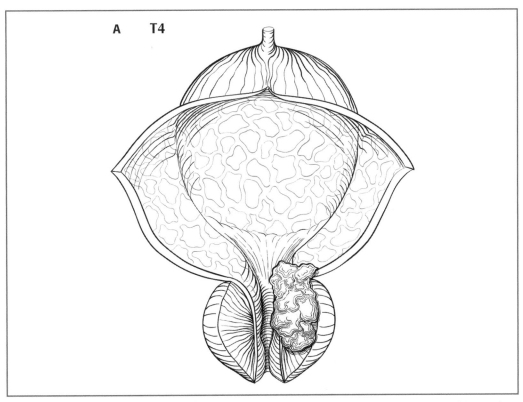

FIGURE 41.9. *(A) T4 is defined as tumor that invades adjacent structures other than seminal vesicles such as bladder, as shown here, external sphincter, rectum, levator muscles, and/or pelvic wall.*

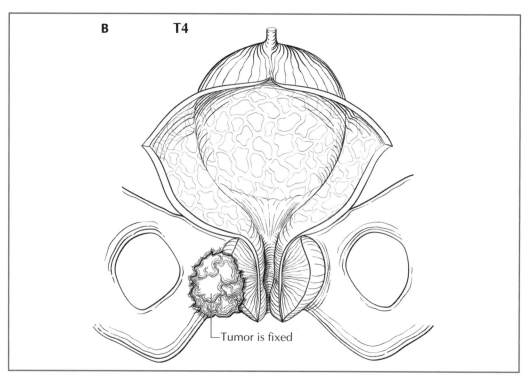

FIGURE 41.9. *(continued) (B) T4 is defined as tumor that is fixed to adjacent structures.*

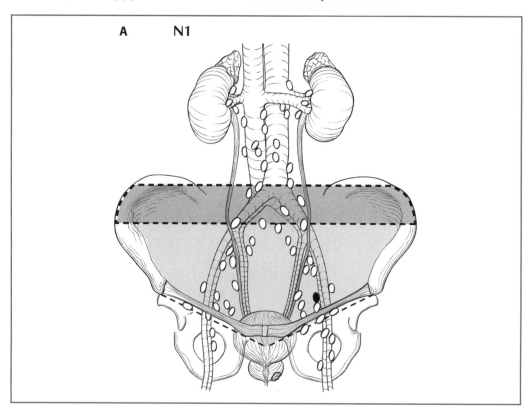

FIGURE 41.10. *(A) N1 is metastasis in regional lymph nodes, here shown unilaterally.*

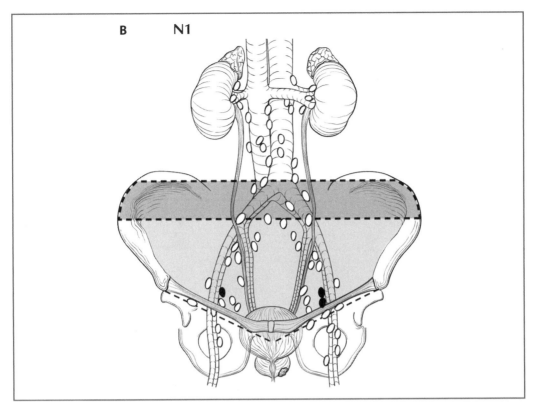

FIGURE 41.10. *(continued) (B) N1 is metastasis in regional lymph nodes, here shown bilaterally.*

PROGNOSTIC FACTORS (SITE-SPECIFIC FACTORS)
(Recommended for Collection)

Required for staging	Prostate-specific antigen Gleason score
Clinically significant	Gleason primary and secondary patterns Gleason tertiary pattern Clinical staging procedures performed Number of biopsy cores examined Number of biopsy cores positive for cancer

Testis
42

ICD-O-3 TOPOGRAPHY CODES

C62.0   Undescended testis
C62.1   Descended testis
C62.9   Testis, NOS

ICD-O-3 HISTOLOGY CODE RANGES

8000–8576, 8590–8670, 8940–8950, 8980–8981, 9060–9090, 9100–9105

ANATOMY

Primary Site. The testes (Figure 42.1) are composed of convoluted seminiferous tubules with a stroma containing functional endocrine interstitial cells. Both are encased in a dense capsule, the tunica albuginea, with fibrous septa extending into the testis and separating them into lobules. The tubules converge and exit at the mediastinum of the testis into the rete testis and efferent ducts, which join a single duct. This duct – the epididymis – coils outside the upper and lower poles of the testicle and then joins the vas deferens, a muscular conduit that accompanies the vessels and lymphatic channels of the spermatic cord. The major route for local extension of cancer is through the lymphatic channels. The tumor emerges from the mediastinum of the testis and courses through the spermatic cord. Occasionally, the epididymis is invaded early, and then the external iliac nodes may become involved. If there has been previous scrotal or inguinal surgery or if invasion of the scrotal wall is found (though this is rare), then the lymphatic spread may be to inguinal nodes.

Regional Lymph Nodes. The following nodes are considered regional (Figures 42.2A, B):

Interaortocaval
Para-aortic (periaortic)
Paracaval
Preaortic
Precaval
Retroaortic
Retrocaval

The left and right testicles demonstrate different patterns of primary drainage that mirror the differences in venous drainage. The left testicle primarily drains to the paraaortic lymph nodes and the right testicle primarily drains to the interaortocaval lymph nodes. The intrapelvic, external iliac, and inguinal nodes are considered regional only after scrotal or inguinal surgery prior to the presentation of the testis tumor. All nodes outside the regional nodes are distant. Nodes along the spermatic vein are considered regional.

Metastatic Sites. Distant spread of testicular tumors occurs most commonly to the lymph nodes, followed by metastases to the lung, liver, bone, and other visceral sites. Stage is dependent on the extent of disease and on the determination of serum tumor markers. Extent of disease includes assessment for involvement and size of regional lymph nodes, evidence of disease in nonregional lymph nodes, and metastases to pulmonary and nonpulmonary visceral sites. The stage is subdivided on the basis of the presence and degree of elevation of serum tumor markers. Serum tumor markers are measured immediately after orchiectomy and, if elevated, should be measured serially after orchiectomy to determine whether normal decay curves are followed. The physiological half-life of AFP is 5–7 days, and the half-life of HCG is 24–48 h. The presence of prolonged half-life times implies the presence of residual disease after orchiectomy. It should be noted that in some cases, tumor marker release may occur (e.g., in response to chemotherapy or handling of a primary tumor intraoperatively) and may cause artificial elevation of circulating tumor marker levels. The serum level of LDH has prognostic value in patients with metastatic disease and is included for staging.

DEFINITIONS OF TNM

Primary Tumor (T)*

The extent of primary tumor is usually classified after radical orchiectomy, and for this reason, a *pathologic stage* is assigned.

pTX	Primary tumor cannot be assessed
pT0	No evidence of primary tumor (e.g., histologic scar in testis)
pTis	Intratubular germ cell neoplasia (carcinoma in situ)
pT1	Tumor limited to the testis and epididymis without vascular/lymphatic invasion; tumor may invade into the tunica albuginea but not the tunica vaginalis (Figure 42.3)
pT2	Tumor limited to the testis and epididymis with vascular/lymphatic invasion, or tumor extending through the tunica albuginea with involvement of the tunica vaginalis (Figure 42.4)
pT3	Tumor invades the spermatic cord with or without vascular/lymphatic invasion (Figure 42.5)
pT4	Tumor invades the scrotum with or without vascular/lymphatic invasion (Figure 42.6)

*Note: Except for pTis and pT4, extent of primary tumor is classified by radical orchiectomy. TX may be used for other categories in the absence of radical orchiectomy.

Regional Lymph Nodes (N)
Clinical

NX	Regional lymph nodes cannot be assessed
N0	No regional lymph node metastasis
N1	Metastasis with a lymph node mass 2 cm or less in greatest dimension; or multiple lymph nodes, none more than 2 cm in greatest dimension (Figure 42.7A, B)
N2	Metastasis with a lymph node mass more than 2 cm but not more than 5 cm in greatest dimension; or multiple lymph nodes, any one mass greater than 2 cm but not more than 5 cm in greatest dimension (Figure 42.8A, B)
N3	Metastasis with a lymph node mass more than 5 cm in greatest dimension (Figure 42.9A, B)

Pathologic (pN)

pNX	Regional lymph nodes cannot be assessed
pN0	No regional lymph node metastasis
pN1	Metastasis with a lymph node mass 2 cm or less in greatest dimension and less than or equal to five nodes positive, none more than 2 cm in greatest dimension (Figure 42.7A, B)
pN2	Metastasis with a lymph node mass more than 2 cm but not more than 5 cm in greatest dimension; or more than five nodes positive, none more than 5 cm; or evidence of extranodal extension of tumor (Figure 42.8A, B, C)
pN3	Metastasis with a lymph node mass more than 5 cm in greatest dimension (Figure 42.9A, B)

Distant Metastasis (M)

M0	No distant metastasis
M1	Distant metastasis
M1a	Nonregional nodal or pulmonary metastasis
M1b	Distant metastasis other than to nonregional lymph nodes and lung

ANATOMIC STAGE/PROGNOSTIC GROUPS

Group	T	N	M	S (Serum Tumor Markers)
Stage 0	pTis	N0	M0	S0
Stage I	pT1–4	N0	M0	SX
Stage IA	pT1	N0	M0	S0
Stage IB	pT2	N0	M0	S0
	pT3	N0	M0	S0
	pT4	N0	M0	S0
Stage IS	Any pT/Tx	N0	M0	S1–3
Stage II	Any pT/Tx	N1–3	M0	SX
Stage IIA	Any pT/Tx	N1	M0	S0
	Any pT/Tx	N1	M0	S1
Stage IIB	Any pT/Tx	N2	M0	S0
	Any pT/Tx	N2	M0	S1
Stage IIC	Any pT/Tx	N3	M0	S0
	Any pT/Tx	N3	M0	S1
Stage III	Any pT/Tx	Any N	M1	SX
Stage IIIA	Any pT/Tx	Any N	M1a	S0
	Any pT/Tx	Any N	M1a	S1
Stage IIIB	Any pT/Tx	N1–3	M0	S2
	Any pT/Tx	Any N	M1a	S2
Stage IIIC	Any pT/Tx	N1–3	M0	S3
	Any pT/Tx	Any N	M1a	S3
	Any pT/Tx	Any N	M1b	Any S

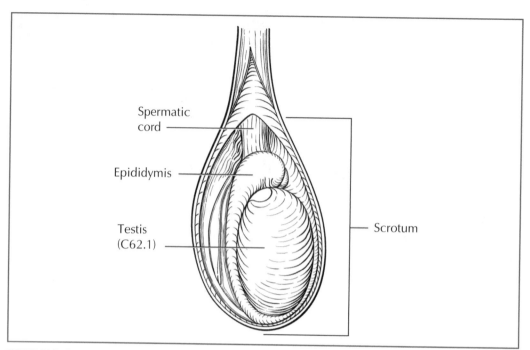

FIGURE 42.1. *Anatomy of the testis.*

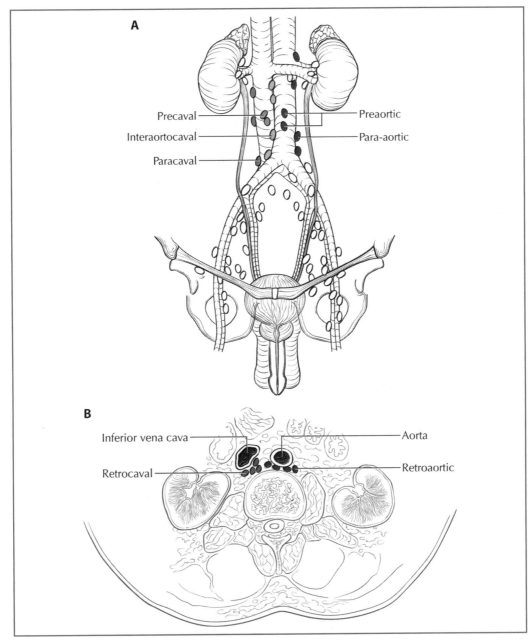

FIGURE 42.2. *(A) Regional lymph nodes of the testis. (B) Regional lymph nodes of the testis.*

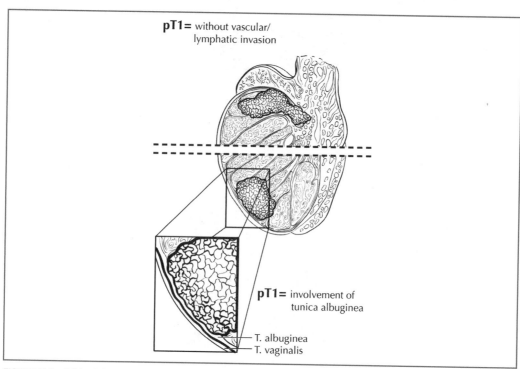

FIGURE 42.3. *pT1 is defined as tumor that is limited to the testis and epididymis without vascular/lymphatic invasion (top illustration). Tumor may invade into the tunica albuginea but not the tunica vaginalis (bottom illustration).*

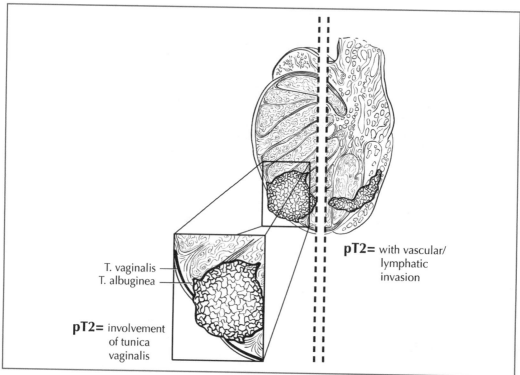

FIGURE 42.4. *pT2 is defined as tumor that extends through the tunica albuginea with involvement of the tunica vaginalis (illustration on left). pT2 is defined as tumor that is limited to the testis and epididymis with vascular/lymphatic invasion (illustration on right).*

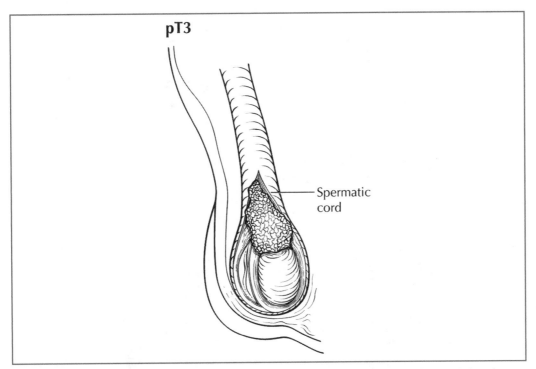

FIGURE 42.5. *pT3 is defined as tumor invades the spermatic cord with or without vascular/lymphatic invasion.*

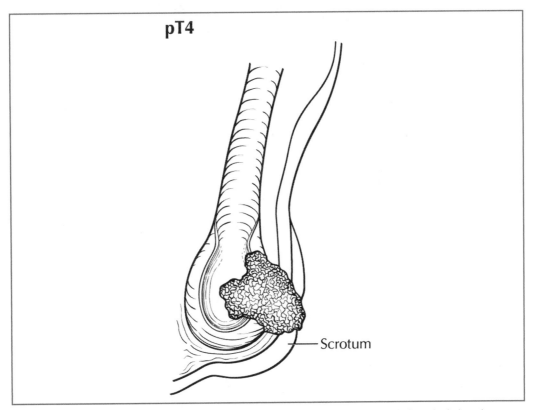

FIGURE 42.6. *pT4 is defined as tumor that invades the scrotum with or without vascular/lymphatic invasion.*

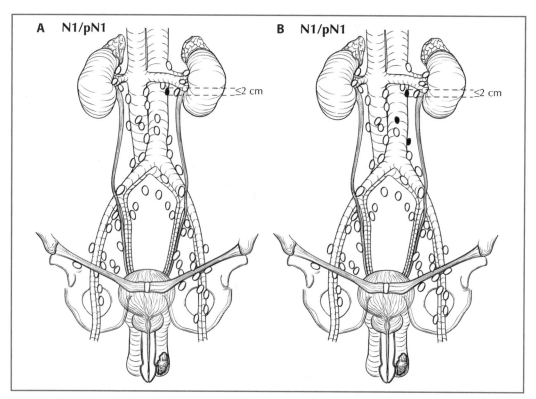

FIGURES 42.7. *(A) N1/pN1 is defined as metastasis with a lymph node mass 2 cm or less in greatest dimension. (B) N1 is defined as metastasis in multiple lymph nodes, none more than 2 cm in greatest dimension, and pN1 is less than or equal to five nodes positive, none more than 2 cm in greatest dimension.*

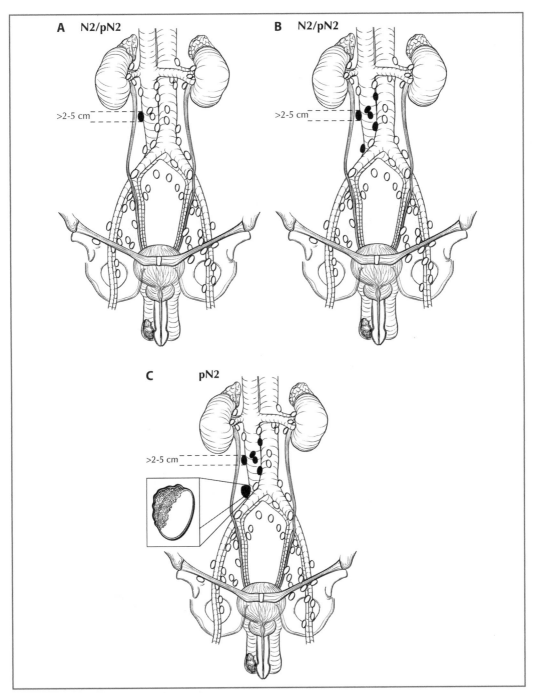

FIGURE 42.8. *(A) N2/pN2 is defined as metastasis with a lymph node mass more than 2 cm but not more than 5 cm in greatest dimension. (B) N2 is defined as metastasis in multiple lymph nodes, any one mass greater than 2 cm but not more than 5 cm in greatest dimension. pN2 is defined as more than five nodes positive, none more than 5 cm. (C) pN2 is defined as evidence of extranodal extension of tumor.*

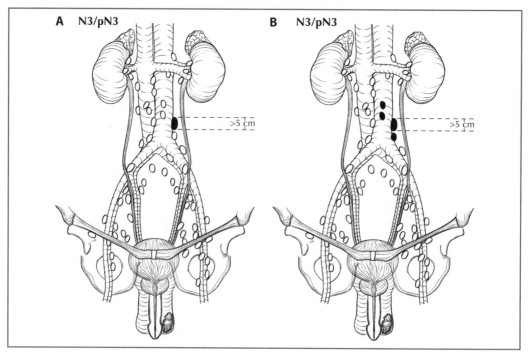

FIGURE 42.9. *N3/pN3 is defined as metastasis with a lymph node mass more than 5 cm in greatest dimension (A), or multiple nodes are involved with one nodal mass exceeding 5 cm (B).*

PROGNOSTIC FACTORS (SITE-SPECIFIC FACTORS)
(Recommended for Collection)

Required for staging	Serum tumor markers (S)

SX   Marker studies not available or not performed
S0   Marker study levels within normal limits
S1 $LDH < 1.5 \times N^*$ *and* hCG (mIu/ml) <5,000 *and* AFP (ng/ml) <1,000
S2 $LDH\ 1.5–10 \times N$ *or* hCG (mIu/ml) 5,000–50,000 *or* AFP (ng/ml) 1,000–10,000
S3 $LDH > 10 \times N$ *or* hCG (mIu/ml) >50,000 *or* AFP (ng/ml) >10,000
* indicates the upper limit of normal for the LDH assay.

Serum tumor marker levels should be measured prior to orchiectomy, but levels after orchiectomy are used for assignment of S category, taking into account the half life of AFP and hCG. Stage grouping classification of Stage IS requires persistent elevation of serum tumor markers following orchiectomy.

The Serum Tumor Markers (S) category comprises the following:

- Alpha fetoprotein (AFP) – half life 5–7 days
- Human chorionic gonadotropin (hCG) – half life 1–3 days
- Lactate dehydrogenase (LDH)

Clinically significant	Size of largest metastases in lymph nodes
	Radical orchiectomy performed

Kidney

43

ICD-O-3 TOPOGRAPHY CODE

C64.9   Kidney, NOS

ICD-O-3 HISTOLOGY CODE RANGES

8000–8576, 8940–8950, 8980–8981

ANATOMY

Primary Site. Encased by a fibrous capsule and surrounded by perirenal fat, the kidney consists of the cortex (glomeruli, convoluted tubules) and the medulla (Henle's loops, collecting ducts, and pyramids of converging tubules). Each papilla opens in the minor calices; these in turn unite in the major calices and drain into the renal pelvis. At the hilus are the pelvis, ureter, and renal artery and vein. Gerota's fascia overlies the psoas and quadratus lumborum muscles. The anatomic sites and subsites of the kidney are illustrated in Figure 43.1.

Regional Lymph Nodes. The regional lymph nodes, illustrated in Figures 43.2A and B, are as follows:

Renal hilar
Caval (paracaval, precaval, and retrocaval)
Interaortocaval
Aortic (paraaortic, preaortic, and retroaortic)

The primary landing zone for right sided tumors is the interaortocaval zone and for left sided tumors the aortic region. The more extended landing zones for RCC are analogous to those for right and left testicular tumors, respectively, although patterns of spread are somewhat more unpredictable. Lymph nodes outside of these templates should be considered distant (metastatic) rather than regional.

Metastatic Sites. Common metastatic sites include the bone, liver, lung, brain, and distant lymph nodes.

C.C. Compton et al. (eds.), *AJCC Cancer Staging Atlas: A Companion to the Seventh Editions of the AJCC Cancer Staging Manual and Handbook*, DOI 10.1007/978-1-4614-2080-4_43, © 2012 American Joint Committee on Cancer

PROGNOSTIC FEATURES AND INTEGRATED ALGORITHMS

Established prognostic factors for various subgroups of patients with RCC include tumor-related factors, patient-related factors, and laboratory biochemical tests. *Integrated algorithms* that incorporate these factors have been validated and have been shown to improve prognostication over anatomic tumor stage alone. The use of these instruments for estimating prognosis and patient counseling can aid in decision-making.

Prognostic Features for RCC

- Tumor related: Stage, tumor size, tumor grade, histologic type, histologic tumor necrosis, sarcomatoid transformation
- Patient related: Asymptomatic vs. local symptoms vs. systemic symptoms, performance status, substantial weight loss, presence of well-defined paraneoplastic syndrome, metastasis free interval, history of prior nephrectomy
- Laboratory biochemical tests: Elevated LDH levels, hypercalcemia, anemia, thrombocytosis, elevated ESR or CRP
- These prognostic and predictive algorithms may be useful in guiding patient counseling and therapy. However, caution should be exercised if used for this purpose as the extent to which the utility of each algorithm has been validated varies. Each used different data sets for development, and the specifics of the data elements used in their application must be precise. In addition, new factors and predictors continue to be discovered and studied. To promote broader use, transparency, and applicability, we hope that future algorithms will utilize the core anatomic elements as specified in the AJCC Staging System.

DEFINITIONS OF TNM

Primary Tumor (T)

TX	Primary tumor cannot be assessed
T0	No evidence of primary tumor
T1	Tumor 7 cm or less in greatest dimension, limited to the kidney
T1a	Tumor 4 cm or less in greatest dimension, limited to the kidney (Figure 43.3)
T1b	Tumor more than 4 cm but not more than 7 cm in greatest dimension limited to the kidney (Figure 43.4)
T2	Tumor more than 7 cm in greatest dimension, limited to the kidney
T2a	Tumor more than 7 cm but less than or equal to 10 cm in greatest dimension, limited to the kidney (Figure 43.5A)
T2b	Tumor more than 10 cm, limited to the kidney (Figure 43.5B)
T3	Tumor extends into major veins or perinephric tissues but not into the ipsilateral adrenal gland and not beyond Gerota's fascia
T3a	Tumor grossly extends into the renal vein or its segmental (muscle containing) branches, or tumor invades perirenal and/or renal sinus fat but not beyond Gerota's fascia (Figure 43.6)
T3b	Tumor grossly extends into the vena cava below the diaphragm (Figure 43.7)
T3c	Tumor grossly extends into the vena cava above the diaphragm or invades the wall of the vena cava (Figure 43.8)
T4	Tumor invades beyond Gerota's fascia (Figure 43.9A) (including contiguous extension into the ipsilateral adrenal gland) (Figure 43.9B)

NX   Regional lymph nodes cannot be assessed

N0   No regional lymph node metastasis

N1   Metastasis in regional lymph node(s) (Figure 43.10)

Distant Metastasis (M)

M0   No distant metastasis

M1   Distant metastasis

ANATOMIC STAGE/PROGNOSTIC GROUPS

Stage I	T1	N0	M0
Stage II	T2	N0	M0
Stage III	T1 or T2	N1	M0
	T3	N0 or N1	M0
StageIV	T4	any N	M0
	Any T	Any N	M1

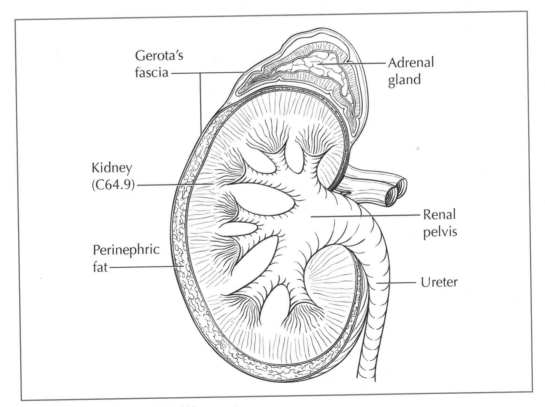

FIGURE 43.1. *Anatomical site of the kidney.*

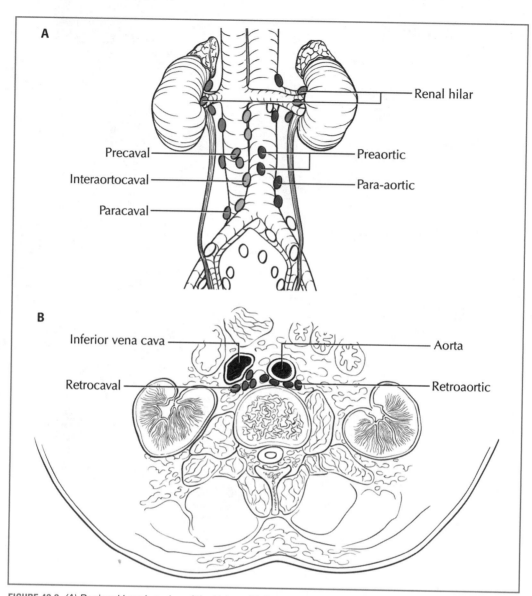

FIGURE 43.2. *(A) Regional lymph nodes of the kidney. (B) Regional lymph nodes of the kidney.*

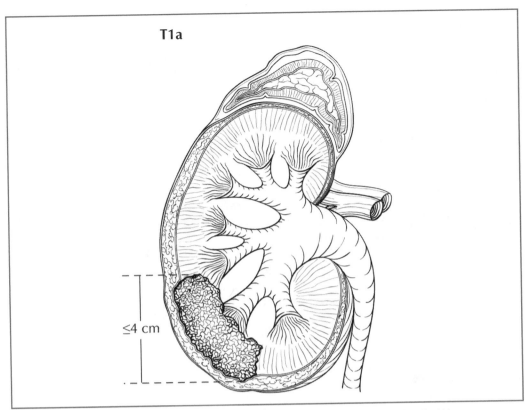

FIGURE 43.3. *T1a is defined as tumor that is 4 cm or less in greatest dimension, limited to the kidney.*

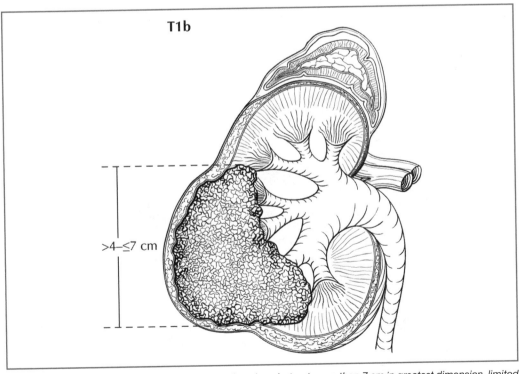

FIGURE 43.4. *T1b is defined as tumor that is more than 4 cm but not more than 7 cm in greatest dimension, limited to the kidney.*

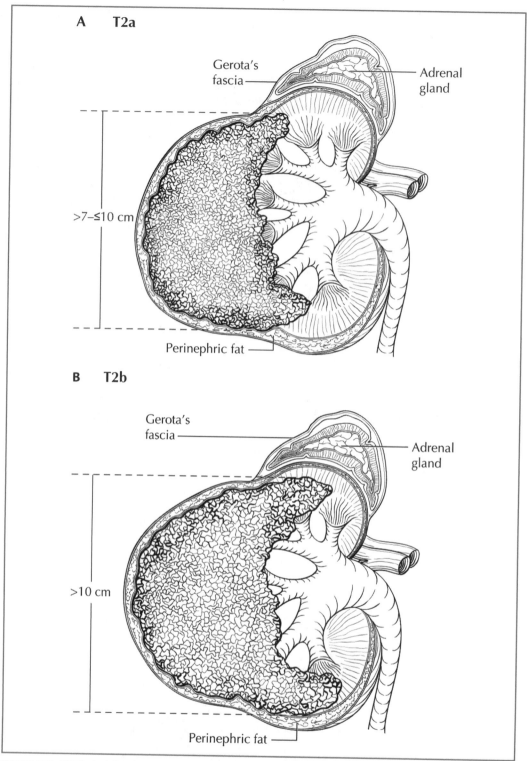

FIGURE 43.5. (A) T2a is defined as tumor that is more than 7 cm but less than or equal to 10 cm in greatest dimension, limited to the kidney. (B) T2b is defined as tumor that is more than 10 cm in greatest dimension, limited to the kidney.

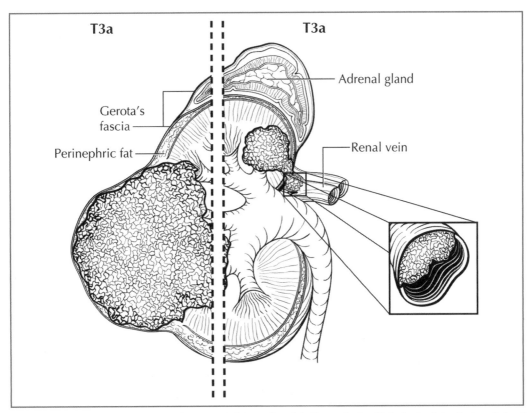

FIGURE 43.6. *T3a is defined as tumor that extends into perinephric tissues but not into the ipsilateral adrenal gland or beyond Gerota's fascia (illustrated on the left) or T3a is tumor that grossly extends into the renal vein (illustrated on the right).*

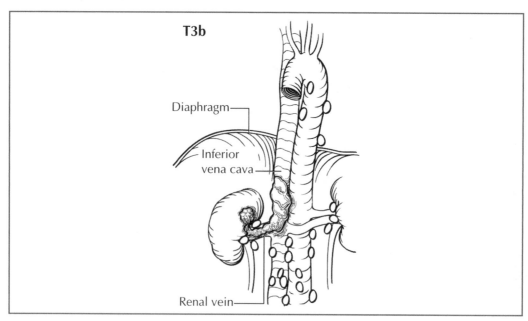

FIGURE 43.7. *T3b is defined as tumor that grossly extends into the vena cava below the diaphragm.*

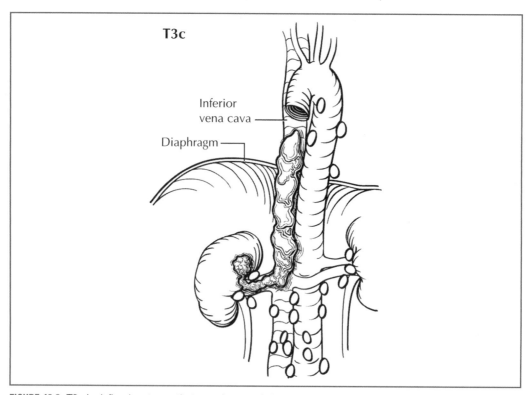

FIGURE 43.8. *T3c is defined as tumor that grossly extends into vena cava above diaphragm or invades the wall of the vena cava.*

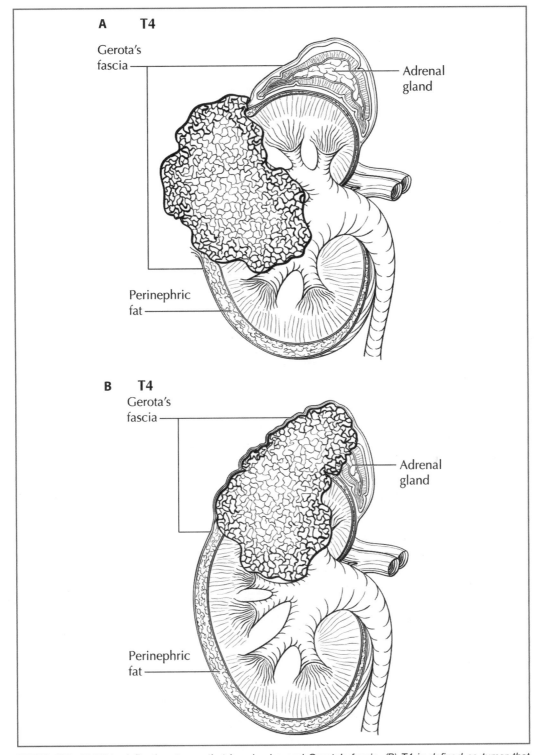

A T4

Gerota's fascia

Adrenal gland

Perinephric fat

B T4

Gerota's fascia

Adrenal gland

Perinephric fat

FIGURE 43.9. *(A) T4 is defined as tumor that invades beyond Gerota's fascia. (B) T4 is defined as tumor that extends contiguously into the ipsilateral adrenal gland.*

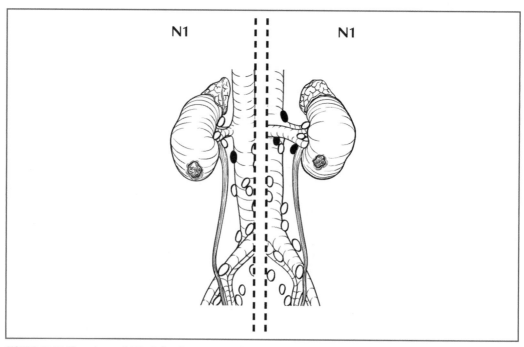

FIGURE 43.10. *Two views of N1, defined as metastasis in regional lymph node(s): N1, on the left, is metastasis in a single regional lymph node. N1, on the right, is metastasis in more than one regional lymph node (here showing three involved regional lymph nodes).*

PROGNOSTIC FACTORS (SITE-SPECIFIC FACTORS) *(Recommended for Collection)*	
Required for staging	None
Clinically significant	Invasion beyond capsule into fat or peri-sinus tissues Venous involvement Adrenal extension Fuhrman grade Sarcomatoid features Histologic tumor necrosis Extranodal extension Size of metastasis in lymph nodes

Renal Pelvis and Ureter

44

SUMMARY OF CHANGES

- The definition of TNM and the Stage Grouping for this chapter have not changed from the Sixth Edition
- Grading: a low- and high-grade designation will replace previous four-grade system to match current World Health Organization/International Society of Urologic Pathology (WHO/ISUP) recommended grading system

---

ICD-O-3 TOPOGRAPHY CODES

C65.9   Renal pelvis
C66.9   Ureter

ICD-O-3 HISTOLOGY CODE RANGES

8000–8576, 8940–8950, 8980–8981

ANATOMY

Primary Site. The renal pelvis and ureter form a single unit that is continuous with the collecting ducts of the renal pyramids and comprises the minor and major calyces, which are continuous with the renal pelvis (Figure 44.1). The ureteropelvic junction is variable in position and location but serves as a "landmark" that separates the renal pelvis and the ureter, which continues caudad and traverses the wall of the urinary bladder as the intramural ureter opening in the trigone of the bladder at the ureteral orifice. The renal pelvis and ureter are composed of the following layers: epithelium, subepithelial connective tissue, and muscularis, which is continuous with a connective tissue adventitial layer. It is in this outer layer that the major blood supply and lymphatics are found.

The intrarenal portion of the renal pelvis is surrounded by renal parenchyma; the extrarenal pelvis, by perihilar fat. The ureter courses through the retroperitoneum adjacent to the parietal peritoneum and rests on the retroperitoneal musculature above the pelvic vessels. As it crosses the vessels and enters the deep pelvis, the ureter is surrounded by pelvic fat until it traverses the bladder wall.

Regional Lymph Nodes. The regional lymph nodes for the renal pelvis are as follows (Figure 44.2):

Renal hilar
Paracaval
Aortic
Retroperitoneal, NOS

The regional lymph nodes for the ureter are as follows (Figure 44.3):

Renal hilar
Iliac (common, internal [hypogastric], external)
Paracaval
Periureteral
Pelvic, NOS

Any amount of regional lymph node metastasis is a poor prognostic finding, and outcome is minimally influenced by the number, size, or location of the regional nodes that are involved.

Metastatic Sites. Distant spread is most commonly to lung, lymph nodes, bone, or liver.

DEFINITIONS OF TNM

Primary Tumor (T)

TX	Primary tumor cannot be assessed
T0	No evidence of primary tumor
Ta	Papillary noninvasive carcinoma (Figure 44.4)
Tis	Carcinoma in situ
T1	Tumor invades subepithelial connective tissue (Figure 44.4)
T2	Tumor invades the muscularis (Figure 44.4)
T3	(For renal pelvis only) Tumor invades beyond muscularis into peripelvic fat or the renal parenchyma T3. (For ureter only) Tumor invades beyond muscularis into periureteric fat (Figure 44.5)
T4	Tumor invades adjacent organs, or through the kidney into the perinephric fat. (Figure 44.6A, B, C)

Regional Lymph Nodes (N)*

NX	Regional lymph nodes cannot be assessed
N0	No regional lymph node metastasis
N1	Metastasis in a single lymph node, 2 cm or less in greatest dimension (Figure 44.7)
N2	Metastasis in a single lymph node, more than 2 cm but not more than 5 cm in greatest dimension; or multiple lymph nodes, none more than 5 cm in greatest dimension (Figure 44.8A, B)
N3	Metastasis in a lymph node, more than 5 cm in greatest dimension (Figure 44.9A, B)

*Note: Laterality does not affect the N classification.

Distant Metastasis (M)

M0	No distant metastasis
M1	Distant metastasis

ANATOMIC STAGE/PROGNOSTIC GROUPS

Stage 0a	Ta	N0	M0
Stage 0is	Tis	N0	M0
Stage I	T1	N0	M0
Stage II	T2	N0	M0
Stage III	T3	N0	M0
Stage IV	T4	N0	M0
	Any T	N1	M0
	Any T	N2	M0
	Any T	N3	M0
	Any T	Any N	M1

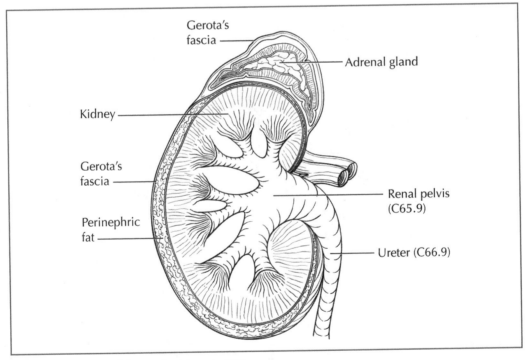

FIGURE 44.1. Anatomy of the renal pelvis and ureter.

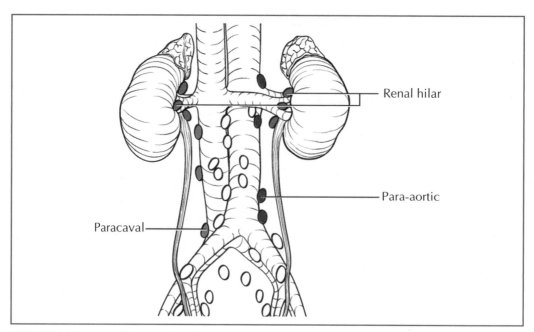

FIGURE 44.2. *The regional lymph nodes of the renal pelvis.*

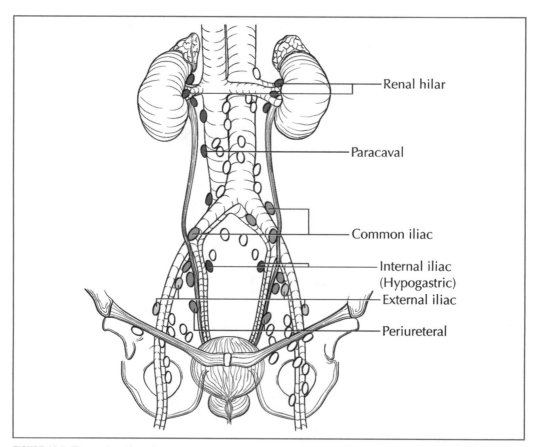

FIGURE 44.3. *The regional lymph nodes of the ureter.*

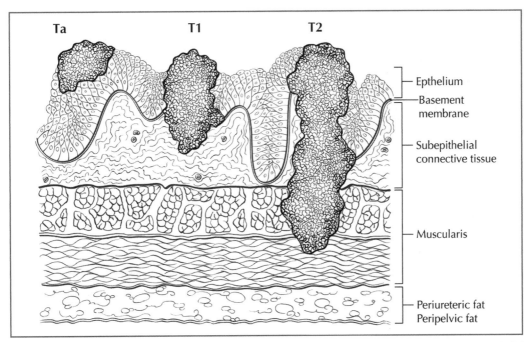

FIGURE 44.4. *Ta is defined as papillary non-invasive carcinoma; T1 is defined as tumor that invades subepithelial connective tissue; T2 is defined as tumor that invades the muscularis.*

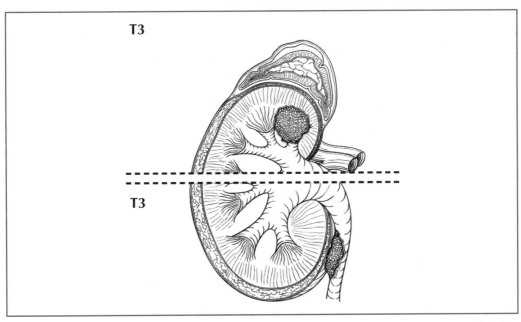

FIGURE 44.5. *T3 for renal pelvis only (top of diagram) is defined as tumor that invades beyond muscularis into peripelvic fat or the renal parenchyma. T3 for ureter only (bottom of diagram) is defined as tumor that invades beyond muscularis into periureteric fat.*

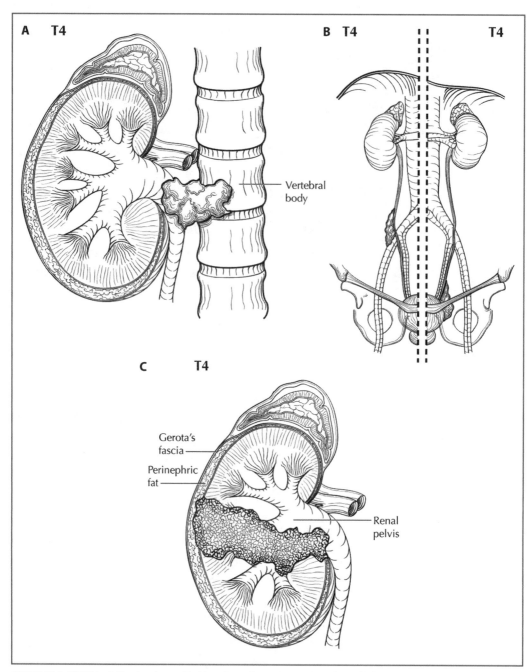

FIGURE 44.6. *(A) T4 is defined as tumor that invades adjacent organs, or through the kidney into the perinephric fat. Here, the tumor invades the vertebral body, (B)T4 for the ureter is defined as tumor that invades adjacent organs. On the left, the tumor invades the iliac vessels. On the right, the tumor invades the bladder. (C) T4 is defined as tumor that invades through the renal parenchyma into the perirenal fat.*

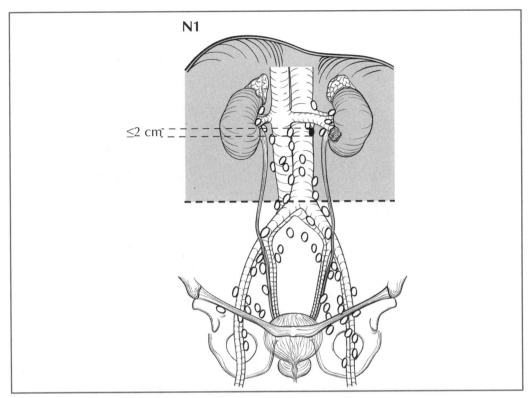

FIGURE 44.7. *N1 is defined as metastasis in a single lymph node, 2 cm or less in greatest dimension.*

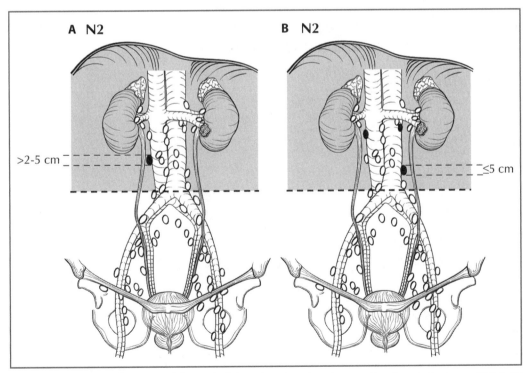

FIGURE 44.8. *(A) N2 is defined as nodal metastasis in a single lymph node, more than 2 cm but not more than 5 cm in greatest dimension, as illustrated. (B) N2 is also defined as multiple lymph nodes involved none more than 5 cm in greatest dimension.*

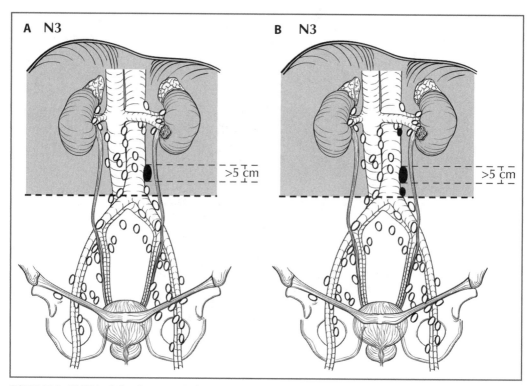

FIGURE 44.9. *(A) N3 is defined as metastasis in a lymph node, more than 5 cm in greatest dimension. As illustrated here, a single nodal mass exceeding 5 cm. (B) N3 is also defined as multiple lymph nodes involved with at least one nodal mass exceeding 5 cm in greatest dimension.*

PROGNOSTIC FACTORS (SITE-SPECIFIC FACTORS)	
(Recommended for Collection)	
Required for staging	None
Clinically significant	Renal parenchymal invasion
	World Health Organization/International Society of Urologic Pathology (WHO/ISUP) grade

Urinary Bladder

45

SUMMARY OF CHANGES

- Primary staging: T4 disease defined as including prostatic stromal invasion directly from bladder cancer. Subepithelial invasion of prostatic urethra will not constitute T4 staging status
- Grading: a low and high grade designation will replace previous 4 grade system to match current World Health Organization/International Society of Urologic Pathology (WHO/ISUP) recom mended grading system
- Nodal classification

  - Common iliac nodes defined as secondary drainage region as regional nodes and not as metastatic disease
  - N staging system change

    - N1: single positive node in primary drainage regions
    - N2: multiple positive nodes in primary drainage regions
    - N3: common iliac node involvement

ICD-O-3 TOPOGRAPHY CODES

C67.0 Trigone of bladder
C67.1 Dome of bladder
C67.2 Lateral wall of bladder
C67.3 Anterior wall of bladder
C67.4 Posterior wall of bladder
C67.5 Bladder neck
C67.6 Ureteric orifice
C67.7 Urachus
C67.8 Overlapping lesion of bladder
C67.9 Bladder, NOS

ICD-O-3 HISTOLOGY CODE RANGES

8000–8576, 8940–8950, 8980–8981

ANATOMY

Primary Site. The urinary bladder consists of three layers: the epithelium and the subepithelial connective tissue (also referred to as lamina propria), the muscularis propria, and the perivesical fat (peritoneum covering the superior surface and upper part). In the male, the bladder adjoins the rectum and seminal vesicle posteriorly, the prostate inferiorly, and the pubis and peritoneum anteriorly. In the female, the vagina is located posteriorly and the uterus superiorly. The bladder is located extraperitoneally (Figure 45.1).

Regional Lymph Nodes. The regional lymph nodes draining the bladder include primary and secondary nodal drainage regions (Figure 45.2). Primary lymph nodes include the external iliac, hypogastric and obturator basins. The presacral lymph nodes are classified as a primary drainage region; however, mapping studies have found this area to be a less frequent site of primary regional metastases. Primary nodal regions drain into the common iliac nodes, which constitute a secondary drainage region. Regional lymph node staging is of significant prognostic importance given the negative impact on recurrence after treatment and long-term survival. The relevant information from regional lymph node staging is obtained from the extent of disease within the nodes (number of positive nodes, extranodal extension) not in whether metastases are unilateral or contralateral. Overall 5-year survival in node positive bladder cancer following definitive local therapy is approximately 33%; however, patients with a greater node burden may be expected to do significantly worse.

Regional nodes include the following:

Primary Drainage
  Hypogastric
  Obturator
  Iliac (internal, external, NOS)
  Perivesical Pelvic, NOS
  Sacral (lateral, sacral promontory [Gerota's])
  Presacral
Secondary Drainage
  Common iliac

The common iliac nodes are considered sites of secondary regionally lymphatic involvement.

Metastatic Sites. Distant spread is most commonly to retroperitoneal lymph nodes, lung, bone, and liver.

PROGNOSTIC FEATURES

Prognostic features for bladder cancer include a variety of pathologic, clinical, and molecular characteristics. Primary tumor stage and grade are important independent predictors of tumor progression and outcome. More recently morphologic prognostic features including lymphovascular invasion and variants of the pattern of tumor growth, such as micropapillary and nested variants, have been found to portend an adverse outcome. Lymph node status has a profound effect on the risk of tumor recurrence and patient survival. Various lymph node parameters demonstrating prognostic significance include the total number of excised lymph nodes, the number of positive lymph nodes, extranodal tumor extension, and the ratio of number of positive lymph nodes to total number of lymph nodes evaluated.

Several molecular factors with prognostic importance have been identified for bladder cancer. These markers are involved in the regulation of the cell cycle, programmed cell death, growth factor signaling, and angiogenesis. Two distinct molecular pathways for bladder tumor progression have been established. Noninvasive tumors appear to progress through a pathway that involves the frequent alteration to chromosome 9, specifically 9q deletions. In contrast high-grade tumors are associated with a loss of heterozygosity of chromosome 17p, 14q, 5q, 3p. Alterations to the TP53 and RB pathways play a central role in the progression of high-grade bladder cancer. Additional regulatory proteins including p21/WAF1, p16, p14ARF, and MDM2 have also been implicated in the dysregulation of cell growth via both TP53/RB-dependent and - independent pathways. Overexpression of tyrosine-kinase receptors that effect signaling of many growth factors including epidermal growth factor (EGF), vascular endothelial growth factor (VEGF), and HER2/neu have been identified as prognostically relevant alterations in bladder cancer.

Ploidy has been investigated as a prognostic factor. In superficial disease, an aneuploid DNA content is associated with shorter disease-free survival and with an increased chance of progression to a higher stage; however, in invasive and metastatic disease, the majority of cases are aneuploid, thus reducing the role of aneuploid DNA content as a discriminant of outcome. In the setting of advanced disease, patient performance status, the presence of visceral metastases, and elevated levels of alkaline phosphatase are important predictors of response to systemic therapy and patient survival.

DEFINITIONS OF TNM

Primary Tumor (T)

TX	Primary tumor cannot be assessed
T0	No evidence of primary tumor
Ta	Noninvasive papillary carcinoma (Figure 45.3)
Tis	Carcinoma in situ: "flat tumor" (Figure 45.3)
T1	Tumor invades subepithelial connective tissue (Figure 45.3)
T2	Tumor invades muscularis propria
pT2a	Tumor invades superficial muscularis propria (inner half) (Figure 45.3)
pT2b	Tumor invades deep muscularis propria (outer half) (Figure 45.3)
T3	Tumor invades perivesical tissue
pT3a	Microscopically (Figure 45.3)
pT3b	Macroscopically (extravesical mass) (Figure 45.3)
T4	Tumor invades any of the following: prostatic stroma, seminal vesicles, uterus, vagina, pelvic wall, abdominal wall
T4a	Tumor invades prostatic stroma, uterus, vagina (Figure 45.3)
T4b	Tumor invades pelvic wall, abdominal wall (Figure 45.3)

Regional Lymph Nodes (N)

Regional lymph nodes include both primary and secondary drainage regions. All other nodes above the aortic bifurcation are considered distant lymph nodes.

NX	Lymph nodes cannot be assessed
N0	No lymph node metastasis
N1	Single regional lymph node metastasis in the true pelvis (hypogastric, obturator, external iliac, or presacral lymph node) (Figure 45.4)
N2	Multiple regional lymph node metastasis in the true pelvis (hypogastric, obturator, external iliac, or presacral lymph node metastasis) (Figure 45.5)
N3	Lymph node metastasis to the common iliac lymph nodes (Figure 45.6)

Distant Metastasis (M)

M0	No distant metastasis
M1	Distant metastasis

Stage 0a	Ta	N0	M0
Stage 0is	Tis	N0	M0
Stage I	T1	N0	M0
Stage II	T2a	N0	M0
	T2b	N0	M0
Stage III	T3a	N0	M0
	T3b	N0	M0
	T4a	N0	M0
Stage IV	T4b	N0	M0
	Any T	N1-3	M0
	Any T	Any N	M1

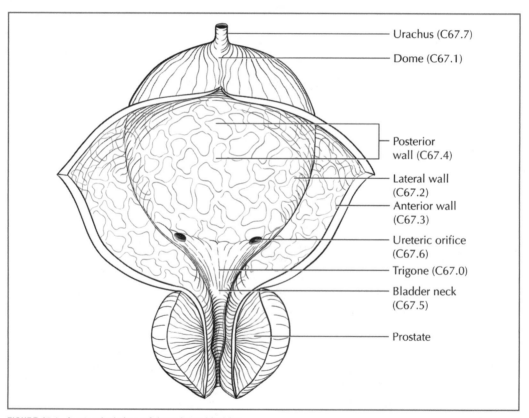

FIGURE 45.1. *Anatomical sites of the urinary bladder.*

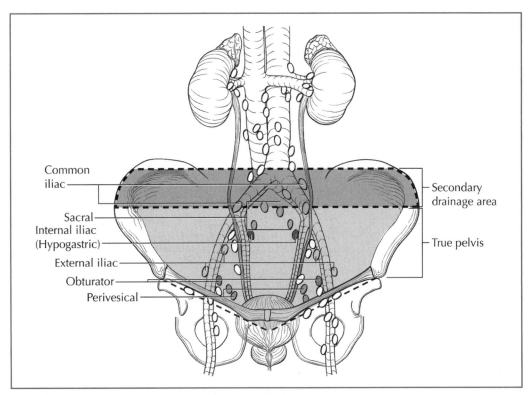

FIGURE 45.2. *Regional lymph nodes of the urinary bladder. The true pelvis is the primary lymphatic drainage area for the urinary bladder. The secondary drainage area superior to the true pelvis includes the common iliac nodes and all nodes up to the level of the aortic bifurcation.*

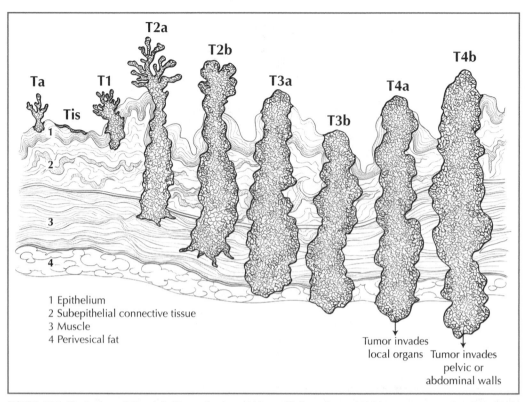

FIGURE 45.3. *Illustration of the definitions of primary tumor (T) for primary bladder cancer, ranging from Ta to T4. Ta is defined as noninvasive papillary carcinoma. Tis is defined as carcinoma in situ. T1 is defined as tumor that invades subepithelial connective tissue. T2a is defined as tumor that invades superficial muscularis propria (inner half). T2b is defined as tumor that invades deep muscularis propria (outer half). T3a is defined as tumor that microscopically invades perivesical fat. T3b is defined as tumor that macroscopically invades perivesical fat. T4a is defined as tumor that invades the prostatic stroma, the uterus, or the vagina. T4b is defined as tumor that invades the pelvic wall or abdominal wall.*

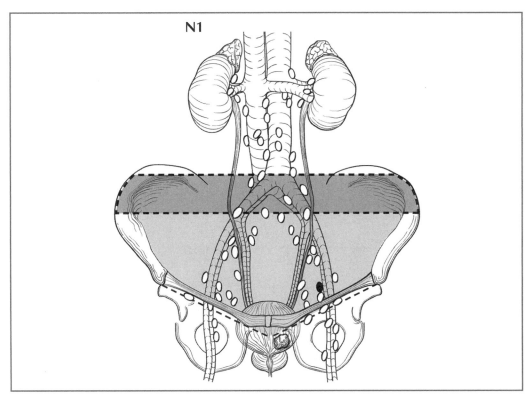

FIGURE 45.4. *N1 is defined as metastasis in a single lymph node in the true pelvis (hypogastric, obturator, external iliac, or presacral lymph node).*

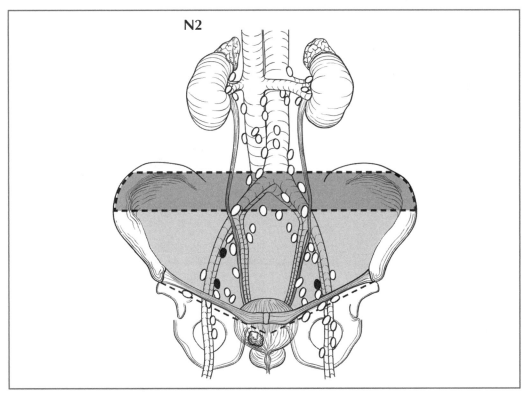

FIGURE 45.5. *N2 is defined as metastasis in multiple regional lymph nodes in the true pelvis (hypogastric, obturator, external iliac, or presacral lymph node metastases).*

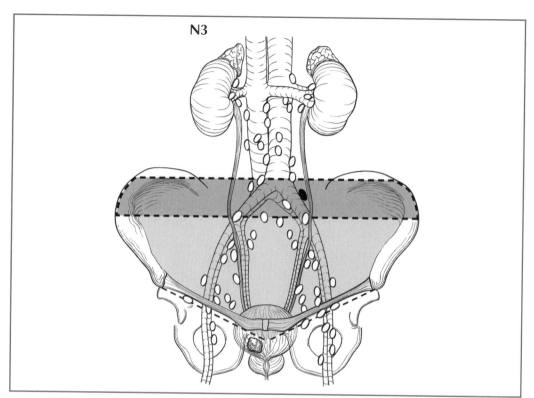

FIGURE 45.6. *N3 is defined as lymph node metastasis to the common iliac lymph node(s) in the secondary drainage area.*

PROGNOSTIC FACTORS (SITE-SPECIFIC FACTORS)
(Recommended for Collection)

Required for staging	None
Clinically significant	Presence or absence of extranodal extension
	Size of the largest tumor deposit in the lymph nodes
	World Health Organization/International Society of Urologic Pathology (WHO/ISUP) grade

Urethra

46

ICD-O-3 TOPOGRAPHY CODE
C68.0   Urethra

ICD-O-3 HISTOLOGY CODE RANGES
8000–8576, 8940–8950, 8980–8981

ANATOMY

Primary Site. The male penile urethra consists of mucosa, submucosal stroma, and the surrounding corpus spongiosum (Figure 46.1 and 46.2). Histologically, the meatal and parameatal urethra are lined with squamous epithelium; the penile and bulbomembranous urethra with pseudostratified or stratified columnar epithelium, and the prostatic urethra with urothelium (transitional epithelium). There are scattered islands of stratified squamous epithelium and glands of Littré liberally situated throughout the entire urethra distal to the prostate portion.

The epithelium of the female urethra is supported on subepithelial connective tissue. The periurethral glands of Skene are concentrated near the meatus but extend along the entire urethra. The urethra is surrounded by a longitudinal layer of smooth muscle continuous with the bladder. The urethra is contiguous to the vaginal wall. The distal two-thirds of the urethra is lined with squamous epithelium, the proximal one-third with urothelium (transitional epithelium). The periurethral glands are lined with pseudostratified and stratified columnar epithelium.

Regional Lymph Nodes. The regional lymph nodes are as follows (Figure 46.3):

Inguinal (superficial or deep)
Iliac (common, internal [hypogastric], obturator, external)
Presacral
Sacral, NOS
Pelvic, NOS

The significance of regional lymph node metastasis in staging urethral cancer lies in the number and size, not in whether unilateral or bilateral.

Metastatic Sites. Distant spread is most commonly to lung, liver, or bone.

C.C. Compton et al. (eds.), *AJCC Cancer Staging Atlas: A Companion to the Seventh Editions of the AJCC Cancer Staging Manual and Handbook*, DOI 10.1007/978-1-4614-2080-4_46,
© 2012 American Joint Committee on Cancer

DEFINITIONS OF TNM

Primary Tumor (T) (Male and Female)

TX	Primary tumor cannot be assessed
T0	No evidence of primary tumor
Ta	Noninvasive papillary, polypoid, or verrucous carcinoma (Figures 46.4, 46.5)
Tis	Carcinoma in situ
T1	Tumor invades subepithelial connective tissue (Figures 46.5, 46.6)
T2	Tumor invades any of the following: corpus spongiosum, prostate, periurethral muscle (Figures 46.5, 46.7A, B)
T3	Tumor invades any of the following: corpus cavernosum, beyond prostatic capsule, anterior vagina, bladder neck (Figure 46.8A, B, C)
T4	Tumor invades other adjacent organs (Figure 46.9)

Urothelial (Transitional Cell) Carcinoma of the Prostate

Tis pu	Carcinoma in situ, involvement of the prostatic urethra (Figure 46.10)
Tis pd	Carcinoma in situ, involvement of the prostatic ducts (Figure 46.11)
T1	Tumor invades urethral subepithelial connective tissue (Figures 46.5, 46.10, 46.11)
T2	Tumor invades any of the following: prostatic stroma, corpus spongiosum, periurethral muscle (Figures 46.11, 46.12)
T3	Tumor invades any of the following: corpus cavernosum, beyond prostatic capsule, bladder neck (extraprostatic extension) (Figure 46.13)
T4	Tumor invades other adjacent organs (invasion of the bladder) (Figure 46.14)

Regional Lymph Nodes (N)

NX	Regional lymph nodes cannot be assessed
N0	No regional lymph node metastasis
N1	Metastasis in a single lymph node 2 cm or less in greatest dimension (Figure 46.15)
N2	Metastasis in a single node more than 2 cm in greatest dimension, or in multiple nodes (Figure 46.16A, B)

Distant Metastasis (M)

M0	No distant metastasis
M1	Distant metastasis

ANATOMIC STAGE/PROGNOSTIC GROUPS

Stage 0a	Ta	N0	M0
Stage 0is	Tis	N0	M0
	Tis pu	N0	M0
	Tis pd	N0	M0
Stage I	T1	N0	M0
Stage II	T2	N0	M0
Stage III	T1	N1	M0
	T2	N1	M0
	T3	N0	M0
	T3	N1	M0
Stage IV	T4	N0	M0
	T4	N1	M0
	Any T	N2	M0
	Any T	Any N	M1

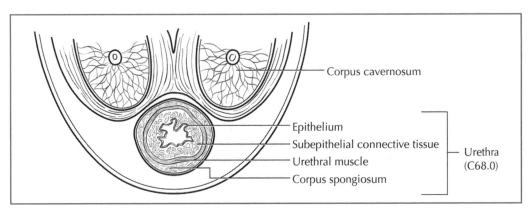

FIGURE 46.1. *Anatomy of the urethra.*

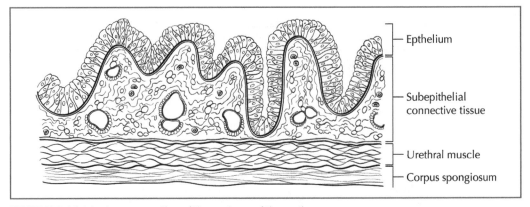

FIGURE 46.2. *Histologic cross-section of the anatomy of the urethra.*

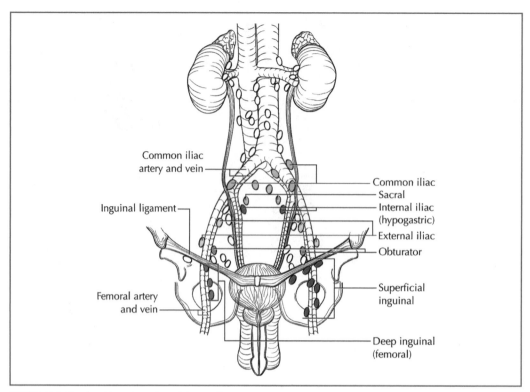

FIGURE 46.3. *Regional lymph nodes of the urethra.*

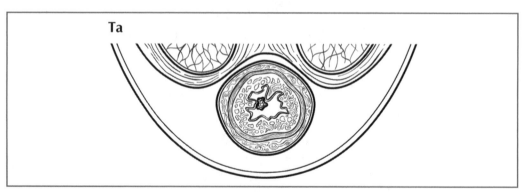

FIGURE 46.4. *Ta is defined as non-invasive papillary, polypoid, or verrucous carcinoma.*

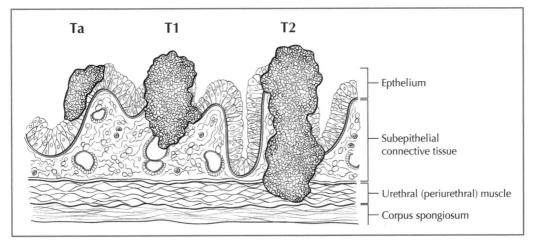

FIGURE 46.5. *Illustrated definitions of primary tumor (T) for Ta, T1, and T2. Ta is defined as noninvasive papillary, polypoid, or verrucous carcinoma. T1 is defined as tumor that invades the subepithelial connective tissue. T2 is defined as tumor that invades the corpus spongiosum, the prostate, or the periurethral muscle (as illustrated).*

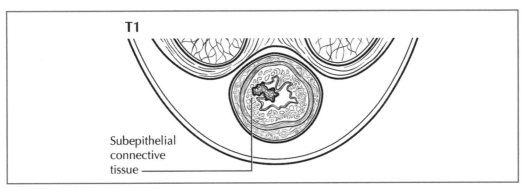

FIGURE 46.6. *T1 is defined as tumor that invades subepithelial connective tissue (includes urothelial carcinoma of the prostate).*

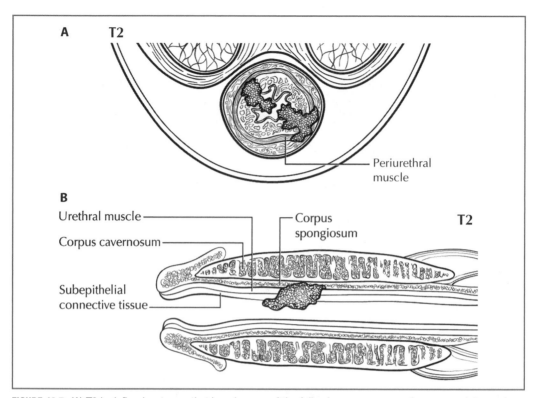

FIGURE 46.7. *(A) T2 is defined as tumor that invades any of the following: corpus spongiosum, prostate, periurethral muscle (as illustrated). (B) T2 is defined as tumor in the male with invasion of the corpus spongiosum.*

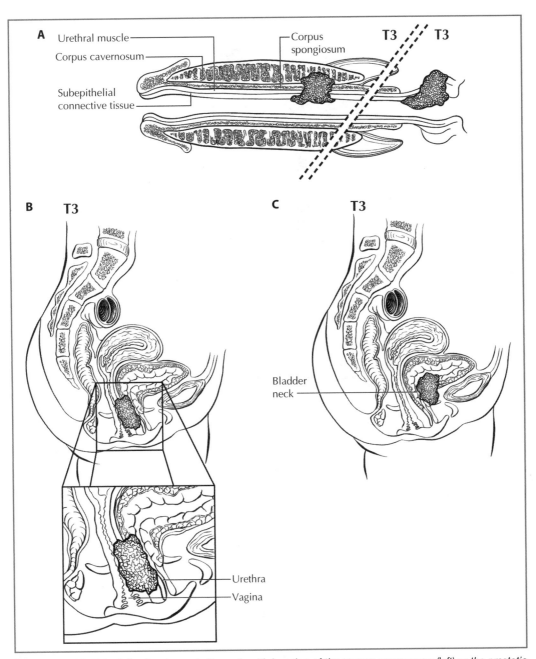

FIGURE 46.8. *(A) T3 is defined as tumor in the male with invasion of the corpus cavernosum (left) or the prostatic capsule (right). (B) T3 is defined as tumor in the female that invades the anterior vagina. (C) T3 is defined as tumor in the female that invades the bladder neck.*

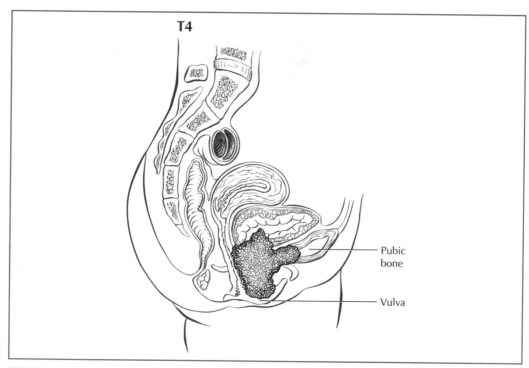

FIGURE 46.9. *T4 is defined as tumor in the female that invades other adjacent organs (illustrated is invasion of the pubic bone and vulva).*

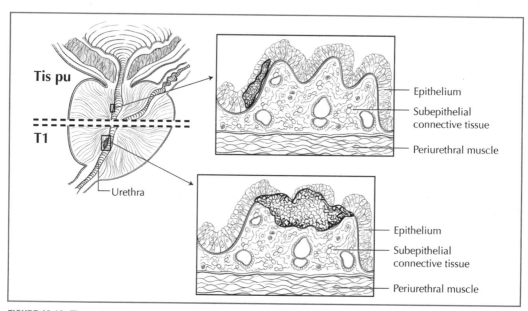

FIGURE 46.10. *The definition of Tis pu for urothelial (transitional cell) carcinoma of the prostate, (above dotted lines) is carcinoma in situ, involvement of the prostatic urethra. T1 (below dotted lines) is defined as tumor that invades subepithelial connective tissue.*

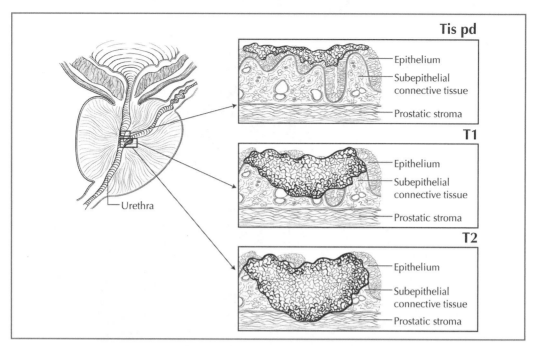

FIGURE 46.11. *Definitions of primary tumor (T) for urothelial (transitional cell) carcinoma of the prostate for Tis pd, T1, and T2 with depth of invasion ranging from the epithelium to the prostatic stroma. Tis pd is defined as carcinoma in situ, involvement of the prostatic ducts. T1 is defined as tumor that invades urethral subepithelial connective tissue. T2 is defined as tumor that invades the prostatic stroma, the corpus spongiosum, or the periurethral muscle.*

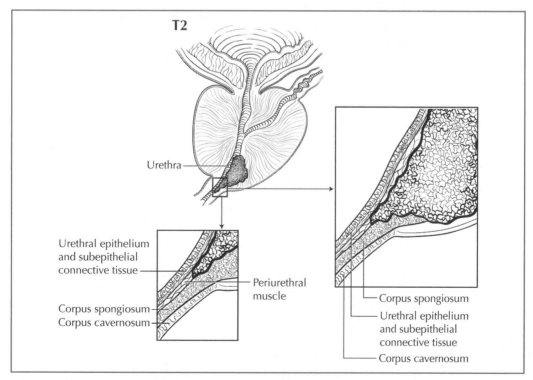

FIGURE 46.12. *T2 for urothelial (transitional cell) carcinoma is defined as tumor that invades any of the following: prostatic stroma, corpus spongiosum (illustrated on right), periurethral muscle (illustrated on left).*

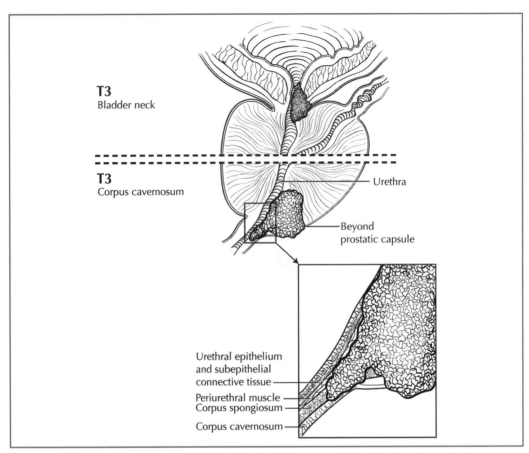

FIGURE 46.13. *Two views of T3 for urothelial (transitional cell) carcinoma. T3 is defined as tumor that invades any of the following: corpus cavernosum, as illustrated below dotted lines; beyond prostatic capsule; bladder neck (extraprostatic extension), as illustrated above dotted lines.*

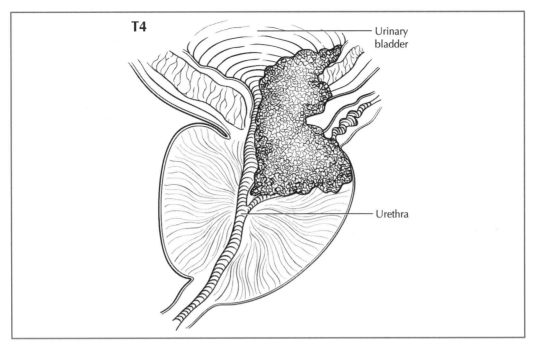

FIGURE 46.14. *T4 is defined as tumor that invades other adjacent organs (invasion of the bladder is illustrated).*

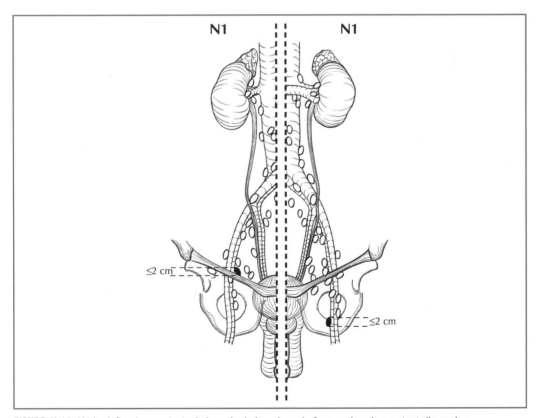

FIGURE 46.15. *N1 is defined as metastasis in a single lymph node 2 cm or less in greatest dimension.*

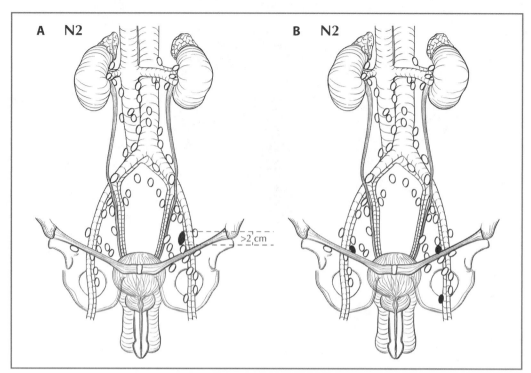

FIGURE 46.16. N2 is defined as metastasis in a single node more than 2 cm in greatest dimension (A), or in multiple nodes (B).

PROGNOSTIC FACTORS (SITE-SPECIFIC FACTORS)
(Recommended for Collection)

Required for staging	None
Clinically significant	World Health Organization/International Society of Urologic Pathology (WHO/ISUP) grade

Adrenal

47

SUMMARY OF CHANGES

- The definition of TNM and the Stage Grouping for this chapter has been created for the first time for the Seventh Edition

---

ICD-O-3 TOPOGRAPHY CODES

C74.0   Cortex of adrenal gland
C74.9   Adrenal gland, NOS

ICD-O-3 HISTOLOGY CODES

8010 (C74.0 only), 8140 (C74.0 only), 8370

ANATOMY

Primary Site. The adrenal glands sit in a supra renal location (retroperitoneal) surrounded by connective tissue and a layer of adipose tissue (Figure 47.1). They are intimately associated with the kidneys and are enclosed within the renal fascia (Gerota's). Each gland has an outer cortex, which is lipid rich and on gross examination appears bright yellow surrounding an inner "gray-white" medullary compartment composed of chromaffin cells. There is a rich vascular supply derived from the aorta, inferior phrenic arteries, and renal arteries. Veins emerge from the hilus of the glands. The shorter right central vein opens into the inferior vena cava and the left central vein opens into the renal vein.

Regional Lymph Nodes. The regional lymph nodes are as follows (Figure 47.2):

Aortic (para-aortic, peri-aortic)
Retroperitoneal, NOS

Metastatic Sites. Common metastatic sites include liver, lung, and retroperitoneum. Metastases to brain and skin are uncommon although cutaneous involvement of the scalp can simulate angiosarcoma.

DEFINITIONS OF TNM

Primary Tumor (T)

TX   Primary tumor cannot be assessed

T0   No evidence of primary tumor

T1   Tumor 5 cm or less in greatest dimension, no extra-adrenal invasion (Figure 47.3)

T2   Tumor greater than 5 cm, no extra-adrenal invasion (Figure 47.4)

T3   Tumor of any size with local invasion, but not invading adjacent organs* (Figure 47.5)

T4   Tumor of any size with invasion of adjacent organs* (Figure 47.6)

*Note: Adjacent organs include kidney, diaphragm, great vessels, pancreas, spleen, and liver.

Regional Lymph Nodes (N)

NX   Regional lymph nodes cannot be assessed

N0   No regional lymph node metastasis

N1   Metastasis in regional lymph node(s) (Figure 47.7)

Distant Metastasis (M)

M0   No distance metastasis

M1   Distance metastasis

ANATOMIC STAGE/PROGNOSTIC GROUPS

Stage I	T1	N0	M0
Stage II	T2	N0	M0
Stage III	T1	N1	M0
	T2	N1	M0
	T3	N0	M0
Stage IV	T3	N1	M0
	T4	N0	M0
	T4	N1	M0
	Any T	Any N	M1

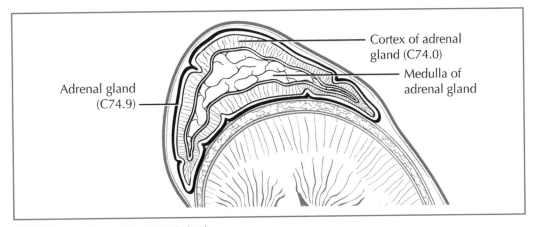

FIGURE 47.1. *Anatomy of the adrenal gland.*

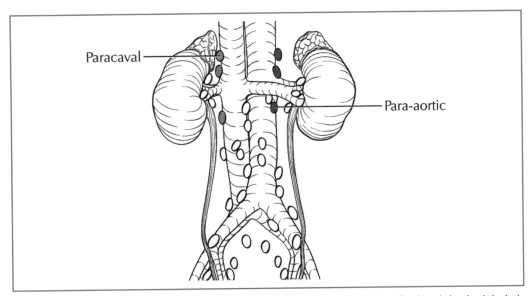

FIGURE 47.2. *Regional lymph nodes of the right adrenal gland. Regional nodes of the left adrenal gland only include the para-aortic.*

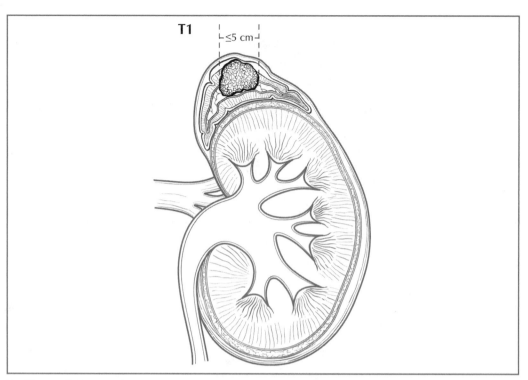

FIGURE 47.3. *T1 is defined as tumor that is 5 cm or less in greatest dimension, no extra-adrenal invasion.*

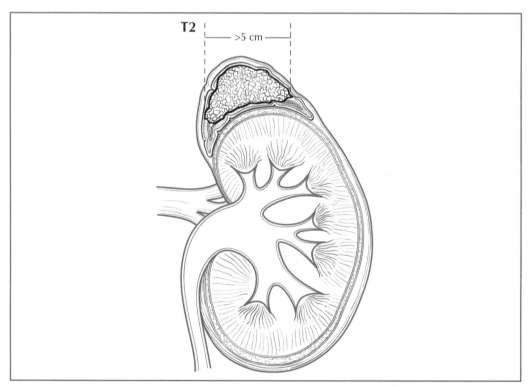

FIGURE 47.4. *T2 is defined as tumor that is greater than 5 cm, no extra-adrenal invasion.*

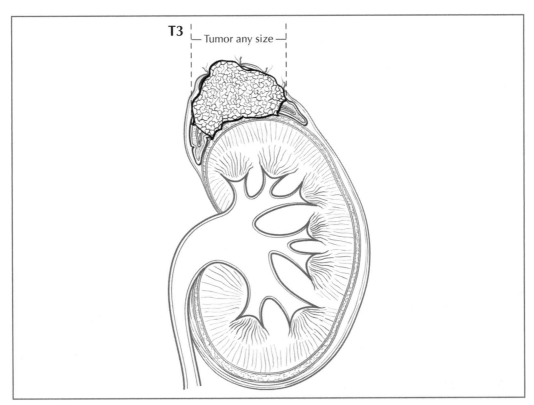

FIGURE 47.5. *T3 is defined as tumor of any size with local invasion, but not invading adjacent organs.*

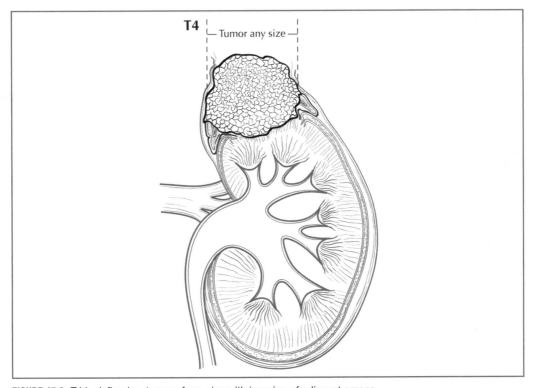

FIGURE 47.6. *T4 is defined as tumor of any size with invasion of adjacent organs.*

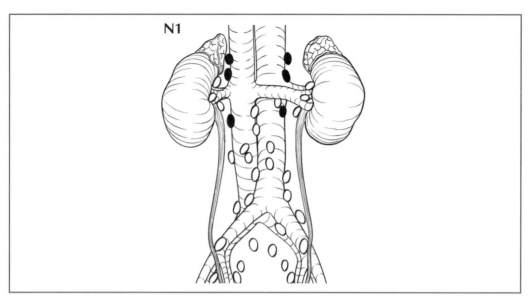

FIGURE 47.7. *N1 is defined as involvement of regional lymph nodes.*

<table>
<tr><td colspan="2">PROGNOSTIC FACTORS (SITE-SPECIFIC FACTORS)
(Recommended for Collection)</td></tr>
<tr><td>Required for staging</td><td>None</td></tr>
<tr><td>Clinically significant</td><td>Tumor weight in grams
Vascular invasion</td></tr>
</table>

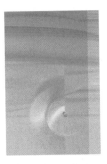

PART X
Lymphoid Neoplasms

INTRODUCTION

Lymphoid malignancies are a diverse group of disorders. These malignancies share derivation from B-cells, T-cells, and NK-cells, but they have a wide range of presentations, clinical course, and response to therapy. The incidence of lymphoid malignancies is significant and increasing. Non-Hodgkin lymphomas occur in more than 63,000 new individuals each year and have been increasing in incidence over the past several decades. Hodgkin lymphoma occurs in approximately 8,000 new individuals each year in the USA and seems stable in incidence. Approximately 20,000 new cases of multiple myeloma and more than 20,000 new cases of lymphoid leukemias occur annually in the USA.

PATHOLOGY

Lymphoid neoplasms are malignancies of B-cells, T-cells, and NK (natural killer) cells. They include Hodgkin lymphoma (Hodgkin disease), non-Hodgkin lymphoma, multiple myeloma, and lymphoid leukemias. Traditionally, classifications have distinguished between *lymphomas*, i.e., neoplasms that typically present with an obvious tumor or mass of lymph nodes or extranodal sites, and *leukemias*, i.e., neoplasms that typically involve the bone marrow and peripheral blood, without tumor masses. However, we now know that many B- and T/NK-cell neoplasms may have both tissue masses *and* circulating cells. Thus, it is artificial to call them different diseases, when in fact they are just different presentations of the same disease. For this reason, we now refer to these diseases as lymphoid neoplasms rather than as lymphomas or leukemias, reserving the latter terms for the specific clinical presentation. In the current classification of lymphoid neoplasms, diseases that typically produce tumor masses are called lymphomas, those that typically have only circulating cells are called leukemias, and those that often have both solid and circulating phases are designated lymphoma/leukemia. Finally, plasma cell neoplasms, including multiple myeloma and plasmacytoma, have typically not been considered *lymphomas*, but plasma cells are part of the B-cell lineage, and, thus, these tumors are B-cell neoplasms, which are now included in the classification of lymphoid neoplasms.

Lymphoid neoplasms are malignancies of lymphoid cells. Lymphoid cells include lymphoblasts, lymphocytes, follicle center cells (centrocytes and centroblasts), immunoblasts, and plasma cells. These cells are responsible for immune responses to infections. Immune responses involve recognition by lymphocytes of foreign molecules, followed by proliferation and differentiation to generate either specific cytotoxic cells (T or NK – natural killer – cells) or antibodies (B-cells and plasma cells). Lymphoid cells are normally found in greatest numbers in lymph nodes and in other lymphoid tissues such as Waldeyer's ring (which includes the palatine and lingual tonsils and adenoids), the thymus, Peyer's patches of the small intestine, the spleen, and the bone marrow (Figure X.1 and Table X.1). Lymphocytes also circulate in the peripheral blood and are found in small numbers in almost every organ of the body, where they either wait to encounter antigens or carry out specific immune reactions. Lymphoid neoplasms may occur in any site to which lymphocytes normally travel. Because lymphocytes normally circulate through the blood as well as the lymphatics – in contrast to epithelial cells, for example – it is often impossible to determine the "primary site" of a lymphoid neoplasm or to use a staging scheme that was developed for epithelial cancers, such as the TNM scheme.

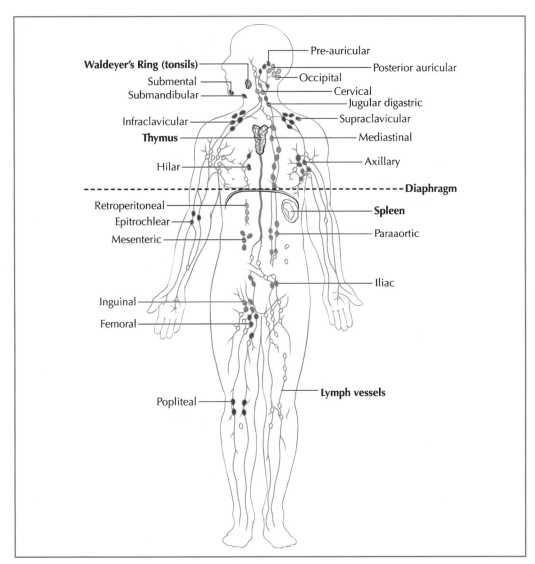

FIGURE X.1. *Lymphatic structures including lymph nodes and lymphatic tissues.*

TABLE X.1. *Lymphatic structures above and below the diaphragm*

Lymph nodes and lymphatic tissue above the diaphragm:

- Waldeyer's ring (palatine tonsils, pharyngeal tonsil, and lingual tonsil)
- Thymus
- Submental
- Submandibular
- Pre-auricular
- Posterior auricular
- Occipital
- Cervical
- Jugular digastric
- Supraclavicular
- Infraclavicular
- Mediastinal
- Hilar
- Axillary
- Epitrochlear

Lymph nodes and lymphatic tissue below the diaphragm:

- Spleen
- Paraaortic
- Mesenteric
- Retroperitoneal
- Iliac
- Inguinal
- Femoral
- Popliteal

Hodgkin and Non-Hodgkin Lymphomas

(Excludes ocular adnexal lymphoma)

48

ICD-O-3 TOPOGRAPHY RANGES

C00.0–C44.0, C44.2–C68.9, C69.1–C69.4, C69.8–C80.9

ICD-O-3 HISTOLOGY CODE RANGES

9590–9699, 9702–9729, 9735, 9737, 9738
9811–9818, 9837 (all sites), 9823, 9827 (excludes C42.0, C42.1, C42.4)

PROGNOSTIC FEATURES

Prognostic Indices Used in Non-Hodgkin and Hodgkin Lymphoma. *International Prognostic Index (IPI).* The International Non-Hodgkin Lymphoma Prognostic Factors Project used pretreatment prognostic factors in a sample of several thousand patients with aggressive lymphomas treated with doxorubicin-based combination chemotherapy to develop a predictive model of outcome for aggressive non-Hodgkin lymphoma. The specific type of lymphoma and the IPI score are the major factors currently used in treatment decisions. On the basis of factors identified in multivariate analysis of the above data set, the International Prognostic Index was proposed. Five pretreatment characteristics were found to be independent statistically significant factors: age in years (≤60 vs. >60); tumor stage I or II (localized) versus III or IV (advanced); number of extranodal sites of involvement (0–1 vs. >1); patient's performance status (ECOG 0 or 1 vs. ≥2); and serum LDH level (normal vs. abnormal). With the use of these five pretreatment risk factors, patients could be assigned to one of the four risk groups on the basis of the number of presenting risk factors: low (0 or 1), low intermediate (2), high intermediate (3), and high (4 or 5). When patients were analyzed by risk factors, they were found to have very different outcomes with regard to complete response (CR), relapse-free survival (RFS), and overall survival (OS). The outcomes indicated that the low-risk patients had an 87% CR rate and an OS rate of 73% at 5 years in contrast to a 44% CR rate and 26% 5-year survival in patients in the high-risk group. A similar pattern of decreasing survival with a number of adverse factors was observed when younger patients only were considered.

The validity of the IPI is less clear in patients with T-cell lymphomas and other classifications have been proposed but none are yet universally accepted.

The Follicular Lymphoma Prognostic Index (FLIPI). The IPI was less useful in follicular lymphomas, and the FLIPI has been proposed. Factors that are included are the number of nodal sites ≤4 vs. >4), serum LDH (normal vs. elevated), age (using 60 years and younger as the cut-off), stage (I–II vs. III–IV), and serum hemoglobin concentration (≥12 vs. <12 g/dL). The three risk groups identified were 0–1 adverse factor, 2 factors, or 3 or more factors. Patients with low-risk disease had a 10-year survival of 71%, 51% with intermediate-risk disease, and only 36% for those with high-risk disease.

C.C. Compton et al. (eds.), *AJCC Cancer Staging Atlas: A Companion to the Seventh Editions of the AJCC Cancer Staging Manual and Handbook*, DOI 10.1007/978-1-4614-2080-4_48,
© 2012 American Joint Committee on Cancer

The International Prognostic Score (IPS). The International Prognostic Score (IPS) has been developed for Hodgkin lymphoma, which predicts outcome based on the following adverse factors: serum albumin <4 g/dL, hemoglobin concentration <10.5 g/dL, male sex, age ≥45 years, stage IV disease, white blood cell count ≥15,000/mm^3, and lymphocytopenia <600/mm^3 or <8%. The rate of freedom from progression by risk category was: 0 factors 84%, 1 – 77%, 2 – 67%, 3 – 60%, 4 – 51%, 5 or higher – 42%. Other factors of note in Hodgkin lymphoma have included the number of sites of disease and the erythrocyte sedimentation rate.

ANATOMIC STAGE/PROGNOSTIC GROUPS

Stage I	Involvement of a single lymphatic site (i.e., nodal region, Waldeyer's ring, thymus or spleen) (I) (Figures 48.1, 48.2); or localized involvement of a single extralymphatic organ or site in the absence of any lymph node involvement (IE) (rare in Hodgkin lymphoma). (Figure 48.3)
Stage II	Involvement of two or more lymph node regions on the same side of the diaphragm (II) (Figures 48.4, 48.5); or localized involvement of a single extralymphatic organ or site in association with regional lymph node involvement with or without involvement of other lymph node regions on the same side of the diaphragm (IIE). (Figure 48.6) The number of regions involved may be indicated by an arabic numeral, as in, for example, II3.
Stage III	Involvement of lymph node regions on both sides of the diaphragm (III) (Figure 48.7), which also maybe accompanied by extralymphatic extension in association with adjacent lymph node involvement (IIIE) (Figure 48.8) or by involvement of the spleen (IIIS) or both (IIIE,S). (Figure 48.9) Splenic involvement is designated by the letter S.
Stage IV	Diffuse or disseminated involvement of one or more extralymphatic organs, with or without associated lymph node involvement (Figure 48.10); or isolated extralymphatic organ involvement in the absence of adjacent regional lymph node involvement, but in conjunction with disease in distant site(s). Stage IV includes any involvement of the liver or bone marrow, lungs (other than by direct extension from another site), or cerebrospinal fluid (Figure 48.11)

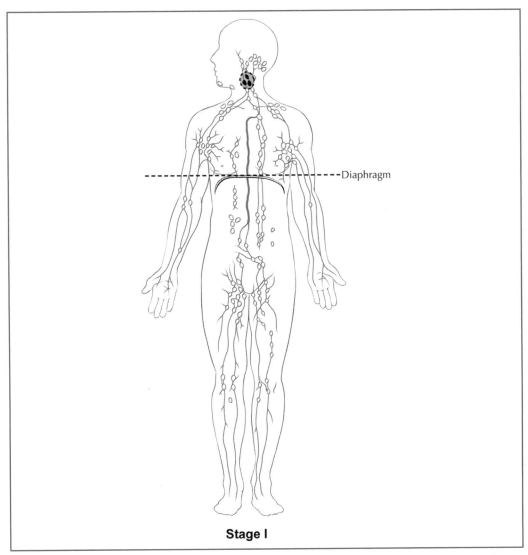

Stage I

FIGURE 48.1. *Stage I is defined as involvement of a single lymphatic site (i.e., nodal region, Waldeyer's ring, thymus or spleen). Illustrated is involvement of the cervical nodal region.*

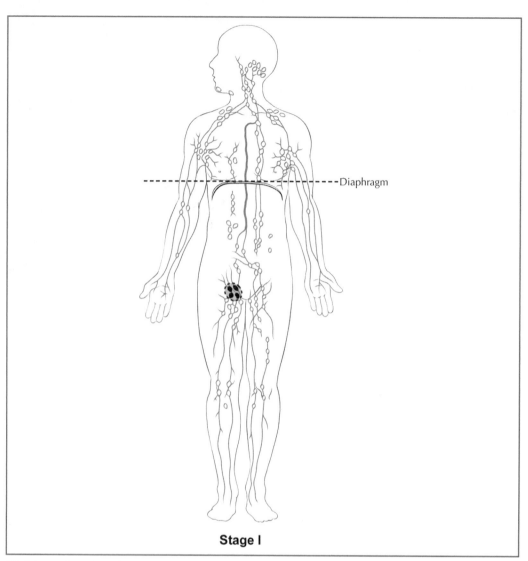

Stage I

FIGURE 48.2. *Stage I is defined as involvement of a single lymphatic site (i.e., nodal region, Waldeyer's ring, thymus or spleen). Illustrated is the inguinal nodal region.*

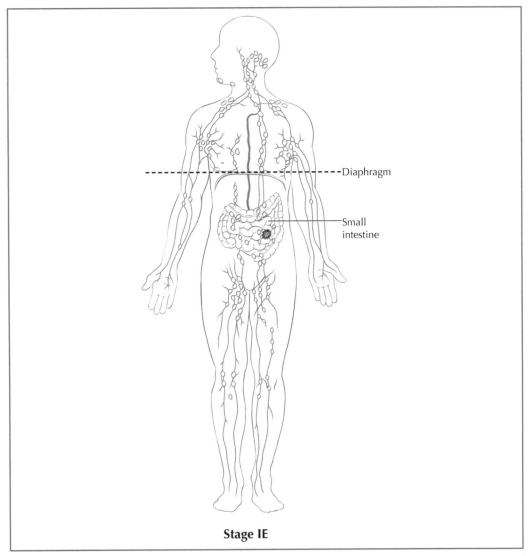

Stage IE

FIGURE 48.3. *Stage IE is defined as localized involvement of a single extralymphatic organ or site in the absence of any lymph node involvement (rare in Hodgkin lymphoma). Illustrated is small intestine involvement.*

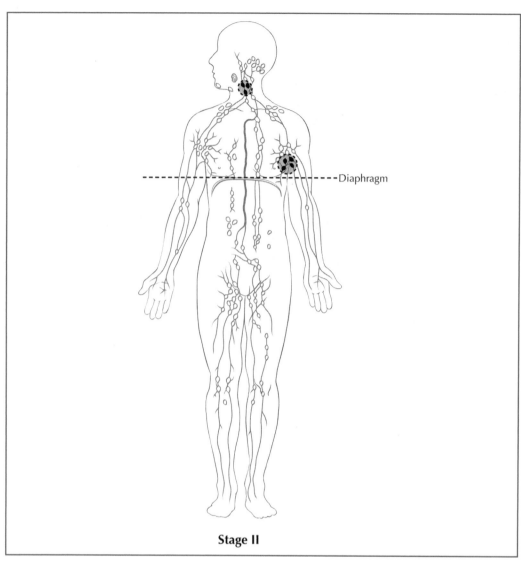

----Diaphragm

Stage II

FIGURE 48.4. *Stage II is defined as involvement of two or more lymph node regions on the same side of the diaphragm. Illustrated are nodes above the diaphragm.*

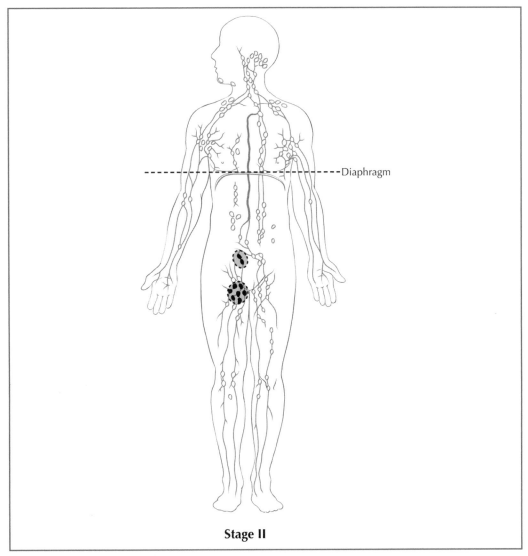

Stage II

FIGURE 48.5. *Stage II is defined as involvement of two or more lymph node regions on the same side of the diaphragm. Illustrated are nodes below the diaphragm.*

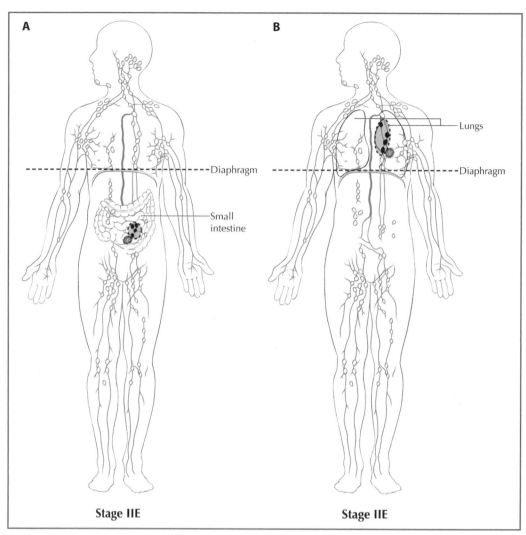

FIGURE 48.6. *(A) Stage IIE is defined as localized involvement of a single extralymphatic organ or site in association with regional lymph node involvement with or without involvement of other lymph node regions on the same side of the diaphragm. Illustrated are involvement of the small intestine and nodes below the diaphragm. (B) Stage IIE is defined as localized involvement of a single extralymphatic organ or site in association with regional lymph node involvement with or without involvement of other lymph node regions on the same side of the diaphragm. Illustrated are involvement of the lung with hilar and mediastinal node involvement.*

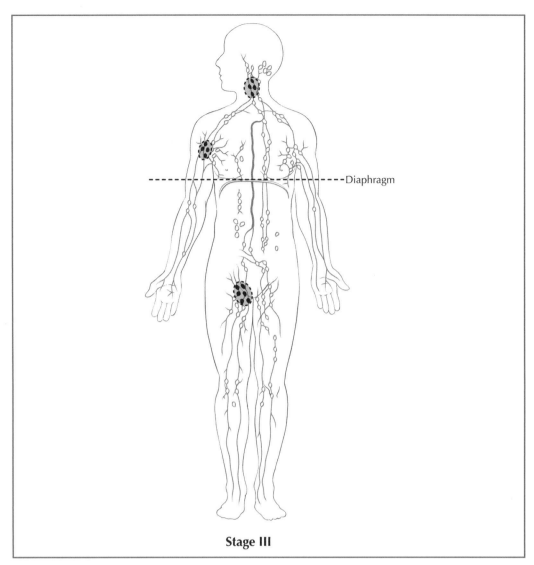

Diaphragm

Stage III

FIGURE 48.7. *Stage III is defined as involvement of lymph node regions on both sides of the diaphragm.*

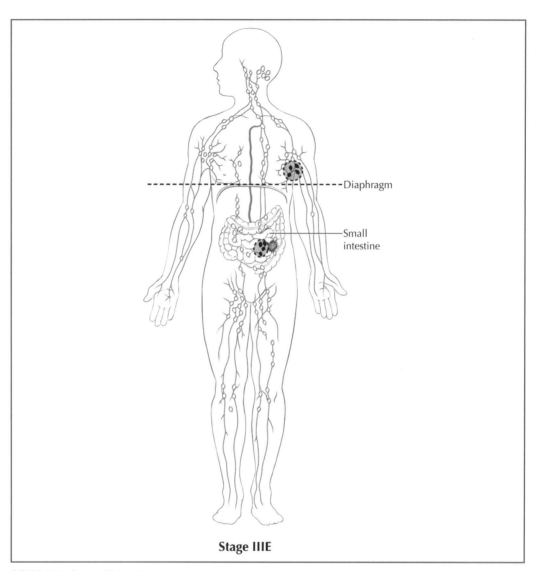

Diaphragm

Small
intestine

Stage IIIE

FIGURE 48.8. *Stage IIIE is defined as involvement of lymph node regions on the opposite side of the diaphragm from the extralymphatic extension in association with adjacent lymph node involvement. Illustrated are nodes on both sides of the diaphragm with the small intestine.*

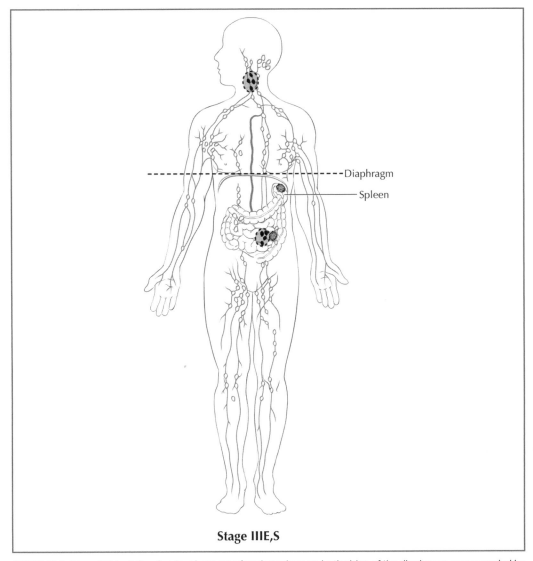

Stage IIIE,S

FIGURE 48.9. *Stage IIIS is defined as involvement of node regions on both sides of the diaphragm accompanied by involvement of the spleen. Stage IIIE,S is defined as involvement of node regions on both sides of the diaphragm, and involving both an extralymphatic organ and the spleen (as illustrated). Splenic involvement is designated by the letter S.*

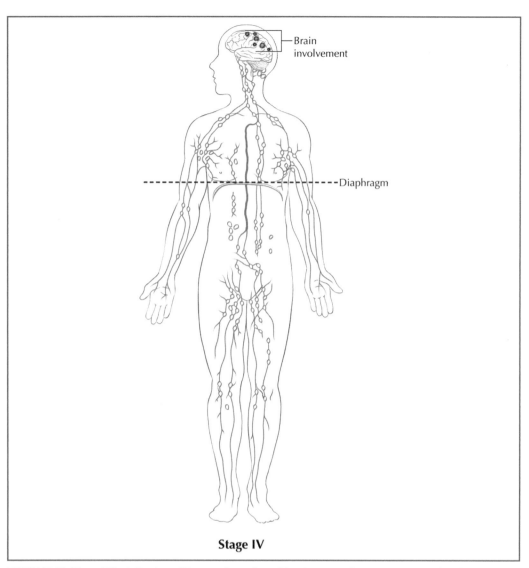

Stage IV

FIGURE 48.10. *Stage IV is defined as diffuse or disseminated involvement of one or more extralymphatic organs, with or without associated lymph node involvement. Illustrated is diffuse involvement of the brain with multiple lesions.*

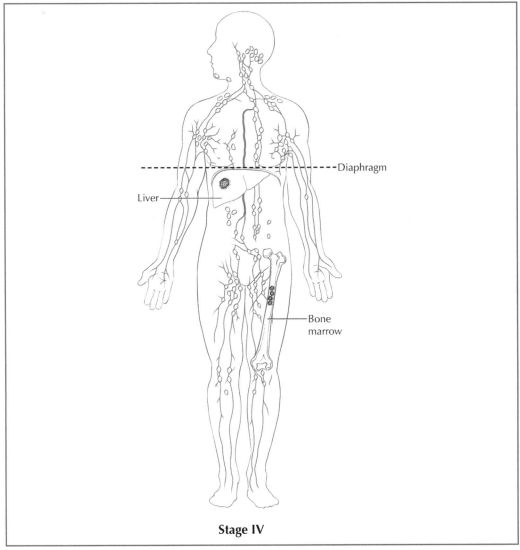

Stage IV

FIGURE 48.11. *Stage IV includes any involvement of the liver (as illustrated), or bone marrow (as illustrated), or lungs (other than by direct extension from another site), or cerebrospinal fluid.*

PROGNOSTIC FACTORS (SITE-SPECIFIC FACTORS)
(Recommended for Collection)

Required for staging	None
Clinically significant	Associated with HIV/AIDS
	Symptoms at diagnosis (B symptoms)
	International Prognostic Index (IPI) score
	Follicular Lymphoma Prognostic Index (FLIPI) score
	International Prognostic Score (IPS)

Primary Cutaneous Lymphomas

49

SUMMARY OF CHANGES

- There are no changes to the stage groups for the seventh edition

ICD-O-3 TOPOGRAPHY RANGES

C44.0–C44.9   Skin
C51.0–C51.9   Vulva
C60.0–C60.9   Penis
C63.2   Scrotum

ICD-O-3 HISTOLOGY CODE RANGES

9700–9701

Primary cutaneous T- and B-cell lymphomas are a heterogeneous group of malignancies with varied clinical presentation and prognosis. The application of molecular, histological, and clinical criteria have allowed for a better characterization of defined entities with distinct features. The World Health Organization and European Organization of Research and Treatment of Cancer (WHO-EORTC) classification for cutaneous lymphomas provides a consensus categorization that allows for more uniform diagnosis and treatment of these disorders. Approximately 80% of the cutaneous lymphomas are of T cell origin. Mycosis fungoides and Sézary syndrome have a formal staging system proposed by the International Society for Cutaneous Lymphomas and EORTC. The other cutaneous non-Hodgkin lymphomas are staged using the same system, described previously, for lymphomas presenting in other anatomic locations.

Mycosis Fungoides. Mycosis fungoides and its variants represent the most common form of cutaneous T cell lymphoma (CTCL). The malignant cell is derived from a post thymic T cell that typically bears a CD4+ helper/memory antigen profile. The disease is characterized by erythematous patches (usually in sun-protected areas) that progress to plaques or tumors. Initial evaluation should include delineation of skin involvement with photographs; skin biopsy (histopathology, immunophenotyping, and T-cell receptor (TCR) gene analysis); CBC with differential, Sézary cell count (peripheral blood); chemistry panel with LDH; and in select instances peripheral blood flow cytometric analysis of T-cell subsets (CD4/CD8 ratio); TCR gene analysis on peripheral blood; lymph node biopsy and bone marrow biopsies (histopathology, immunophenotyping and TCR gene analysis); CT/PET scans; and serologic tests (HTLV-1 and HIV). Skin directed and systemic therapies are determined by the patient's stage and symptoms. Prognosis is stage dependent.

Sézary Syndrome. Sézary syndrome is the aggressive leukemic, and erythrodermic form of CTCL, which is characterized by circulating atypical, malignant T lymphocytes with cerebriform nuclei (Sézary cells), and lymphadenopathy. The Sézary cells also have a mature memory T-cell phenotype (CD3+, CD4+) with loss of CD7 and CD26.

C.C. Compton et al. (eds.), *AJCC Cancer Staging Atlas: A Companion to the Seventh Editions*
of the AJCC Cancer Staging Manual and Handbook, DOI 10.1007/978-1-4614-2080-4_49,
© 2012 American Joint Committee on Cancer

ISCL/EORTC Revision to the Classification of Mycosis fungoides and Sézary Syndrome

Skin

T1	Limited patches,* papules, and/or plaques** covering less than 10% of the skin surface. May further stratify into T1a (patch only) vs. T1b (plaque ± patch) (Figures 49.1A, 49.1B, 49.2A, and 49.2B)
T2	Patches, papules or plaques covering 10% or more of the skin surface. May further stratify into T2a (patch only) vs. T2b (plaque ± patch) (Figures 49.1A, 49.1B, 49.2A, and 49.2B)
T3	One or more tumors*** (1≥-cm diameter) (Figures 49.3A and 49.3B)
T4	Confluence of erythema covering 80% or more of body surface area

Node

N0	No clinically abnormal peripheral lymph nodes****; biopsy not required
N1	Clinically abnormal peripheral lymph nodes; histopathology Dutch grade 1 or NCI LN0-2
N1a	Clone negative*****
N1b	Clone positive*****
N2	Clinically abnormal peripheral lymph nodes; histopathology Dutch grade 2 or NCI LN3
N2a	Clone negative*****
N2b	Clone positive*****
N3	Clinically abnormal peripheral lymph nodes; histopathology Dutch grades 3–4 or NCI LN4; clone positive or negative
Nx	Clinically abnormal peripheral lymph nodes; no histologic confirmation

Visceral

M0	No visceral organ involvement
M1	Visceral involvement (must have pathology confirmation^ and organ involved should be specified)

Peripheral Blood Involvement

B0	Absence of significant blood involvement: 5% or less of peripheral blood lymphocytes are atypical (Sézary) cells^^
B0a	Clone negative*****
B0b	Clone positive*****
B1	Low blood tumor burden: more than 5% of peripheral blood lymphocytes are atypical (Sézary) cells but does not meet the criteria of B2

Peripheral Blood Involvement (*continued*)

B1a   Clone negative*****

B1b   Clone positive*****

B2   High blood tumor burden: 1000/µL Sézary cells^^ or more with positive clone*****

*For skin, patch indicates any size skin lesion without significant elevation or induration. Presence/absence of hypo- or hyperpigmentation, scale, crusting, and/or poikiloderma should be noted. (Figures 49.1A and 49.1B)

**For skin, plaque indicates any size skin lesion that is elevated or indurated. Presence or absence of scale, crusting, and/or poikiloderma should be noted. Histologic features such as folliculotropism or large-cell transformation (>25% large cells), CD30+ or CD30−, and clinical features such as ulceration are important to document (Figures 49.2A and 49.2B).

***For skin, tumor indicates at least one 1-cm diameter solid or nodular lesion with evidence of depth and/or vertical growth. Note total number of lesions, total volume of lesions, largest size lesion, and region of body involved. Also note if histologic evidence of large-cell transformation has occurred. Phenotyping for CD30 is encouraged (Figures 49.3A and 49.3B).

****For node, abnormal peripheral lymph node(s) indicates any palpable peripheral node that on physical examination is firm, irregular, clustered, fixed or 1.5 cm or larger in diameter. Node groups examined on physical examination include cervical, supraclavicular, epitrochlear, axillary, and inguinal. Central nodes, which are not generally amenable to pathologic assessment, are not currently considered in the nodal classification unless used to establish N3 histopathologically.

*****A T-cell clone is defined by PCR or Southern blot analysis of the T-cell receptor gene.

^ For viscera, spleen and liver may be diagnosed by imaging criteria.

^^ For blood, Sézary cells are defined as lymphocytes with hyperconvoluted cerebriform nuclei. If Sézary cells are not able to be used to determine tumor burden for B2, then one of the following modified ISCL criteria along with a positive clonal rearrangement of the TCR may be used instead: (1) expanded CD4+ or CD3+ cells with CD4/CD8 ratio of 10 or more, (2) expanded CD4+ cells with abnormal immunophenotype including loss of CD7 or CD26.

Histopathologic Staging of Lymph Nodes in *Mycosis fungoides* and Sézary Syndrome

Updated ISCL/ EORTC classification	Dutch system	NCI-VA classification
N1	Grade 1: dermatopathic lymphadenopathy (DL)	LN0: no atypical lymphocytes
		LN1: occasional and isolated atypical lymphocytes (not arranged in clusters)
		LN2: many atypical lymphocytes or in 3–6 cell clusters
N2	Grade 2: DL; early involvement by MF (presence of cerebriform nuclei >7.5 µm)	LN3: aggregates of atypical lymphocytes; nodal architecture preserved
N3	Grade 3: partial effacement of LN architecture; many atypical cerebriform mononuclear cells (CMCs)	LN4: partial/complete effacement of nodal architecture by atypical lymphocytes or frankly neoplastic cells
	Grade 4: complete effacement	

ANATOMIC STAGE/PROGNOSTIC GROUPS

ISCL/EORTC Revision to the Staging of Mycosis fungoides and Sézary Syndrome

	T	N	M	Peripheral Blood Involvement
Stage IA	1	0	0	0, 1
Stage IB	2	0	0	0, 1
Stage IIA	1,2	1,2	0	0, 1
Stage IIB	3	0–2	0	0, 1
Stage III	4	0–2	0	0, 1
Stage IIIA	4	0–2	0	0
Stage IIIB	4	0–2	0	1
Stage IVA1	1–4	0–2	0	2
Stage IVA2	1–4	3	0	0–2
Stage IVB	1–4	0–3	1	0–2

From Olsen E, Vonderheid E, Pimpinelli N, et al. Revisions to the staging and classification of mycosis fungoides and Sézary syndrome: a proposal of the International Society for Cutaneous Lymphomas (ISCL) and the cutaneous lymphoma task force of the European Organization of Research and Treatment of Cancer (EORTC). Blood. 2007;110(6):1713–22, with permission of the American Society of Hematology.

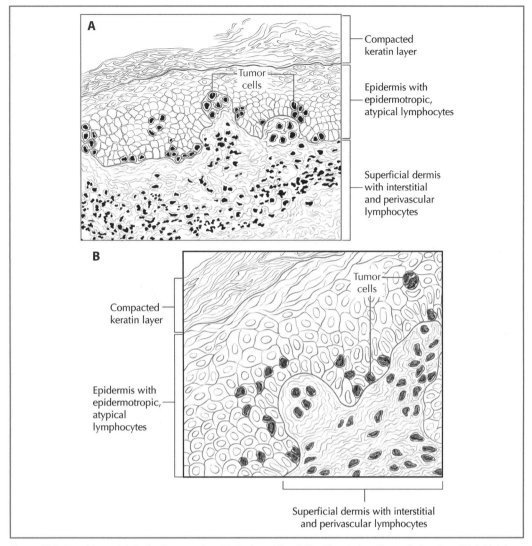

Figure 49.1. *For skin, patch indicates any size skin lesion without significant elevation or induration. (A) A histology slide with 4× magnification power is illustrated showing the compacted keratin layer; the epidermis with epidermotrophic, atypical lymphocytes; and the superficial dermis with interstitial and perivascular lymphocytes. (B) A histology slide with 40× magnification power is illustrated showing the compacted keratin layer, the epidermis with epidermotrophic, atypical lymphocytes; and the superficial dermis with interstitial and perivascular lymphocytes.*

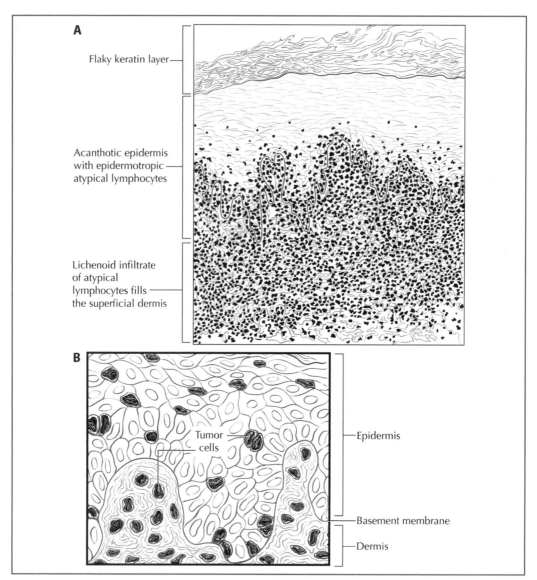

Figure 49.2. *For skin, plaque indicates any size skin lesion that is elevated or indurated. (A) A histology slide with 10× magnification power is illustrated showing the flaky keratin layer, the acanthotic epidermis with epidermotropic atypical lymphocytes, and the lichenoid infiltrate of atypical lymphocytes fills the superficial dermis. (B) A histology slide with 40× magnification power is illustrated showing the epidermis; the basement membrane, and the dermis.*

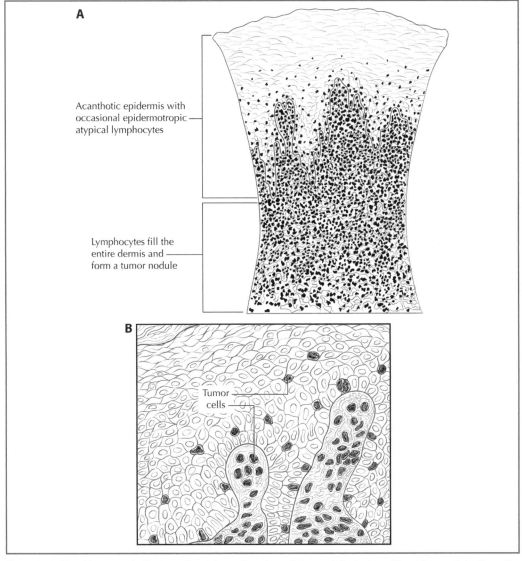

Figure 49.3. *For skin, tumor indicates at least 1 cm diameter solid or nodular lesion with evidence of depth and/or vertical growth. (A) A histology slide with 4× magnification power is illustrated showing acanthotic epidermis with occasional epidermotropic atypical lymphocytes; and lymphocytes fill the entire dermis and form a tumor nodule. (B) A histology slide with 40× magnification power is illustrated showing fewer cells in the epidermis with progression to tumor stage.*

Primary Cutaneous CD30+ Lymphoproliferative Disorders. Primary cutaneous CD30+ lymphoproliferative disorders are the second most common group of CTCL. This spectrum of diseases includes lymphomatoid papulosis, anaplastic large cell lymphoma and borderline cases. The distinction between these entities can be challenging and is often determined by clinical behavior. Lymphomatoid papulosis represents a benign, chronic recurrent, self-healing, papulonodular, and papulonecrotic CD4+, CD30+ skin eruption. Primary cutaneous anaplastic large cell lymphoma typically presents with solitary or localized nodules.

Follicle Center Cell Lymphoma. Follicle center cell lymphoma is the most common cutaneous B cell lymphoma (CBCL). Erythematous nodules or plaques are comprised of a proliferation of centrocytes (small to large cleaved cells) and centroblasts (large round cells with prominent nuclei). The clinical course is usually indolent even when the infiltrate is composed of predominantly large cells.

Marginal Zone Lymphoma. Marginal zone lymphoma is an indolent CBCL. It has the histologic appearance of a MALT lymphoma and shows a nodular or diffuse dermal infiltrate with a heterogeneous cellular infiltrate of small lymphocytes, lymphoplasmacytoid cells, plasma cells, intranuclear inclusions (Dutcher bodies), and reactive germinal centers that may be infiltrated by neoplastic cells. They are often localized and usually follow an indolent course.

Large B-Cell Lymphoma of the Leg. Large B-cell lymphoma of the leg is an aggressive lymphoma most commonly seen in elderly women. Patients present with tumors that may ulcerate. The histologic evaluation shows a diffuse dermal infiltrate comprised of predominantly centroblasts often with multilobulated nuclei.

Index

A

Accurate microscopic diagnosis, 7
Adenocarcinomas, 133
  exocrine and endocrine pancreas, 298–299
  lung, 316
Adenosarcoma, corpus uteri, 482–483, 489–493
Adjacent hepatic parenchyma, 270, 273
Adrenal
  anatomic stage/prognostic groups, 596
  distant metastasis (M), 596
  metastatic sites, 595
  primary site, 595, 597
  primary tumor (T), 596, 598, 599
  prognostic factors, 600
  regional lymph nodes, 595–597, 600
Adventitia, 132, 138
AFP. *See* Alpha fetoprotein
AJCC Cancer Staging Manual, 16, 17, 22
AJCC staging system, 558
Alpha fetoprotein (AFP), 496, 556
Amalgamate lymph node, 312
American College of Radiology Appropriateness
    Criteria, 8
American Joint Committee on Cancer (AJCC), 441
Ampulla
  distant metastases (M), 224
  primary tumor (T), 224, 233–235
  regional lymph nodes (N), 224, 235, 236
Ampulla of Vater
  anatomic stage/prognostic groups, 289
  distant metastasis, 289, 294, 295
  duodenal wall, 288, 291
  location, 287, 289
  metastatic sites, 287
  pancreas, 288, 292
  papilla, 287
  peripancreatic soft tissues, 288, 292
  prognostic factors, 295
  prognostic features, 288
  regional lymph nodes, 287, 288, 290, 293, 294
  sphincter of Oddi, 288, 291
Anaplastic carcinoma, 115
Anatomical subsites
  lip, 42, 46
  oral cavity, 42, 47, 48
Anorectal lymph nodes, 204
Anus
  anatomic stage/prognostic groups, 205
  distant metastasis (M), 205

metastatic sites, 204
primary site, 203–204, 206
primary tumor (T), 205, 207, 208
prognostic features, 204
regional lymph nodes (N), 204–206, 209–212
Aortic lymph nodes
  adrenal, 595
  kidney, 557
  prostate, 536
  renal pelvis, 567
Appendix
  carcinoid (*see* Carcinoid)
  carcinoma (*see* Carcinomas)
  metastatic sites, 170
  primary site, 170, 174
  prognostic features, 170
  regional lymph nodes, 170, 174
Atlas of Tumor Pathology, 8
Autoimmune deficiency syndrome (AIDS), 464
Axillary ipsilateral lymph nodes, 422

B

B-cells, 601–602
Bilateral para-aortic lymph nodes, 478
Bone
  anatomic stage/prognostic groups, 344
  distant metastasis (M), 343, 347, 348
  Ewing's sarcoma, 341–342
  EWS-FLI1 type 1 fusion gene, 342
  HER2/erbB-2 expression, 342
  HLA class I expression, 343
  MDR1, 342
  P-glycoprotein, 342
  platelet-derived growth factor-AA expression, 343
  P53, p16INK4A, and p14ARF expression, 342
  primary site, 341, 344
  primary tumor (T), 343, 345, 346
  prognostic factors, 348
  pulmonary metastases, 341
  regional lymph nodes, 341, 343
  secondary bone metastases, 341
  soft tissue sarcomas, 342
Bowen's disease, 362
Breast
  anatomic stage/prognostic groups, 426–427
  cancer, 24, 29
  chest wall, 421
  distant metastases, 426
  macrometastases, 422

Breast (*continued*)
  metastatic sites, 422
  nodal metastases, 422
  posttreatment ypM classification, 426
  posttreatment ypN, 426
  posttreatment ypT, 423–424
  primary site, 421, 427
  primary tumor (T), 423, 428–432
  prognostic factors, 440
  prognostic features, 421
  regional lymph nodes (N), 421–422, 424–425,
    428, 432–439
Bronchioloalveolar carcinomas, 316
Buccal mucosa, 42

C

Cancer Bioinformatics Grid (caBIG), 8
Cancer staging data form, 17
Cancer survival analysis
  actuarial method, 24
  cause-adjusted survival rate, 25, 26
  confidence intervals, 27
  Kaplan–Meier method, 25
  life table method, 24, 25, 29, 30
  long rank test, 28
  patient-, disease-, and treatment-specific,
    25, 29–31
  regression methods, 27
  relative survival rate, 26
  risks competition, 26
  SEER Program, 24
  standard error, 27
  starting time, 28
  survival curve and rate, 23
  time intervals, 28–29
  uncensored and censored cases, 23
  vital status, 28
CAP Cancer Protocols, 8, 18
Carcinoembryonic antigen (CEA), 313
Carcinoid
  anatomic stage/prognostic groups, 173
  distant metastasis (M), 172
  primary tumor (T), 172, 181–183
  regional lymph nodes (N), 172, 184
Carcinomas
  anus, 204
  appendix, 171, 175–180
  breast, 421
  colon and rectum, 188
  fallopian tube, 505
  hepatocellular, 252
  liver, 242
  lung, 311
  small intestine, 155
  stomach, 144, 145, 147
  uterine, 479–480, 484–487
Carotid space (CS), 56
Caval lymph nodes, 557

Cervical esophagus, 130
Cervical lymph nodes, 536
Cervix uteri
  anatomic stage/prognostic groups, 466
  distant metastasis (M), 465
  metastatic sites, 464
  primary site, 463, 466
  primary tumor (T), 464–465, 467–474
  prognostic factors, 475
  prognostic features, 464
  regional lymph nodes, 463–465, 467, 474
Child-Pugh class B and C liver disease, 242
Cholangiocarcinoma, 269
Chondrosarcoma, 343
Circulating tumor cells (CTCs), 422
Clinicopathologic tumor, 359
Collaborative Stage Data Collection System, 8
Colon and rectum
  anatomic boundary, 190
  anatomic stage/prognostic groups, 192
  circumferential resection margins, 188–189, 196
  distant metastasis (M), 192, 201, 225
  divisions of, 186, 193
  independent prognostic factors, 190–191
  isolated tumor cells, 189
  KRAS, 189
  metastatic sites, 187
  molecular markers, 190–191
  molecular node involvement, 189
  primary site, 186
  primary tumor (T), 191, 196–198, 224, 237–239
  prognostic factors, 190–191
  regional lymph nodes (N), 187, 191–192, 194,
    199, 200, 225, 239
  residual tumor (R), 189
  TNM stage of disease, 190
  tumor regression grade, 188
Common iliac lymph nodes
  cervix uteri, 463
  corpus uteri, 478
  fallopian tube, 505
  ovary and primary peritoneal carcinoma, 495
  prostate, 536
  urethra, 583
  urinary bladder, 576
Contralateral mediastinal nodes, 329
Corpora cavernosa penis, 523
Corpus spongiosum penis, 523
Corpus uteri
  adenosarcoma, 482–483, 489–493
  leiomyosarcoma and endometrial stromal sarcoma,
    481, 488–491
  metastatic sites, 478
  primary site, 477, 483
  prognostic factors, 493
  prognostic features, 478–479
  regional lymph nodes (N), 478, 484
  uterine carcinomas, 479–480, 484–487
  uterine sarcomas, 481, 483

Major salivary glands (*continued*)
  parotid, submandibular, and sublingual glands, 105, 108
  regional lymph nodes, 105–106
  T2, 106, 109
  T4a, 106, 111
  T4b, 106, 112
  T3, extraparenchymal extension, 106, 110
  tumor, greatest dimension, 106, 108
Malignant cells, 477
Masticator space, 56
Maxillary sinus, 91, 93, 96–98
MCC. *See* Merkel cell carcinoma
Median survival time, 24
Mediastinal nodes, cervix uteri, 463
Medullary carcinoma, 115
Merkel cell carcinoma (MCC)
  anatomic stage/prognostic groups, 374
  distant metastasis (M), 373
  extracutaneous invasion, 372
  metastatic sites, 372
  microscopic *vs.* macroscopic metastases, 372
  primary sites, 371
  primary tumor (T), 373, 377–379
  prognostic factors, 383
  prognostic features and survival results, 372
  regional lymph nodes, 371–376, 380–382
  regional metastases, 372
Microsatellites, 386
Mucosal lip, 42
Mucosal melanoma
  anatomic stage/prognostic groups, 122
  anatomy, 121
  distant metastasis, 122
  prognostic factors, 125
  regional lymph nodes, 122
  T4a and T4b, 122, 124
  T3, mucosal disease, 122, 123
Multidrug resistance 1 gene (MDR1), 342
Multiple primary melanomas, 389
Multiple regression analysis, 27
Muscularis propria, 132, 138
Mycosis fungoides
  anatomic stage/prognostic groups, 622
  CTCL, 619
  histopathologic staging, lymph nodes, 621
  node, 620
  peripheral blood involvement, 620–621, 623–625
  skin, 619, 620
  visceral, 620
Myometrium, 477

N

Nasal cavity and paranasal sinuses
  anatomic stage/prognostic groups, 94
  distant metastases, 92
  ethmoid sinus, 93, 94, 99–103
  maxillary sinus, 91, 93, 96–98

prognostic features, 92
  regional lymph nodes, 92, 94
  Zubrod/ECOG performance scale, 93
Nasopharynx, 56
  T1 tumors, 58, 63, 64
  T2 tumors, 58, 64
  T3 tumors, 58, 65
  T4 tumors, 58, 66
National Comprehensive Cancer Network (NCCN), 8
Natural killer (NK) cells, 601–602
Neuroendocrine tumors, 299
  anatomic stage/prognostic groups, 225
  duodenal, 222–223
  gastric, 222
  jejunoileal, 223
  metastatic sites, 222
  primary site, 221
  rectal, 223
  regional lymph nodes, 221–222, 227–229
Nodal metastases, 515
Nodal micrometastases, 386, 388, 390, 393

O

Observed survival rate, 26
Obturator iliac lymph nodes, 583
Obturator lymph nodes
  cervix uteri, 463
  corpus uteri, 478
  fallopian tube, 505
  ovary and primary peritoneal carcinoma, 495
  prostate, 535
  urinary bladder, 576
  vagina, 455
Oral tongue, 42
Oropharynx, 56, 62, 63
  T4a tumor, 59, 70
  T4b tumor, 59, 71
  T1 tumors, 59, 67
  T2 tumors, 59, 68
  T3 tumors, 59, 69
Osteosarcoma, 341–343
Ovary and primary peritoneal carcinoma
  anatomic stage/prognostic groups, 498
  distant metastasis (M), 497
  metastatic sites, 496
  primary site, 495, 498
  primary tumor (T), 496–497, 499–503
  prognostic factors, 504
  prognostic features, 496
  pTNM pathologic classification, 497
  regional lymph nodes, 495, 497, 499, 504
Oviducts, 477

P

Pancoast tumors, 316
Papillary/follicular, 115
Para-aortic lumbar, 536

V

W

Z